Mastitis control

Mastitis control
From science to practice

Proceedings of international conference

30 september - 2 October 2008

The Hague, the Netherlands

edited by:

T.J.G.M. Lam

Wageningen Academic
Publishers

ISBN 978-90-8686-085-2

First published, 2008

Wageningen Academic Publishers
The Netherlands, 2008

Preface

Mastitis has been one of the most studied diseases in the dairy industry in recent decades. The reasons for this interest are obvious. Mastitis affects the health of dairy cows. A large proportion of cows suffer from mastitis and it is one of the most important reasons for culling. Mastitis is thus responsible for a decrease in farm profitability, a decline in animal welfare and a reduction in the farmer's job satisfaction. Moreover, mastitis negatively influences milk quality and this affects dairy processing.

Since 2005 a great number of mastitis research projects have been started in the Netherlands. The scope of each of these projects is different but they have one thing in common, they are all directed towards the improvement of on-farm udder health: from science to practice. And that is why the Dutch dairy industry took the initiative to organise an International Conference on Mastitis Control with this 'science to practice' theme.

This book reflects the latest knowledge on mastitis control. Out of more than 120 abstracts, the Scientific Committee selected 42 oral presentations. This book contains the six-page papers of each oral presentation given during the conference and the abstracts of each poster presentation.

Because we believe that scientific evidence is an important foundation for effective mastitis control, the conference was aimed at science that is useful in practice. The International Conference entitled 'Mastitis Control: From science to practice', was held from 30 September to 2 October, 2008. Approximately 350 people attended the conference.

Finally, we would like to acknowledge all the people that have been involved in the organisation of the conference.

The Organising Committee

International Conference on Mastitis Control 2008: From science to practice

Organising Committee

Dr. Ir. Henk Hogeveen, chairman
Faculty of Veterinary Medicine, Utrecht University

Marie-Louise Bögemann, secretary, treasurer
Netherlands National Committee of the International Dairy Federation

Dr. Theo Lam, scientific affairs
UGCN Dutch Udder Health Centre

Couzijn Bos, sponsoring
GD Animal Health Service

Ir. Jolanda Jansen, public relations
Chair group Communication Science, Wageningen University

Ir. Wilma Steeneveld, conference program manager
Faculty of Veterinary Medicine, Utrecht University

Scientific Program Committee

Dr. Theo Lam
UGCN Dutch Udder Health Centre, the Netherlands

Prof. Dr. Julie Fitzpatrick
Moredun Research Institute, United Kingdom

Prof. Dr. Martin Green
University of Nottingham, United Kingdom

Prof. Dr. Bonnie Mallard
University of Guelph, Canada

Prof. Dr. Graeme Mein
Werribee, Australia

Dr. Ir. Francesca Neijenhuis
Animal Sciences Group, Wageningen UR, the Netherlands

Dr. Mirjam Nielen
Faculty of Veterinary Medicine, Utrecht University, the Netherlands

Prof. Dr. Pamela Ruegg
University of Wisconsin, USA

Ing. Otlis Sampimon
GD Animal Health Service, the Netherlands

Dr. Ir. Gerdien van Schaik
GD Animal Health Service, the Netherlands

Dr. Tine van Werven
Faculty of Veterinary Medicine, Utrecht University, the Netherlands

Table of contents

Keynote

Infectious pressure

Detection, diagnosis and treatment

Milking and milking machine

Management, planning and control

Keynote

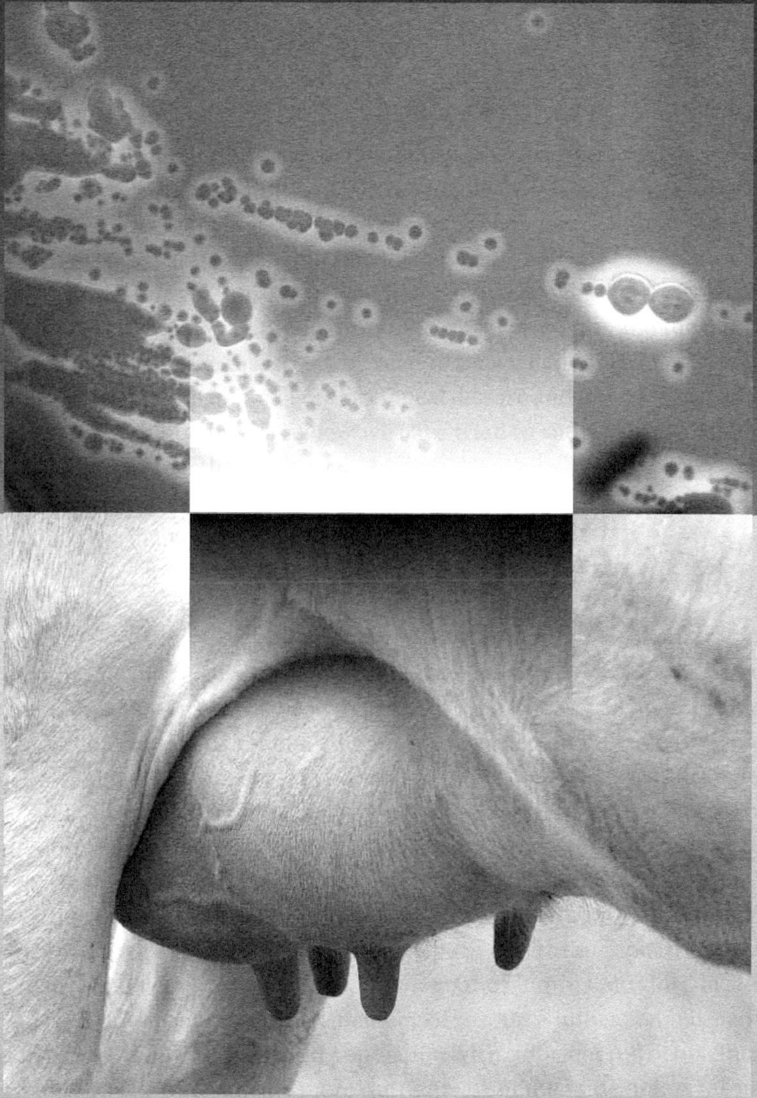

been implemented in the Norwegian cattle population. As described by Østerås *et al.* (2007), both subclinical and clinical mastitis increased in the population from 1975 to 1990 (Figure 1A, 1B), but showed an important decrease thereafter. The 3 main reasons for the large decrease in mastitis were described by the authors as effects of preventative management programs, improvements due to genetic changes and an effect of changing the attitude of the dairy producers towards treatment. The authors also argue that many of the actions taken to bring about improvements would not have been possible without a functioning and practical disease recording system. Although many individual farms record diseases, the Nordic countries are still the only ones using a National disease recording database.

The specific prevention program used in Norway was not described in full detail in the paper by Østerås *et al.* (2007). However the usual 10-point NMC udder health program was generally advised with the exception of the standard use of dry-cow therapy. A lot of credit has been given to the introduction of a strong genetic selection for udder health (Steine *et al.*, 2008), as the introduction of this program coincided with the start of the decreasing trend in both clinical and subclinical mastitis (Heringstad *et al.*, 2003). The availability of Nation wide

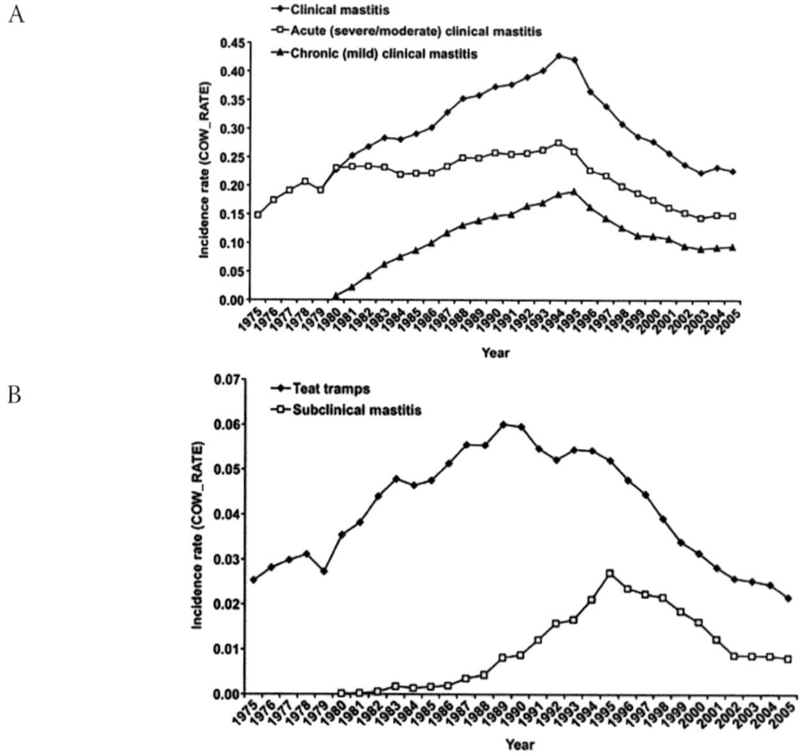

Figure 1. Incidence rate of Clinical (A) and Subclinical (B) mastitis in Norwegian dairy cows (from Østerås et al., *2007).*

data lend a lot of credibility to the observed patterns and this is further strengthened by a reduction in intramammary antibiotic sales coinciding with the reduction in clinical mastitis cases (Østerås *et al.*, 2007).

Other milk quality improvement programs are in operation throughout the world. Some of the well publicised programs include the Dutch Udder Health Center (UGCN), the Australian 'Count-down down under' program, the Canadian Bovine Mastitis Research Network, the Milk money program in Wisconsin, the Quality count$ in Minnesota and the Quality Milk Production Services in New York State. This list is by no means complete and several other programs exist throughout the world. Some of these programs are temporary in nature and a response to increasing udder health problems, others are more permanent and aim to provide long-term services to the dairy industry. The general premise of these programs is to promote excellent milk quality and to support the dairy farmers to reach this goal. Most, if not all of these programs work with a generic format for problem solving. This format, known as the herd health circle consists of goal setting, risk assessment & problem analysis, execution and finally evaluation & monitoring (see Figure 2). Often this herd health circle is preceded by an effort to immediately resolve the problem at hand using some short term relief measures. Briefly, the steps involved in improvement of udder health and production of high quality milk will be explained. This will also provide a framework to discuss the important outstanding questions in milk quality research.

Step 1. Resolve udder health issues to acceptable levels with (usually) short term solutions. This often involves treatment of selected cows with subclinical mastitis, dumping milk of the worst quality offenders or culling of some problem cows. Rapid identification of cows with poor milk quality remains an issue. Tests like the California Mastitis Test (CMT) or somatic cell count (SCC) are valuable but not easy for daily use. Further research into automated detection system of milk of poor quality would be of great value.

Step 2. Goal setting involves identifying realistic goals with the herd owner, the manager and the staff. Although this appears to be straightforward given that milk is the preeminent product that leaves the dairy, this is often neglected and motivating the herd owner and staff

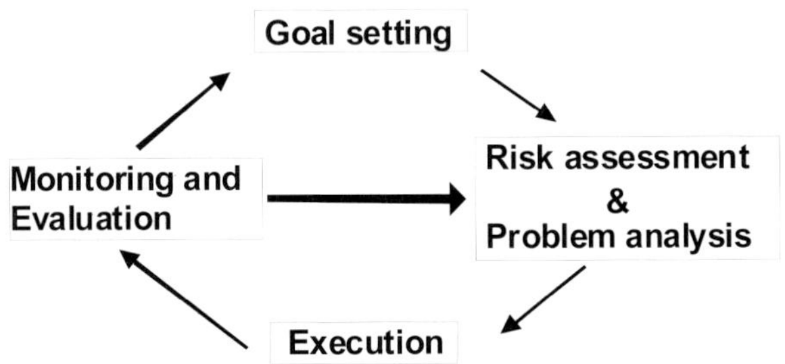

Figure 2. The Herd Health circle as it is applied to udder health programs on dairy farms.

to improve is at times very difficult. The processes underlying the motivation of the herd owner and staff are complex and not well understood. Using existing knowledge on mastitis control, an average reduction of 20% in mastitis incidence and prevalence can be achieved but the success of control programs depends on the level of adoption by dairy producers (Green *et al.*, 2007b).Research into motivational aspects of udder health programs is expected to be of great value for future success of udder health programs. Both economic incentive policies and producer motivation are important areas of research (Valeeva *et al.*, 2007; Jansen *et al.*, 2008; Nightingale *et al.*, 2008).

Step 3. Actual problem investigation and Risk assessment. Problem investigation obviously depends on the herd problem. We will focus here on two main issues: high incidence of clinical mastitis and SCC that are higher than the established herd goal. Often problem analysis depends on the availability of udder health data (Bulk milk quality data, data from Dairy Health Improvement Association (DHIA) or similar schemes, clinical disease records), conduct of on-farm risk assessment using questionnaire data, scoring results (hygiene scoring, teat end scoring, body condition scoring), on-farm measurements (e.g. milk flow patterns, milking equipment vacuum testing, equipment washing analysis, timing of parlor routines) and farm observations.

A. High incidence of clinical mastitis. Incidence of clinical mastitis is to some extent farm specific. This is the case because diagnostic efficacy may differ between farms depending on the diagnostic tools and diagnostic procedures used. Milking procedures that include fore stripping will likely detect more cases than procedures that rely on other detection methods. Use of automated in-line diagnostic tools such as conductivity or enzymatic measurement will increase diagnostic accuracy if their specificity is acceptable. A schematic protocol for analysis of clinical mastitis problems is shown in Figure 3. Clinical mastitis problems can be divided into two main areas: high incidence of first cases and high rate of reoccurrence of clinical symptoms.

A1. High incidence of first cases. An incidence of less than 20% of cows getting a first case of clinical mastitis is a realistic goal on most farms. To investigate first cases of clinical mastitis, it is necessary to describe the patterns of disease occurrence: high post partum incidence or high mid lactation incidence (pointing at dry cow versus lactating cow problems), a high incidence in a single parity (particularly first lactation heifers versus cows), evaluating whether there is evidence for point source outbreaks, evidence of seasonality, or any other discernable pattern. The distribution of pathogens associated with first clinical cases is very valuable as well as the presence of a high proportion of culture negative cases. Further research into prevention of first clinical mastitis cases through improving management, improved treatment protocols, genetic selection or vaccination will be necessary. Particularly the very high incidence of first cases of clinical mastitis in heifers in early lactation is an area in need of further development (Svensson *et al.*, 2006).

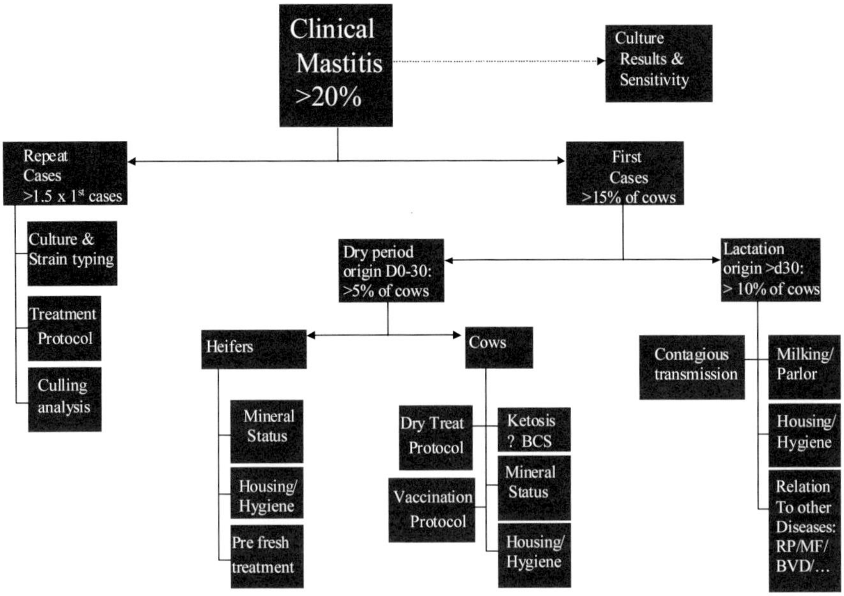

Figure 3. Schematic protocol for clinical mastitis evaluation.

A2. High incidence of repeat cases. When the incidence of repeat cases, i.e. subsequent clinical cases in cows that already had a first case of clinical mastitis, is twice as high as the incidence of first cases among all cows in the herd, a more detailed investigation of the causes underlying the occurrence of repeat cases should be performed. Key areas of investigation include the pathogen distribution of repeat cases, antimicrobial sensitivity patterns, presence of dominant strains within a bacterial species in repeat cases using strain typing techniques (Zadoks and Schukken, 2006), and the presence of specific risk factors for cows experiencing multiple cases of mastitis. Investigation of the recommended treatment protocols and the protocols executed on the farm is of great importance. A formal treatment evaluation may be valuable in order to obtain quantitative cure data for each treatment protocol used on the farm. Further research into the biology of bacterial host adaptation, more successful treatment strategies and the underlying reasons for susceptibility to repeat cases will need to be conducted (Steeneveld *et al.*, 2008).

B. High somatic cell counts. High SCC issues can generally be split into three main areas: high new intra-mammary infection (IMI) risk in lactation, high prevalence of chronic infections and high post partum infection prevalence. In all these cases 'infection' is defined as a SCC value above the threshold for normal milk SCC concentration. Generally this threshold is set at 200,000 cells per ml. A schematic protocol for analysis of high SCC problems is shown in Figure 4.

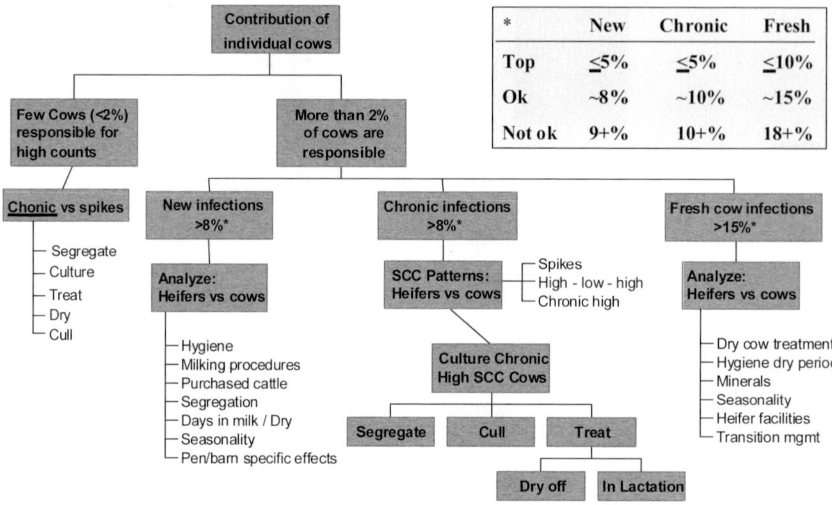

*	New	Chronic	Fresh
Top	≤5%	≤5%	≤10%
Ok	~8%	~10%	~15%
Not ok	9+%	10+%	18+%

Figure 4. Schematic protocol for high SCC evaluation.

B1. High new 'infection' risk in lactation. Herds that aim to have a bulk milk SCC of approximately 150,000 cells/ml should aim for <5% new infection risk per month, at 250,000 this would approximately be <8%. Investigation of high new IMI risks that exceed targets would focus on milking parlor hygiene and milking procedures, quality of post milking teat disinfection, hygiene in stalls and walkways, transmission of infection between cows (no segregation of cows infected with contagious pathogens), purchasing of cows without testing and an increased susceptibility of cows to infection due to other infectious diseases or metabolic disorders. Further research into cow susceptibility to infection, management associated with reduced exposure and (emerging) bacterial pathogens responsible for high new infections risk is needed.

B2. High prevalence of chronic infections. When high milk quality is the objective of the dairy, less than 5% of cows should have persistent high SCC. For a bulk milk SCC around 250,000 cells/ml the objective should be less than 10% of cows with persistent high SCC. Investigation into persistent high SCC will need to identify parity groups with high risk, seasonal effects, time of start of persistent infections (dry period, early lactation, late lactation), pathogen distribution and when necessary strain typing of identified pathogens. Evaluation of treatment protocols of subclinical mastitis during lactation is valuable. Percentage contribution to the bulk tank may be calculated for the persistent high SCC cows. Evaluation of culling strategies is of importance for the group of animals with persistent high SCC. Further research into host adaptation of strains within bacterial species, targeted clinical and sub-clinical treatment strategies, and the importance of so called 'minor pathogens' is of value to better understand the dynamics of persistent high SCC cows.

B3. High prevalence of postpartum infections. For high milk quality, 10% or less of cows should have an increased SCC post partum. For bulk milk SCC values around 250,000, a goal of less than 15% of cows with high SCC post partum should be the objective. Further investigation into parity specific problems, dry cow treatment and teat seal protocols, transition management, and dry cow hygiene are warranted. Further research into pre-calving treatment of cows and heifers (De Vliegher *et al.*, 2004), the patho-biology of teatsealants, the immune response in the dry period and optimal vaccination strategies is warranted.

Step 4. Execution of proposed solutions. Training of individuals involved in execution of the proposed solutions is of great importance. In many countries non-native speakers perform many of the repetitive but important tasks in harvesting milk. Pictorial displays of best management practices may be essential for proper execution. Again, understanding motivation of herd owners, managers and staff will turn out to be of great value for adequate implementation and continuation of suggested best management practices. Given the large variation of mastitis patterns between farms (Olde Riekerink *et al.*, 2008), farm specific solutions are anticipated.

Step 5. Evaluation and monitoring. Several evaluation and monitoring options exits. Bulk milk monitoring can be a good starting point as it is relatively cheap and includes most of the milk produced in the dairy (Lievaart *et al.*, 2007). Other parameters that are important to monitor include clinical mastitis incidence, monitoring new and chronic subclinical infections, and monitoring culling due to udder health reasons. Monitoring programs can work at herd level (Schukken *et al.*, 2003), regional level or national level (Østerås *et al.*, 2007).

Recent developments in mastitis research

Bacterial pathogens

Many of the recent developments in our understanding of the bacterial pathogens involved in IMI come from the emergence of molecular epidemiology. This discipline has provided many tools for more precise study of pathogens. A recent review (Zadoks and Schukken, 2006) summarised the most frequently used methods and applications. With the tools provided by molecular typing, the epidemiology of bacterial pathogens causing IMI has radically changed. Our classic concept of environmental and contagious mastitis pathogens has been challenged by several publications showing that some strains of previously defined environmental organisms behave in a contagious manner while some strains of previously defined contagious organisms do not show any signs of cow-to-cow transmission (Zadoks *et al.*, 2003; Munoz *et al.*, 2007; Haveri *et al.*, 2007; Fournier *et al.*, 2008). For this reason, the terms host-adapted as it refers to strains that easily transmit between cows and opportunistic IMI that cause single more severe infections have been introduced. It has become clear that this terminology should be used for individual strains and describe their behavior in the host and that these definitions are not adequate to describe bacterial species. The use of comparative genomic analyses allows us to identify a set of molecular genetic features that distinguish clones of host adapted bovine-associated strains optimised for mastitis pathogenesis from those that infect other hosts or are only infrequently recovered from bovine mastitis cases. It is expected that in the next few years many of the genes associated with host adaptation to the bovine mammary gland will be identified, as is already being done for *Staphylococcus aureus* (Herron-Olson *et al.*, 2007). Obviously, these genes would be of value as potential vaccine targets. Host adaptation of bacterial pathogens to the bovine mammary gland has now been described for numerous bacterial pathogens. This includes *Escherichia coli* (Blum *et al.*, 2008; Dogan *et al.*, 2006), *Staphylococcus aureus* (Herron-Olson *et al.*, 2007), *Klebsiella* spp. (Munoz *et al.*, 2007), *Streptococcus uberis* (Zadoks, 2007) and *Streptococcus agalactiae* (Bisharat *et al.*, 2004). As indicated above, host-adapted strains would be more likely to be involved in mastitis outbreaks and more likely result in persistent infections and repeated cases of clinical mastitis. It is now recognised that repeated cases of clinical mastitis form a major component of clinical mastitis events on many dairy farms (Steeneveld *et al.*, 2008). For an example, see Figure 5. Hence our increased understanding of the genomic correlates of host-adaptation may have an important impact on reduction of clinical and sub-clinical mastitis on dairy farms.

The developments in bacterial genomics and molecular diagnostic technology will also result in an increased use of molecular diagnostics for rapid and accurate detection of mastitis

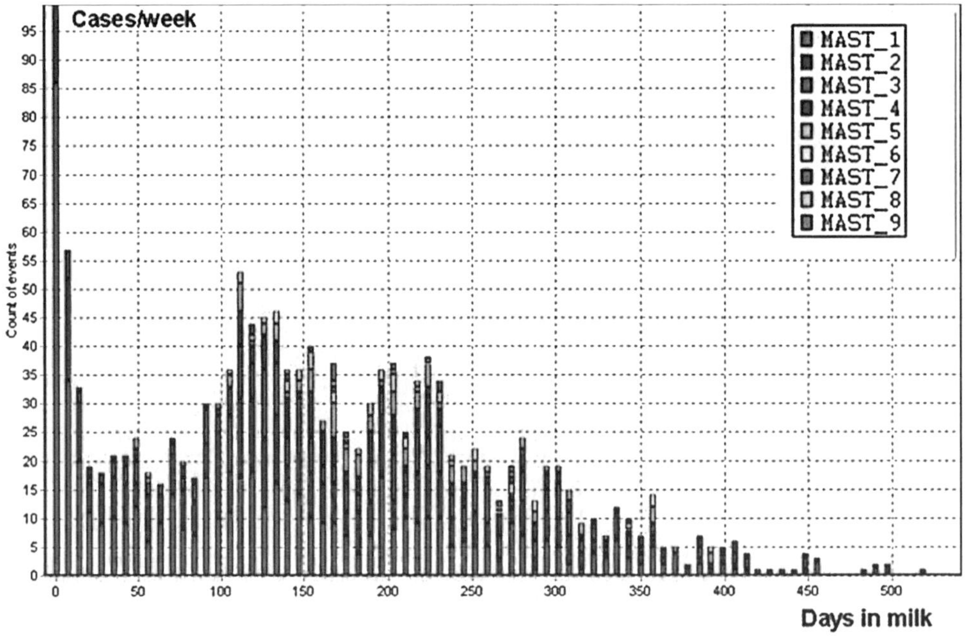

Figure 5. A farm with a predominance of repeated cases of mastitis.

pathogens (Lee *et al.*, 2008). It is likely that some of these technologies will be implemented in the next few years in routine diagnostics of bovine IMI.

An increasing number of pathogens is gaining recognition as emerging causes of mastitis. In some situations pathogens capable of causing IMI are described that were not recognised before, as in the case of *Coxiella burnetii* (Barlow *et al.*, 2008). In other situations, bacterial pathogens emerge as a more frequent cause of mastitis as in the case of *Klebsiella* spp. (Munoz *et al.*, 2007) or are now recognised as a more important contributor to herd problems as in the case of coagulase negative staphylococci (Sampimon *et al.*, 2007; Taponen *et al.*, 2007).

Producer, management and environment

A highly underestimated field in mastitis research is the field of communication sciences. In many situations the biology and management factors resulting in mastitis and milk quality problems on a dairy farm are well known and can be relatively easily resolved. The main problem on such dairies is communication to the herd owner and motivation of the herd owner to implement known successful strategies. This area of motivational research is now developing and showing great promise. It will be necessary to understand the important motivators of dairy farmers to be able to successfully bring knowledge and technology to the dairy farm (Jansen *et al.*, 2008). In a recent study by Valeeva *et al.* (2007), it was observed that factors that are internal to the farm performance and the individual farmer provided more motivation than external factors related to esteem and recognition within the dairy sector. The authors identified 3 distinct clusters that were driving motivation of dairy farmers with regard to mastitis management: milk price premium - or penalty - oriented motivation, motivation to have an efficient (well-organised) farm that easily complies with regulatory requirements, and basic economic motivation. Nightingale *et al.* (2007) recently also established the importance of premium programs in reducing bulk milk SCC. As to the basic economic motivation, the total economic losses of mastitis (subclinical and clinical) per cow present on the farm were recently estimated between 65 and 182 Euro per cow per year depending on the bulk tank SCC (Huijps *et al.*, 2008). However, the authors also showed that most farmers expected their economic losses to be lower than those calculated from their actual data. Underestimating the economic losses of mastitis appears to be a problem and it may be important to more accurately provide economic data to dairy farmers to increase their motivation for implementation of control procedures (Huijps *et al.*, 2008).

An important control procedure for both clinical and subclinical mastitis is the rational use of antimicrobial therapy for these two types of mastitis. A number of recent papers addressed the efficacy and economic value of subclinical mastitis treatment (Steeneveld *et al.*, 2007; Swinkels *et al.*, 2005a,b). Their research indicated that profitability of treatment of chronic subclinical *S. aureus* and *S. uberis* mastitis depended on farm-specific factors such as average cure rate and the value of discarded milk and cow-specific factors such as duration of infection and the likelihood of transmission to other cows. It was shown by Swinkels *et al.* (2005a,b) that treatment of subclinical mastitis is particularly valuable to reduce duration of infection. Treatment of IMI with long durations may have an important impact on the risk of new infections in the herd. Quantification of the direct and indirect effects of treatment of IMI is important to provide economic motivation for the use of rational antimicrobial treatment protocols. Furthermore, adequate treatment of the initial case of clinical mastitis may reduce the incidence and related costs of repeated cases (Bar *et al.*, 2008).

Cows

In the last years, major advances in host genetics and genomics have had an important impact on bovine mastitis. Mastitis has an unfavourable genetic correlation with milk production (Heringstad *et al.*, 2003), and selection for increased milk production is therefore expected to increase the incidence of the disease. In observational studies high producing herds typically shower higher rates of clinical mastitis (Sato *et al.*, 2008). However, it was shown that if selection against mastitis is included in a total merit index, the genetic level of mastitis may be kept constant or even improved (Heringstad *et al.*, 2003). Selection can be either direct using clinical mastitis (CM) records, or indirect via information on traits that are genetically correlated to mastitis, such as SCC, or both. Denmark, Finland, Norway, and Sweden are the only countries having national recording systems for CM (Østerås *et al.*, 2007), whereas SCC is routinely recorded in many countries. In the latter, genetic improvement of udder health relies mainly on selection for reduced SCC. It was argued that direct selection for reduced incidence of CM would be 23 to 43% more efficient in terms of reducing incidence of clinical mastitis among second-crop daughters, than indirect selection using linear somatic cell score. However, De Haas *et al.* (2008) recently argued that indirect selection using SCC peak patterns would be equally efficient in reducing incidence of clinical mastitis when compared to direct selection against clinical mastitis.

More detailed analysis of the bovine genome has become available since the publication of the full bovine genome (Miller *et al.*, 2007). With the completion of the bovine genome sequence assembly, single nucleotide polymorphism (SNP) assays spanning the whole bovine genome has become possible. It is expected that relating the bovine genome to observed data on clinical and subclinical mastitis will result in identification of specific genes or gene mutations that relate to a higher or lower mastitis incidence. Recent work by Sugimoto *et al.* (2006) is a good example of this. They observed that cows that were more susceptible to mastitis had a three-base insertion in the forebrain embryonic zinc finger-like (FEZL) gene. Recognition of this mutation provides an opportunity for directed genetic selection against mastitis susceptibility. The combination of quantitative genetics with full utilisation of the bovine genome will provide major tools for genetic improvement with regard to mastitis susceptibility if genetic and genomic data can be correlated to phenotypic data on disease, i.e. data on clinical and subclinical mastitis. This is expected to have an important impact on clinical mastitis incidence and the risk of new IMI on dairy farms world wide.

The innate immune response to bacterial penetration of the mammary gland is evoked within hours of infection and the rapidity and magnitude of this response have been demonstrated to influence the resolution of this disease (Bannerman *et al.*, 2004a). Pathogen specific recognition is accomplished by a series of receptors known as Toll-like receptors (Yang *et al.*, 2008). These receptors recognise bacterial signals and their activation regulates cytokine expression in the host immune cells. Cytokines and other mediators of inflammation are known to play critical roles in the innate immune response to intramammary infection. The ability of bacteria to establish infection is determined, in part, by the nature and rapidity of the corresponding host innate immune response. Over the past decade, understanding of the innate immune response to intramammary infection has increased, and there is mounting evidence that suggests that immune modulators (e.g. recombinant cytokines) that influence the innate immune response may be therapeutically beneficial (Bannerman *et al.*, 2004a,b,c). Cytokines also may be useful biomarkers of disease severity and outcome. For example, the highest concentrations of milk C5a were detected in cows infected with strains of *K. pneumoniae* and *S. uberis* that induced very severe clinical mastitis (Bannerman *et al.*, 2004b,c). In contrast, IMI with pathogens that induced less severe symptoms of clinical mastitis were accompanied by lower milk concentrations of C5a (Bannerman *et al.*, 2004a). Hence early information on cytokine response may prove to be useful as an early prognostic indicator, and it may guide the selection of treatment of clinical bovine mastitis.

A particularly interesting period with regard to the risk factors for IMI and the cow's immune response to IMI is the dry period. Several studies have now established the late dry period as an important period of new IMI as shown in Figure 6, although the host does not show a visible response to these IMI (Green *et al.*, 2007a; Bradley and Green, 2004). Further studies on the immune response to IMI in the dry period are necessary to develop prevention strategies that will eventually lead to a reduced incidence of clinical mastitis and a lower prevalence of increased SCC at the first test post-partum.

The impact of nutrition during the dry period and transition to lactation is expected to be large. Energy intake, trace element and vitamin intake and fiber in the diet appear of importance to reduce clinical disease post partum (Beever, 2006). More information is becoming available about other factors affecting the cow's immune response. In a recent study it was shown that herds that became free of Bovine Virus Diarrhea Virus infection had a reduced incidence of clinical mastitis compared to infected control herds (Berends *et al.*, 2008). Similarly, a Danish study recently showed a relationship between lameness and an increased risk of clinical mastitis (Sato *et al.*, 2008). These studies are helpful in the development of integrated control programs to reduce the incidence of clinical mastitis.

Very little is known about cow well-being, pain and pain relief as it related to mastitis, but its importance is increasingly recognised (Anil *et al.*, 2005). Detection of pain in dairy cows as an objective measurable parameter is in its infancy (Fitzpatrick *et al.*, 1998). Without objective parameters the impact of mastitis on animal well-being and the potential use of

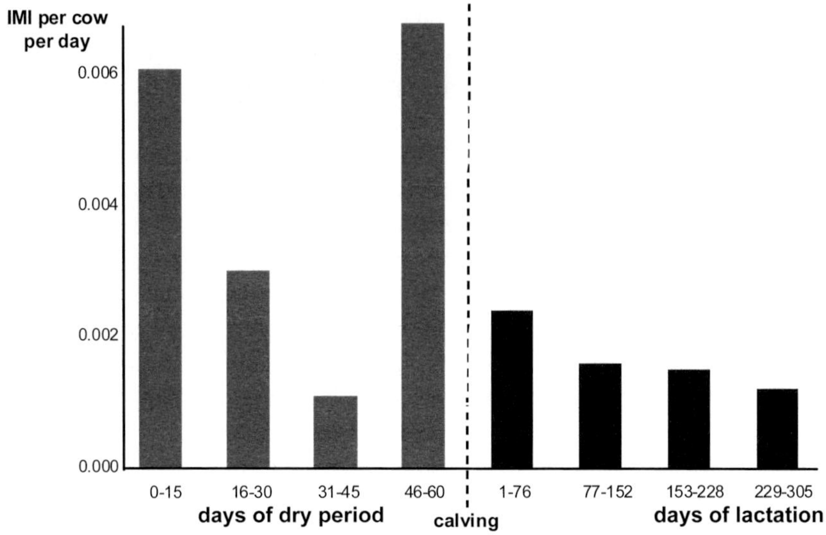

Figure 6. Incidence of new IMI during dry period and lactation (adjusted from Burvenich et al., *2008).*

pain relieving and anti-inflammatory drugs remain difficult to study. Clearly, more work in this area will be needed.

Future perspectives

Milk quality is manageable. Knowledge and tools are available to produce milk of high quality. In contrast, knowledge and tools for reduction of incidence of clinical mastitis on dairy farms are lacking. In fact, the components for a 'perfect storm' of escalating mastitis incidence are in place: first, bacterial pathogens increasingly show an adaptation to the bovine host; second, host susceptibility to clinical mastitis is increasing due to a positive correlation with milk production; and third, producer motivation to implement mastitis control programs appears to be decreasing. To mitigate the occurrence of this 'perfect clinical mastitis storm', progress needs to be made in research and on-farm application of knowledge in these three areas. A key issue is to steer producer motivation such that our increased knowledge and improved tools are applied in day-to-day management. Research on the success of implementation of comprehensive milk quality programs is needed to better understand producer motivation. A successful clinical mastitis reduction program will undoubtedly include a genetic selection component. Bacterial mammary pathogen research is now making full use of the molecular genetic tools that have become available. Further research into host or niche adaptation of mastitis pathogens will likely provide opportunities for early diagnosis, vaccination, treatment and prevention programs. Host response to mastitis pathogens has been studied in great detail in the last years. Particularly the pathogen specific innate immune response was elucidated for many bacterial IMI. These studies will likely lead to developments in early detection, prognostic indicators and symptomatic treatment. A better understanding of host response during the dry period will be needed to implement control programs for IMI during this crucial period. The cellular immune response to IMI remains poorly understood and more research in this area is needed.

Above all, it is important to maintain a connection between on-farm control programs and the direction of research in mastitis. Ultimately the research will need to be applied on farms and lead to an increase in milk quality, reduction in clinical disease and improvement of animal well-being and farm efficiency and profitability.

References

Anil, L., Anil S.S. and Deen, J., 2005. Pain Detection and Amelioration in Animals on the Farm: Issues and Options. J. Appl. Animal Welfare Sci., 8: 261-278.

Bannerman, D.D., Paape, M.J., Lee, J.W., Zhao, X., Hope, J.C. and Rainard, P., 2004a. *Escherichia coli* and *Staphylococcus aureus* elicit differential innate immune responses following intramammary infection. Clin. Diagn. Lab. Immunol. 11: 463-472.

Bannerman, D.D., Paape, M.J., Goff, J.P., Kimura, K., Lippolis, J.D. and Hope, J.C., 2004b. Innate immune response to intramammary infection with *Serratia marcescens* and *Streptococcus uberis*. Vet. Res. 35: 681-700.

Bannerman, D.D., Paape, M.J., Hare, W.R. and Hope, J.C., 2004c. Characterization of the bovine innate immune response to intramammary infection with *Klebsiella pneumoniae*. J. Dairy Sci. 87: 2420-2432.

Bar, D., Gröhn, Y.T., Bennett, G., González, R.N., Hertl, J.A., Schulte, H.F., Tauer, L.W., Welcome, F.L. and Schukken, Y.H., 2008. Effects of repeated episodes of generic clinical mastitis on mortality and culling in dairy cows. J. Dairy Sci. 91: 2196-2204.

Barlow, J., Rauch, B., Welcome, F., Kim, S.G., Dubovi, E. and Schukken, Y., 2008. Association between *Coxiella burnetii* shedding in milk and subclinical mastitis in dairy cattle. Vet. Res. 39: 23.

Beever, D.E., 2006. The impact of controlled nutrition during the dry period on dairy cow health, fertility and performance. Anim. Reprod. Sci. 96: 212-226.

Berends, I.M., Swart, W.A., Frankena, K., Muskens, J., Lam, T.J.G.M. and Van Schaik, G., 2008. The effect of becoming BVDV-free on fertility and udder health in Dutch dairy herds. Prev. Vet. Med. 84: 48-60.

Bisharat, N., Crook, D.W., Leigh, J., Harding, R.M., Ward, P.N., Coffey, T.J., Maiden, M.C., Peto, T. and Jones, N., 2004. Hyperinvasive neonatal group B streptococcus has arisen from a bovine ancestor. J. Clin. Microbiol. 42: 2161-2167.

Blum, S., Heller, E.D., Krifucks, O., Sela, S., Hammer-Muntz, O. and Leitner, G., 2008. Identification of a bovine mastitis *Escherichia coli* subset. Vet. Microbiol. (in press).

Bradley A.J. and Green M.J. 2004. The importance of the nonlactating period in the epidemiology of intramammary infection and strategies for prevention. Vet. Clin. North Am. Food Anim. Pract. 20: 547-568.

Burvenich, C., De Spiegeleer, B., Peelman and L. Paape, M.J., 2008. Innate immunobiology of the bovine mammary gland and *E. coli* infections. Hungarian Veterianary Journal 130: 25-28 (suppl. I).

De Haas Y., De Jong G. and Lam T.J.G.M., 2008. Udder health: breeding. Tijdschr Diergeneeskd. 133: 464-468.

De Vliegher, S., Barkema, H.W., Stryhn, H., Opsomer, G. and De Kruif, A., 2004. Impact of early lactation somatic cell count in heifers on somatic cell counts over the first lactation. J. Dairy Sci. 87: 3672-3682.

Dogan, B., Klaessig, S., Rishniw, M., Almeida, R.A., Oliver, S.P., Simpson, K. and Schukken, Y.H., 2006. Adherent and invasive *Escherichia coli* are associated with persistent bovine mastitis. Vet. Microbiol. 116: 270-282.

Fitzpatrick, J.L., F.J. Young, D. Eckersall, D.N. Logue, C.J. Knight and A. Nolan, 1998. Recognising and controlling pain and inflammation in mastitis. Proceedings of the British Mastitis Conference 1998, Axient/Institute for Animal Health, Milk Development Council/Novartis Animal Health, pp. 36-44.

Fournier, C., Kuhnert, P., Frey, J., Miserez, R., Kirchhofer, M., Kaufmann, T., Steiner, A. and Graber, H.U., 2008 Bovine *Staphylococcus aureus*: Association of virulence genes, genotypes and clinical outcome. Res. Vet. Sci. (in press).

Green, M.J., Bradley, A.J., Medley, G.F. and Browne, W.J., 2007a. Cow, farm, and management factors during the dry period that determine the rate of clinical mastitis after calving. J. Dairy Sci. 90: 3764-3776.

Green, M.J., Leach, K.A., Breen, J.E., Green, L.E. and Bradley, A.J., 2007b. National intervention study of mastitis control in dairy herds in England and Wales. Vet. Rec. 160: 287-293.

Haveri, M., Roslöf, A., Rantala, L. and Pyörälä, S., 2007. Virulence genes of bovine *Staphylococcus aureus* from persistent and nonpersistent intramammary infections with different clinical characteristics. J. Appl. Microbiol. 103: 993-1000.

Heringstad, B., Rekaya, R., Glanola, D., Klemetsdal, G. and Welgel, K.A., 2003. Genetic change for clinical mastitis in Norwegian cattle: a threshold model analysis. J. Dairy Sci. 86: 369-375.

Herron-Olson, L., Fitzgerald, J.R., Musser, J.M. and Kapur, V. 2007. Molecular correlates of host specialization in *Staphylococcus aureus*. PLoS ONE. 2:e1120.

Huijps, K., Lam, T.J.G.M. and Hogeveen, H., 2008. Costs of mastitis: facts and perception. J. Dairy Res. 75: 113-120.

Jansen, J., Van den Borne, B.H.P., Renes, R.J., Van Schaik, G., Lam T.J.G.M. and Leeuwis, C., 2008. Mastitis incidence explained by farmers' attitude and behaviour. Proceedings SVEPM 2008 Liverpool, UK, pp. 117-129.

Lee, K.H., Lee, J.W., Wang, S.W., Liu, L.Y., Lee, M.F., Chuang, S.T., Shy, Y.M., Chang, C.L., Wu, M.C. and Chi, C.H., 2008. Development of a novel biochip for rapid multiplex detection of seven mastitis-causing pathogens in bovine milk samples. J. Vet. Diagn. Invest. 20: 463-471.

Lievaart, J.J., Kremer, W.D. and Barkema, H.W., 2007. Comparison of bulk milk, yield-corrected, and average somatic cell counts as parameters to summarize the subclinical mastitis situation in a dairy herd. J. Dairy Sci. 90: 4145-4148.

Miller, W., Rosenbloom, K., Hardison, R.C., Hou, M., Taylor, J., Raney, B., Burhans, R., King, D.C., Baertsch, R., Blankenberg, D., Kosakovsky Pond, S.L., Nekrutenko, A., Giardine, B., Harris, R.S., Tyekucheva, S., Diekhans, M., Pringle, T.H., Murphy, W.J., Lesk, A., Weinstock, G.M., Lindblad-Toh, K., Gibbs, R.A., Lander, E.S., Siepel, A., Haussler, D. and Kent, W.J. 2007. 28-way vertebrate alignment and conservation track in the UCSC Genome Browser. Genome Res. 12: 1797-1808.

Munoz, M.A., Welcome, F.L., Schukken, Y.H. and Zadoks, RN., 2007. Molecular epidemiology of two *Klebsiella pneumoniae* mastitis outbreaks on a dairy farm in New York State. J. Clin. Microbiol. 45: 3964-3971.

Nightingale, C., Dhuyvetter, K., Mitchell, R. and Schukken, Y., 2008. Influence of variable milk quality premiums on observed milk quality. J. Dairy Sci. 91: 1236-1244.

Olde Riekerink, R.G., Barkema, H.W., Kelton, D.F. and Scholl, D.T., 2008. Incidence rate of clinical mastitis on Canadian dairy farms. J. Dairy Sci. 91: 1366-1377.

Østerås, O., Solbu, H., Refsdal, A.O., Roalkvam, T., Filseth, O. and Minsaas, A., 2007. Results and evaluation of thirty years of health recordings in the Norwegian dairy cattle population. J. Dairy Sci. 90: 4483-4497.

Sato, K., Bartlett, P.C., Alban, L., Agger, J.F. and Houe, H. 2008. Managerial and environmental determinants of clinical mastitis in Danish dairy herds. Acta Vet. Scand. 50: 4-11.

Sampimon, O.C., Vernooij, J.C., Mevius, D.J. and Sol, J., 2007. Sensitivity to various antibiotics of coagulase-negative staphylococci isolated from samples of milk from Dutch dairy cattle. Tijdschr. Diergeneeskd. 132: 200-204.

Schukken, Y.H., Wilson, D.J., Welcome, F., Garrison-Tikofsky, L., González, R.N., 2003. Monitoring udder health and milk quality using somatic cell counts. Vet. Res. 34: 579-596.

Steeneveld, W., Swinkels, J. and Hogeveen, H., 2007. Stochastic modelling to assess economic effects of treatment of chronic subclinical mastitis caused by *Streptococcus uberis*. J. Dairy Res. 74: 459-467.

Steeneveld, W., Hogeveen, H., Barkema, H.W., Van den Broek, J. and Huirne, R.B., 2008. The influence of cow factors on the incidence of clinical mastitis in dairy cows. J. Dairy Sci. 91: 1391-1402.

Steine, G., Kristofersson, D., Guttormsen, A.G., 2008. Economic evaluation of the breeding goal for Norwegian Red dairy cattle. J. Dairy Sci. 91: 418-426.

Sugimoto, M., Fujikawa, A., Womack, J.E. and Sugimoto, Y., 2006. Evidence that bovine forebrain embryonic zinc finger-like gene influences immune response associated with mastitis resistance. Proc. Natl. Acad. Sci. USA. 103: 6454-6459.

Svensson, C., Nyman, A.K., Persson Waller, K. and Emanuelson, U., 2006. Effects of housing, management, and health of dairy heifers on first-lactation udder health in southwest Sweden. J. Dairy Sci. 89: 1990-1999.

Swinkels, J.M., Rooijendijk, J.G., Zadoks, R.N. and Hogeveen, H., 2005a. Use of partial budgeting to determine the economic benefits of antibiotic treatment of chronic subclinical mastitis caused by *Streptococcus uberis* or *Streptococcus dysgalactiae*. J. Dairy Res. 72: 75-85.

Swinkels, J.M., Hogeveen, H. and Zadoks, R.N., 2005b. A partial budget model to estimate economic benefits of lactational treatment of subclinical *Staphylococcus aureus* mastitis. J. Dairy Sci. 88: 4273-87.

Taponen, S., Koort, J., Björkroth, J., Saloniemi, H. and Pyörälä, S., 2007. Bovine intramammary infections caused by coagulase-negative staphylococci may persist throughout lactation according to amplified fragment length polymorphism-based analysis. J. Dairy Sci. 90: 3301-3307.

Valeeva, N.I., Lam, T.J.G.M. and Hogeveen, H., 2007. Motivation of dairy farmers to improve mastitis management. J. Dairy Sci. 90: 4466-4477.

Yang, W., Zerbe, H., Petzl, W., Brunner, R.M., Günther, J., Draing, C., Von Aulock, S., Schuberth, H.J. and Seyfert, H.M. 2008. Bovine TLR2 and TLR4 properly transduce signals from *Staphylococcus aureus* and *E. coli*, but *S. aureus* fails to both activate NF-kappaB in mammary epithelial cells and to quickly induce TNFalpha and interleukin-8 (CXCL8) expression in the udder. Mol. Immunol. 45: 1385-1397.

Zadoks, R.N., 2007. Sources and epidemiology of *Streptococcus uberis*, with special emphasis on mastitis in dairy cattleCAB Reviews: Perspectives in Agriculture, Veterinary Science, Nutrition and Natural Resources 2, No. 030

Zadoks, R.N. and Schukken, Y.H., 2006. Use of molecular epidemiology in veterinary practice. Vet. Clin. North Am. Food Anim. Pract. 22: 229-261.

Zadoks, R.N., Gillespie, B.E., Barkema, H.W., Sampimon, O.C., Oliver, S.P. and Schukken, Y.H., 2003. Clinical, epidemiological and molecular characteristics of *Streptococcus uberis* infections in dairy herds. Epidemiol. Infect. 130: 335-349.

Infectious pressure

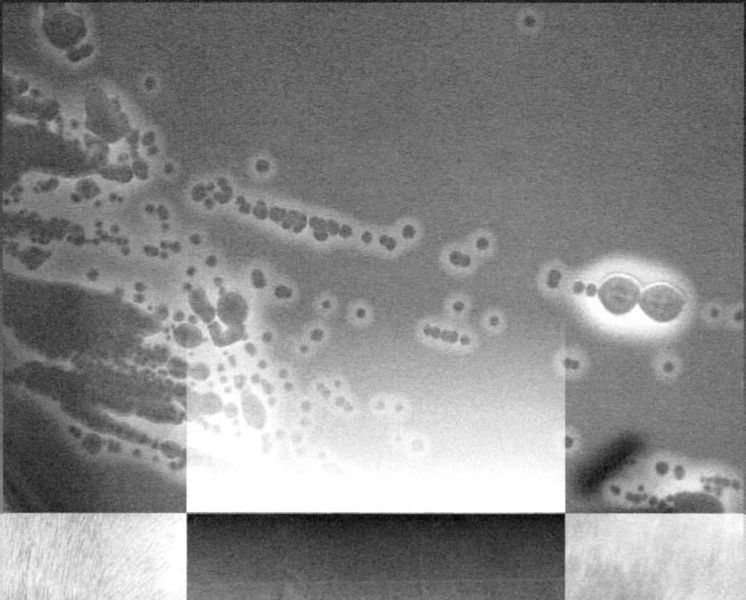

Prevalence of subclinical mastitis pathogens and adoption of udder health management practices on Dutch dairy farms: preliminary results

O.C. Sampimon[1], R.G.M. Olde Riekerink[1] and T.J.G.M. Lam[1,2]
[1]GD Animal Health Service, P.O. Box 9, 7400AA, Deventer, the Netherlands
[2]Dutch Udder Health Centre, P.O. Box 2030, 7420AA, Deventer, the Netherlands
Corresponding author: o.sampimon@gddeventer.com

Abstract

A changing distribution of mastitis pathogens over time and an increasing herd size may have an effect on the execution and effect of udder health management practices in dairy farms. In this study 200 herds were visited to study the prevalence and distribution of subclinical mastitis pathogens and estimate the adoption of udder health management practices. A total of 11,225 quarters of 2,873 cows were sampled and cultured. Cows with increased SCC were selected for sampling based on Dutch DHI data. Of the sampled quarters, 4,612 had a high SCC (≥200,000 cells/ml). Bacterial growth occurred in 1,691 (3%) of these milk samples. Coagulase-negative staphylococci and *Staphylococcus aureus* were the most prevalent pathogens and were isolated in 566 (12%) and 411 (8.6%) milk samples, respectively. *Staphylococcus aureus* was found to be penicillin-resistant in 68 (1.5%) milk samples. Management practices were divided in six categories, general management, housing conditions, young stock management, nutrition, milking procedures and therapy. In this study, 22% of the farmers wore gloves during milking. Checking the first streams of milk before attaching the milking unit was carried out by 49% of the milkers. Post milking teat disinfection was performed by 81% of the farmers. Antibiotic treatment for all cows at drying-off, treatment of the first symptoms of clinical mastitis, and treatment of high SCC was done by 87%, 69%, and 47% of farmers, respectively. Coagulase-negative staphylococci, and *Staph. aureus* were most frequently isolated pathogens in subclinical mastitis. Most recommended management practices were used on most farms, but there is room for improvement.

Keywords: management, pathogens, subclinical mastitis

Introduction

Mastitis is one of the most important diseases in dairy cattle, resulting in significant economic losses for dairy farmers (Halasa *et al.*, 2007). It is a multifactorial disease which is a challenge to manage, and in which numerous management factors are involved, such as housing facilities, milking procedures, feeding programmes, treatment regimes and others. More than 100 bacterial species can cause bovine mastitis (Smith and Hogan, 2001). At the herd level it is important to know which pathogens are involved in clinical and subclinical mastitis, to be able to implement the correct management practices in case of an udder health problem. Also at the population level, it is important to know which pathogens are most frequently causing mastitis and what their antimicrobial sensitivity pattern is.

The prevalence of intramammary infection (IMI) and distribution of mastitis pathogens were determined in The Netherlands in 1973, 1975, 1980 and in 1985 (Vecht *et al.*, 1989). In the 70's, *Streptococcus agalactiae* was the predominant mastitis pathogen (6.9% infected quarters), while in the 80's *Staph. aureus* became the most frequently isolated pathogen (3.7% infected quarters). Average BMSCC in The Netherlands decreased from 331,000 cells/ml in 1985 to 219,000 cells/ml in 2007. A decrease in prevalence of subclinical mastitis and a shift in pathogen distribution involved in IMI can therefore be expected.

The objectives of this study were to determine the prevalence of subclinical mastitis pathogens and the pathogens involved, and the adoption of udder health management practices on 200 randomly selected Dutch dairy farms.

Materials and methods

Herd and cow selection

A total of 400 herds were selected of which 210 participated in the study. In total 10 herds decided not to participate in the study, reasons for not participating were lack of time (9 herds) and no DHIA available (1 herd). All herds were sampled between August 2007 and February 2008. Based on the currently used cut-off levels in the Netherlands by the Dutch DHI, all quarters of cows (SCC>250,000 cells/ml) and heifers (SCC>150,000 cells/ml) were sampled once. The milk samples were collected within one week after arrival of the milk recording results on the farm. Selected cows were sampled immediately before milking. Dry and treated cows were excluded from sampling. All samples were collected according to the NMC guidelines by trained personnel of the GD Animal Health Service (GD) in Deventer, the Netherlands. The milk samples were transported on ice to the GD and stored frozen for culture and SCC.

Laboratory analyses

At arrival at the GD laboratory milk samples were split. In the first sample SCC was determined using a Fossomatic cell counter (Foss Electric, Hillerød, Denmark). If the SCC was above 200,000 cells/ml bacteriological culturing was carried out according to NMC guidelines (Harmon *et al.*, 1990). A milk sample was considered culture-positive if ≥100 cfu/ml of a major pathogen (i.e. *Staph. aureus, Streptococcus uberis, Strep. agalactiae, Streptococcus dysgalactiae* and *E. coli*) or ≥500 cfu/ml of a minor pathogen (i.e. CNS, *Bacillus* spp. and *Corynebacterium bovis*) were cultured. Milk samples that were culture-positive for more than two bacteria species were considered to be contaminated.

Questionnaire

A questionnaire was conducted on farm by GD staff to obtain information on management factors of the farms such as housing facilities, milking procedures, feeding and treatment regimes. The questionnaire was tested before use at 2 dairy farms. The questions were aimed at the year preceding the sampling date.

Results

In total, 11,225 quarter milk samples were collected of 2,873 cows. Of the sampled quarters, 4,612 had a high SCC (≥200,000 cells/ml). Bacterial growth occurred in 1,691 (37%) of these milk samples. Coagulase-negative staphylococci and *Staph. aureus* were the most prevalent pathogens and were isolated in 566 (12%) and 411 (8.6%) milk samples respectively (Table 1). Penicillin-resistant *Staph. aureus* was found in 68 (1.4%) milk samples. Mean herd size was 72 lactating cows (ranging from 20 to 267).

The most common barn types was the free-stall barns (95%). Herringbone milking parlors (75%) were most frequently used followed by side-by-side (8%) and rotary parlors (6%). An automatic milking system was used on 4% of the farms. A number of relevant udder health management parameters that were surveyed in the questionnaire are summarised in Table 2.

Table 1. Distribution of the pathogens from 200 random selected dairy farms.

Pathogen	**n**	**Of all samples (n=4,612)**	**Of all isolates (n=1,691)**
Coagulase-negative staphylococci	566	11.9	30.5
Staphylococcus aureus	411	8.6	22.2
Penicillin sensitive	(343)	(7.2)	(18.5)
Penicillin resistant	(68)	(1.4)	(3.7)
Streptococcus uberis	272	5.7	14.7
Streptococcus dysgalactiae	239	5.0	12.9
Corynebacterium spp.	171	3.6	9.2
Other streptococci	119	2.5	6.4
Coliform	51	1.1	2.8
Yeast	20	0.4	1.1
Streptococcus agalactiae	17	0.4	0.9
Arcanobacterium pyogenes	8	0.2	0.4
Culture negative	2,914	61.1	-
Contaminated	7	0.2	-

Table 2. Udder health management factors in 200 random selected Dutch dairy farms.

Management factor		**% of herds**
Bedding in stalls	rubber mats	38%
	mattresses	31%
Separate calving area available		78%
Cleaning calving area after each calving		17%
Calving area also used as sick-pen		71%
Drinking water indoor season	water well	62%
	tap water	34%
	ditch water	2%
Cows pastured in summer	day and night	21%
	daytime only	55%
	not at all	21%
Wearing gloves during milking		21%
Fore-stripping		49%
Wiping before attachment	dry cloths	43%
	paper towel	40%
	wet disinfecting wipes	6%
	not at all	4%
Flushing liners with water	after every cow	13%
	after high SCC cow	63%
Bacteriology on a regular base	clinical cases	26%
	high SCC cows	17%
Postmilking teat disinfection practiced		82%
Clinical mastitis treatment	at first signs	69%
	postponed	31%
Change therapy after unsuccessful treatment		74%
Treatment subclinical mastitis		47%
Dry cow treatment with antibiotics	blanket (all cows)	87%
	selective	11%
	no antibiotics	2%
Milk containing antibiotic residues fed to calves		48%
Dry cows managed in two groups		44%
Teat disinfection dry cows		11%
Heifers precalving	housed with dry cows	47%
	housed with lactating cows	31%
	separate group	20%
Teat disinfection heifers precalving		8%

Rubber mats and mattresses were most common base for bedding in the stalls, sand boxes were not present. Mattresses and use of lime or bedding sanitizers were associated with *Staph. aureus* prevalence (P=0.03 and P<0.01, respectively). Drinking water sources other than tap water tended to be associated with *Strep. uberis* prevalence.

Stripping teats to detect clinical mastitis and to increase milk let down was practiced by 49% of the farmers, with a minority of them wearing milkers' gloves. Wiping udders before milking cluster attachment was most of the times carried out with cloths or paper towels. Only a minority did not wipe the udder before attachment. It was not possible to inventory the time between pretreatment and attachment in the questionnaire.

Clinical mastitis, clots in the milk and or a swollen quarter, was treated with antibiotics as soon as the first symptoms were observed in most of the farms (69%). In all other cases, farmers postponed treatment until the next milking, discarded milk a few times during daytime or used homeopathic treatment. If in cases of clinical mastitis, antibiotic treatment was not successful, most of the farmers (74%) changed to a different treatment. In our study, 8% of the farms had one or more sucklers in the group of heifers last year.

Discussion

In our study, all quarters of lactating cows with an elevated SCC were sampled. Coagulase-negative staphylococci, *Staph. aureus*, and *Strep. uberis* were most frequently isolated. Most recommended management practices were used on most farms. Ideally, every lactating animal in the participating herds should be sampled, as was done in earlier Dutch studies (Vecht *et al.*, 1989), and in some international studies (González *et al.*, 1988; Pitkälä *et al.*, 2004). However, by selecting cows we were able to reduce costs of the survey, as was done in other studies in Norway and in England and Wales (Østerås *et al.*, 2006, Bradley *et al.*, 2007).

Vecht *et al.* (1989) did not mention CNS as a distinct group of bacteria and named them 'other bacteria'. Coagulase-negative staphylococci were the most frequently isolated group of organisms isolated in most recent mastitis surveys (Pitkälä *et al.*, 2004; Bradley *et al.*, 2007). Prevalence of *Strep. agalactiae* IMI has decreased considerably in the last 30 years coinciding with the introduction of a penalty system for elevated bulk milk SCC in The Netherlands. Subsequently, the bulk milk SCC decreases in the same period (Nightingale *et al.*, 2008), probably as a result of an increased adoption of udder health management practices. Sol (2002) also found a decreased prevalence of *Strep. agalactiae* and *Staph. aureus* IMI and an increase of *Strep. uberis* IMI between 1975 and 2000 in milk samples submitted to the GD. Milk samples submitted to the GD were mainly samples of cows with an elevated SCC, therefore these results were not comparable with the survey results of Vecht *et al.* (1989).

Some other factors may also influence udder health. Hygiene can be measured by doing a hygiene score of cows and environment. Given the peak of clinical mastitis cases in the early lactation period, cleanliness of the maternity pen is assumed to be of great importance (Barkema *et al.*, 1998). In our study only 17% of farms cleaned the maternity pen after each calving. Drinking water from another source than tap water during the indoor season increased prevalence of CNS IMI (Sampimon *et al.*, 2008). In our study 66% used another water source than tap water. These 'other' water sources may increase the exposure to dirt which seems to be associated with *Strep. uberis* prevalence on these farms. Summer is the time when flies are most active. In our study fly control was practiced in some way on 86% of the farms. Flies, especially the hornfly *Haematobia irritans* which is very common in the Netherlands, can transmit *Staph. aureus* (Owens *et al.*, 1998).

Transmission of *Staph. aureus* and especially *Strep. agalactiae* can be influenced by milking procedures and the milking machine. In the Netherlands, the number of automatic milking systems and the size of milking parlors are increasing. Udder preparation is time consuming and some farmers in growing farms stopped practicing it. Wearing gloves, in our study 21% of the farmers, decreases bacterial load on hands and will reduce the exposure of bacteria on teats (Olde Riekerink *et al.*, 2008). Wet udder preparation was not practiced on a large scale in our study, 14%, but can increase clinical cases of *E. coli* (Schukken *et al.*, 1990). Post-milking teat disinfection is an important procedure to prevent IMI, which is practiced by 82% of our farms. The percentage of post milking teat disinfection in 1985 was considerably lower, namely 60% (Vecht *et al.*, 1989).

In our study, 17% of the farms collected milk samples for culturing. Culturing milk samples from cows with an elevated SCC is necessary to select the correct quarter for treatment. Additionally regular sampling of quarter milk samples of cows with an elevated SCC in a dairy herd is also useful to evaluate the distribution of pathogens on a herd-level. Mastitis control programs can subsequently be adjusted accordingly.

Drying off cows with antibiotics is meant to prevent new IMI and to cure existing IMI during the dry period. In our study more than 80% of the farmers used blanket dry cow therapy. In 1985 this was 58% (Vecht *et al.*, 1989). Forming two groups of dry cows, far-off and close-up, is necessary to avoid problems with milk leaking and to support a better feeding program (Barkema *et al.*, 1999). When farms manage dry cows as a single group, in our study 56% of the farms, heifers and close-up cows were often housed in the lactating group for several weeks before parturition. This may increase prevalence of milk leaking, and may increase incidence of udder edema due to high protein intake. This may have an unfavourable effect on udder health, because heifers with udder edema are 1.65 times more likely to develop clinical mastitis (Waage *et al.*, 2001).

Coagulase-negative staphylococci, *Staph. aureus*, and *Strep. uberis* were most frequently isolated pathogens in subclinical mastitis. Most recommended management practices were used on most farms, but there is room for improvement.

Acknowledgements

This study is part of the five-year udder health program of the Dutch Udder Health Centre and was financially supported by the Dutch Dairy Board. We thank the participating farmers for their time and special thanks to Ms. Vera Eerland, Ms. Sarienke Barneveld and the students who did the sampling work.

References

Barkema, H.W., Schukken, Y.H., Lam, T. J.G.M., Beiboer, M. L., Wilmink, H., Benedictus, G. and Brand, A., 1998. Incidence of clinical mastitis in dairy herds grouped in three categories by bulk milk somatic cell counts. J. Dairy Sci. 81: 411-419.

Barkema, H.W., Schukken, Y.H., Lam, T.J.G.M., Beiboer, M.L., Benedictus, G. and Brand, A., 1999. Management practices associated with the incidence rate of clinical mastitis. J. Dairy Sci. 82:1643-1654.

Bradley, A.J., Leach, K.A., Breen, J.E., Green, L.E. and Green, M.J., 2007. Survey of the incidence and aetiology of mastitis on dairy farms in England and Wales. Vet. Rec. 160: 253-258.

Gonzalez R.N., Jasper, D.E., Farver, T.B., Bushnell, R.B. and Franti, C.E., 1988. Prevalence of udder infections and mastitis in 50 California dairy herds. J. Am. Vet. Med. Ass. 193: 323-328.

Halasa, T., Huijps, K., Østerås, O. and Hogeveen, H., 2007. Economic effects of bovine mastitis and mastitis management: A review. Vet. Quart. 29: 18-31.

Harmon, R.J., Eberhart, R.J., Jasper, D.E., Langlois, B.E. and Wilson, R.A., 1990. Microbiological procedures for the diagnosis of udder infection. National Mastitis Council Inc., Arlington, VA, USA.

Nightingale, C., Dhuyvetter, K., Mitchell, R. and Schukken, Y.H., 2008. Influence of variable milk quality premiums on observed milk quality. J. Dairy Sci. 91: 1236-1244.

Olde Riekerink, R.G.M., Sampimon, O.C., Eerland, V.J., Swarts, M.J. and Lam, T.J.G.M., 2008. Comparing bacterial counts on bare hands with gloved hands during milking. In: Mastitis control – From science to practice. Wageningen Academic Publishers, the Netherlands, pp. 77-82

Østerås, O., Sølverød, L. and Reksen, O., 2006. Milk culture results in a large Norwegian survey – effects of season, parity, days in milk, resistance, and clustering. J. Dairy Sci. 89: 1010-1023.

Owens, W.E., Oliver, S.P., Gillespie, B.E., Ray, C.H. and Nickerson, S.C., 1998. Role of horn flies (*Haematobia irritans*) in *Staphylococcus aureus*-induced mastitis in dairy heifers. Am. J. Vet. Res. 59: 1122-1124.

Pitkälä, A., Haveri, M., Pyörälä, S., Myllys, V. and Honkanen-Buzalski, T., 2004. Bovine mastitis in Finland 2001 – prevalence, distribution of bacteria, and antimicrobial resistance. J. Dairy Sci. 87: 2433-2441.

Sampimon, O.C., Barkema, H.W. Berends, I.M.G.A., Sol, J. and Lam, T.J.G.M., 2008. Prevalence and herd-level risk factors for intramammary infection with coagulase-negative staphylococci in Dutch dairy herds. Vet. Microbiol. (in press).

Schukken, Y.H., Grommers, F.J., Van der Geer, D., Erb, H.N. and Brand, A., 1990. Risk factors for clinical mastitis in herds with a low bulk milk somatic cell count. 1. Data and risk factors for all cases. J. Dairy Sci. 73: 3463-3471.

Smith, K.L. and Hogan, J.S., 2001. The world of mastitis. Proc. 2nd Intern. Symp. mastitis and milk quality, Vancouver, BC, Canada, September 13-15, pp. 1-12.

Sol, J., 2002. Cure of *Staphylococcus aureus* mastitis in Dutch dairy cows. PhD-thesis, Utrecht University, the Netherlands.

Vecht, U., Wisselink, H.J. and Defize, P.R., 1989. Dutch national mastitis survey. The effect of herd and animal factors on somatic cell count. Neth. Milk Dairy J. 43: 425-435.

Waage, S., Odegaard, S.A., Lund, A., Brattgjerd, S., Rothe, T., 2001. Case-control study of risk factors for clinical mastitis in postpartum dairy heifers. J. Dairy Sci. 84:392-399.

Prevalence of mastitis pathogens in milk samples from Portuguese dairy cattle

L. Pinho[1,2], J. Ferreira[3], C. Cabral[3], R. Lameira[3], P. Meireles[3], F. Vaz[3], J. Carvalheira[1,4] and G. Thompson[1,2]
[1]Instituto de Ciências Biomédicas de Abel Salazar (ICBAS), Universidade do Porto, Rua Padre Armando Quintas, 4480-661 Vairão, Vila do Conde, Portugal
[2]Unidade Multidisciplinar de Investigação Biomédica (UMIB), Universidade do Porto, Largo Professor Abel Salazar, 4100 Porto, Portugal
[3]Serviços Veterinários Associados – SVA, Rua Dom Sancho I, 3202, 4760-485 Fradelos, Portugal
[4]Centro de Investigação em Biodiversidade e Recursos Genéticos (CIBIO), Universidade do Porto, Rua Padre Armando Quintas, 4480-661 Vairão, Vila do Conde, Portugal
Corresponding author: luis.pinho@mail.icav.up.pt

Abstract

Prevalence of contagious and environmental etiologic agents of bovine mastitis was obtained from 15,046 milk samples of subclinical and clinical mastitis submitted for bacteriologic culture. Milk samples were obtained between January 2005 and January 2008 in the Northwest Portugal from 373 dairy farms. Environmental agents were the most prevalent (69.4%) compared to contagious agents (30.3%). *Streptococcus* spp. non-*agalactiae* (16.5%) were the most frequent agent followed by coagulase-negative *Staphylococcus* (12.9%). On the other hand, the most frequent contagious agents found were *Corynebacterium* spp. (16.2%), followed by *Staphyloccus aureus* (12.6%), and *Streptococcus agalactiae* (0.9%). No growth and contaminated samples represented, respectively, 10.6% and 11.6% of the total samples. Comparisons between dairy farms enrolled or not, in milk quality programs were made. We conclude that the development and implementation of milk quality programs to control both environmental and contagious organisms should be mandatory in this region of the country.

Keywords: aetiology, pathogens, prevalence

Introduction

Mastitis is the most frequent and costly disease in dairy production and is associated with both direct (e.g. veterinary treatments, increased labour, loss of production), and indirect costs (e.g. premature culling, reduced milk price due to increased bulk milk SCC) (Fetrow, 2000; Ruegg, 2001; Ødegård, 2006). This disease is primarily caused by organisms, such as bacteria, yeasts, algae and mycoplasma. However, from the total 137 different organisms that has been identified as possible aetiological agents of mastitis, the majority of infections are caused by staphylococci, streptococci, and gram-negative bacteria (Bradley, 2002). Bacterial pathogens that cause mastitis are generally classified as either contagious or environmental based upon their primary reservoir and mode of transmission. Contagious mastitis pathogens are found in the udder of the cow, and they are commonly transmitted among cows by contact with infected milk. The most important contagious mastitis pathogens include *Streptococcus agalactiae, Staphylococcus aureus, Corynebacterium bovis,* and *Mycoplasma* spp. On the other hand, cows are continuously exposed to environmental mastitis pathogens because the primary route of exposure is contact with moisture, mud, and manure. Unlike mastitis caused by contagious pathogens, environmental mastitis cannot be eradicated from a dairy herd.

Since the implementation of the Five-Point Plan in the 1960s (Neave *et al.*, 1966), there has been a dramatic decrease in bulk milk somatic cell counts, clinical mastitis and the importance of the contagious mastitis pathogens. However, the absolute as well relative incidence of environmental pathogens has increased over the same period of time. *S. aureus* continues to be a major cause of sub-clinical mastitis though there appears to be some evidence that pathogens previously considered to be purely environmental may also be capable of causing persistent infections (Bradley, 2002; Ruegg, 2001).

Prevalence and seasonal trends have been examined in different studies, and different trends were identified for various pathogens (Wilson *et al.*, 1997; Myllys *et al.*, 1998; Makovec and Ruegg, 2003; Tenhagen *et al.*, 2006; Østerås et al, 2006). Information about the prevalence of mastitis pathogens in Portugal is scarce, and the last epidemiological survey showed that more than 50% of the total infected quarters were caused by subclinical infections due to *S. aureus* and *Streptococcus uberis* (Louzã *et al.*, 1986). For the last years, the somatic cell count has decreased in Portuguese dairy herds but the relationship with mastitis pathogens was not studied.

The objective of this study was to determine the prevalence of the mastitis pathogens organisms in dairy herds from Northwest Portugal, in milk samples from dairy cows submitted to a veterinary laboratory between January 2005 and January 2008.

Material and methods

Submitted samples belonged to 373 farms and were obtained from January 2005 to January 2008. Milk samples were cultured using standard microbiologic methods as described by the National Mastitis Council (1999). Briefly, 0.01 ml of milk was streaked on a portion of a blood agar plate (Biomérieux, Portugal), MacConkey plate (Biomérieux, Portugal), and Sabouraud-dextrose-agar plate (Biomérieux, Portugal) and incubated at 37 °C overnight. Plates were examined for growth at 24 and 48 h. Bacteria were identified by colony morphology and growth, and Gram stain. For gram-positive cocci, catalase tests were performed to distinguish catalase-negative *Streptococcus* spp. from catalase-positive *Staphylococcus* spp. The CAMP test and growth on Edwards modified agar (Luis Esteve Nuez, Spain) were used to differentiate *S. agalactiae* from other streptococci. Catalase-positive gram-positive cocci were further identified using a coagulase test, hemolysis patterns, and observation under optic microscope. Gram-positive bacilli were further identified using the catalase test and biochemical reactions as needed. Gram-negative bacilli were identified by the oxidase test (Biomérieux, Portugal), motility test, triple sugar-iron agar, and Simmons citrate (Luis Esteve Nuez, Spain). Contaminated samples were defined as a mixture of more than two different species of organisms. Samples were classified as No Growth when no colonies were observed at 48 h of incubation.

Results

Milk samples submitted for microbiological diagnostic (n=15,046) were characterised as No growth (n=2,009), contaminated (n=2,209), or with the presence of mastitis pathogens (n=10,828). Twenty three farms were part of a mastitis control program during the same period of study. The number of isolates per year ranged from 3,178 to 6,735 (Figure 1).

As expected, no growth or contaminated samples represented 22.2% of the total submitted samples. Environmental agents were the most prevalent (69.4%) compared to contagious agents (30.3%). *Streptococcus* spp. non-*agalactiae* (20.7%) were more frequently isolated followed by coagulase-negative *Staphylococcus* (14.7%), coliforms (14.3%), yeast (9.4%), *Enterococcus* spp. (4.3%), *Bacillus* spp. (3.5%) and fungi (0.2%). Contagious agents most frequently found were *Corynebacterium* spp. (16.5%), followed by *S. aureus* (12.9%), and *S. agalactiae* (0.9%) (Table 1).

Pure samples (n=8,472) and multiple samples (n=2,356) yielded the total number of bacterial results (n=14,761). A higher percentage of milk samples with no microbiologic results (19.2%) and a lower percentage of contaminated samples (9.9%) were found in milk samples originated from dairy farms enrolled in a milk quality program when compared to the total samples

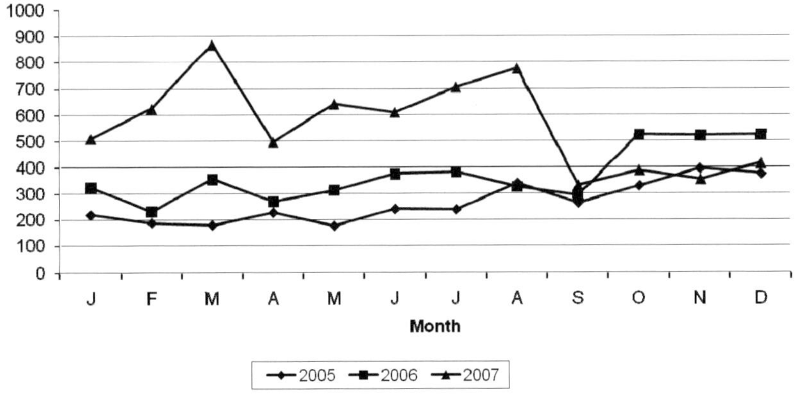

Figure 1. Number of isolates per year from January to December.

Table 1. Results of submitted milk samples.

Isolate	Number of isolates	% of results	% of positive culture samples
No growth	2,009	10.59	-
Contaminated	2,209	11.64	-
Streptococcus spp.[1]	3,053	16.09	20.68
Corynebacterium spp.	2,438	12.85	16.52
Staphylococcus coagulase-negative	2,208	11.63	14.96
Coliformes	2,112	11.13	14.31
Staphylococcus aureus	1,899	10.01	12.86
Yeast	1,391	7.33	9.42
Enterococcus spp.	631	3.32	4.27
Bacillus spp.	514	2.71	3.48
Prototheca spp.	155	0.82	1.05
Arcanobacterium pyogenes	145	0.76	0.98
Streptococcus agalactiae	138	0.73	0.93
Others	40	0.21	0.27
Fungi	37	0.19	0.25

[1] Not including *Strep. agalactiae.*

analysed. *Corynebacterium* spp. was the contagious pathogen most frequently found (17.5%), while *Streptococcus* spp. was the environmental agent with a higher number of isolates. When comparing milk samples from the milk quality program to the total submitted samples, no significant differences were observed in the percentage of environmental pathogens (68.1%) as well as in the percentage of contagious agents (31.8%) (Table 2).

Discussion

Milk samples analysed in this study were originated from clinical and subclinical cases of mastitis, whole herd checks and from surveillance programs. Samples submitted to the laboratory tend to be biased towards problem cows and herds, thus the results may only transmit a part of the region reality. The short period of the study (January 2005 to January 2008) was not sufficient to take conclusions about trends of mastitis pathogens. The lack of information regarding parity, days in milk and farm management practices may affect negatively the significance of the results implying the need of further studies.

Table 2. Results of milk samples from dairy farms enrolled in a milk quality program.

Isolate	Number of isolates	% of results	% of positive culture samples
No growth	742	19.25	-
Contaminated	381	9.89	-
Streptococcus spp.[1]	658	17.07	24.09
Corynebacterium spp.	477	12.38	17.47
Staphylococcus coagulase-negative	412	10.69	15.09
Staphylococcus aureus	356	9.24	13.04
Coliformes	348	9.03	12.74
Yeast	256	6.64	9.37
Enterococcus spp.	110	2.85	4.03
Bacillus spp.	38	0.99	1.39
Streptococcus agalactiae	36	0.93	1.32
Arcanobacterium pyogenes	24	0.62	0.88
Prototheca spp.	9	0.23	0.33
Fungi	5	0.13	0.18
Others	2	0.05	0.07

[1] Not including *Strep. agalactiae.*

Samples with no microbiologic results represented a small percentage of the total results when compared to other identical studies (Bradley, 2002; Makovec and Ruegg, 2003). This fact may be explained by improper hygiene measures when collecting milk samples. Moreover, the clinician's perception is that the majority of samples are usually submitted to the laboratory only after failure of the first therapy, which may mask the original cause of mastitis. Therefore, results from this study may differ from reality emphasising more the microbiological environment at the time of sampling.

Growth inhibitors were not evaluated in samples with no growth which may introduce some bias in the results. In addition, some of the samples characterised as no growth may be attributed to *Mycoplasma* spp. or to other fastidious microorganisms, which have specific growth requirements, and were out of the scope of this work. The real importance of these agents as a cause of mastitis in the country is not yet known and will be the objective of further studies.

The results showed that environmental pathogens were the predominant group of microorganisms isolated from milk samples which is in agreement with other authors (Bradley,

A comparison of the occurrence of mastitis in Dutch primi- and multiparous cows

B.H.P. van den Borne[1], G. van Schaik[2], T.J.G.M. Lam[2,3] and M. Nielen[1]
[1]Utrecht University, Faculty of Veterinary Medicine, Marburglaan 2, 3584 CL Utrecht, the Netherlands
[2]Animal Health Service (GD), P.O. Box 9, 7400 AA Deventer, the Netherlands
[3]Dutch Udder Health Centre, P.O. Box 2030, 7420 AA Deventer, the Netherlands
Corresponding author: b.vandenborne@uu.nl

Abstract

Accurate estimates of the occurrence of mastitis in either heifers or multiparous cows are important to set goals and to select animals to focus on in a mastitis control program, both at the farm and national level. Because no recent estimates were available in the Netherlands, the goal of this study was to determine (sub)clinical mastitis prevalence and incidence in Dutch primi- and multiparous cows. A study on 396 dairy farms with 45,322 cows was conducted from July 2004 till June 2005. Composite somatic cell counts (CSCC) were gathered from the test day recording to calculate subclinical mastitis (SCM) prevalence as the proportion animals with a CSCC >200,000 cells/ml. SCM incidence rate was calculated as the number of new infections divided by the number of cow days at risk. Additionally, clinical mastitis (CM) was recorded by a subset of 205 farmers on 25,879 cows. CM incidence rate was calculated similarly to SCM. Negative binomial models were used separately for primi- and multiparous cows to correct for overdispersion. Average SCM prevalence was 13.2% for primi- and 27.6% for multiparous cows. SCM prevalence was the highest in August 2004 and the lowest in February 2005 for both primi- and multiparous cows. SCM incidence rate was higher in multiparous cows (1.17/365 days at risk) compared to primiparous cows (0.81/365 days at risk). Additionally, CM incidence rate was also higher in multiparous cows (0.41/365 days at risk) compared to primiparous cows (0.20/365 days at risk). This study gives insight in the current prevalence and incidence rate of mastitis in Dutch primi- and multiparous cows. It is a good starting point for further research, to set goals for mastitis control and to monitor the influence of control measures.

Keywords: clinical mastitis, monitoring, parity, subclinical mastitis

Introduction

Mastitis causes economic losses due a decreased milk production, usage of antibiotics, discarded milk, increased culling and extra labour (Halasa *et al.*, 2007). Furthermore, mastitis decreases animal welfare and frustrates the farmer's routine during milking.

Parity is an important factor for the occurrence of both subclinical and clinical mastitis, besides other cow associated risk factors such as milk production, stage of lactation and breed. A higher occurrence of (sub)clinical mastitis is generally seen in multiparous cows, but a higher incidence is seen in early lactation in primiparous cows. Barkema *et al.* (1998) estimated the incidence rate of clinical mastitis (CM) in Dutch primiparous cows to be 0.16 (/365 days at risk) while increasing incidence rates of (+/-) 0.22 to 0.51 (/365 days at risk) were observed in multiparous cows with increasing parity. However, these estimates are based on data collected in 1993 and 1994 and no recent estimates on the occurrence of clinical mastitis in the Netherlands are available.

A study has therefore been conducted to determine the current (sub)clinical mastitis prevalence and incidence rate in both primi- and multiparous cows in the Netherlands. With these estimates, goals can be set in a mastitis control program for primi- and multiparous cows, both at the farm and national level.

Material and methods

An extensive survey on 408 randomly selected dairy farms was performed from July 1st, 2004 till June 30th, 2005 to collect data on (sub)clinical mastitis occurrence. To focus on farms that were expected to stay in business the next five years, farms had to have more than 50 dairy cows, had to participate in the Dutch test day recording with intervals from three to six weeks and the age of the farmer had to be below 57 years of age.

Composite somatic cell counts (CSCC) were gathered from the regular test day recording from all 396 participating dairy herds to calculate prevalence and incidence rate of subclinical mastitis (SCM). Additionally, 205 farmers recorded date of mastitis and the infected quarter of all CM cases in their herds. A CM case was diagnosed by the farmer as a cow with visual abnormalities in the milk and/or quarter. Farms with five or less test day recordings (n=8) and with no clinical mastitis occurring in the study period (n=4) were excluded from the analysis.

Mastitis indicators

CSCC are commonly used as a reflection of the udder health status of a cow as they reflect an inflammatory response, although they do not truly identify an intramammary infection (Schukken *et al.*, 2003). Nevertheless, a cow was assumed to have subclinical mastitis (SCM) in this study when it had an elevated CSCC. SCM prevalence was therefore calculated as the proportion animals at a test day with a CSCC above a certain threshold. The threshold of 200,000 cells/ml was chosen as the default because this threshold is commonly used internationally. But, as sensitivity and specificity differ for different thresholds and different thresholds do exist worldwide, the thresholds of 250,000 cells/ml, 150,000 cells/ml and 100,000 cells/ml were also evaluated to observe differences between thresholds.

SCM prevalence was calculated as the proportion of animals with a CSCC above the threshold at a certain test day. SCM incidence rate was calculated as the number of new cases of SCM divided by the number of days at risk. SCM prevalence and incidence rate were both calculated at the herd level. A new case of SCM at cow level was defined to be an elevation in CSCC above a certain threshold after two consecutive CSCC measurements below that threshold, regardless of the dry period. The number of cow (or heifer) days at risk was defined at cow level as the number of days with a CSCC below the threshold, as illustrated in Figure 1. The days between calving and the first CSCC measurement after calving were also considered to be at risk if the first CSCC measurement after calving was below the threshold, as were the days between the last CSCC measurement before drying off and the first expected test day record in the dry period, assessed at the herd level, if the CSCC was below the threshold. The remaining days during the dry period were not considered to be at risk for increased CSCC. The number of new SCM cases and the number of days at risk within a herd were added up to calculate herd level SCM incidence rate. SCM incidence was expressed as the number of CSCC elevations in 365 cow (or heifer) days at risk when calculated at the herd level. The four different thresholds were used to define new SCM cases and time at risk in four separate analyses. Incidence rate of CM was similarly calculated as the number of quarter cases of mastitis divided by the number of cow (or heifer) days at risk, both assessed at farm level. Every CM case diagnosed by the farmer was assigned to be a new case of CM with the exception of clinical mastitis events occurring within 14 days in the same quarter. Those were not considered a new case and were therefore deleted. The number of days at risk was assessed as the number of days an animal was present at the farm during the study period, with the exception for heifers, who became at risk at their first calving.

Statistical analysis

To estimate SCM prevalence at herd level, negative binomial models with repeated measures and the autoregressive correlation structure, to correct for repeated measures, were used in PROC GENMOD (SAS Institute, Cary, USA). Herd level SCM and CM incidence rates were also estimated using negative binomial models in PROC GENMOD (SAS Institute, Cary, USA), although no repeated effect was used in these models. Separate models were made for primi- and multiparous cows. Model fit for all models was evaluated by checking for normality of the residuals. All models showed a good fit.

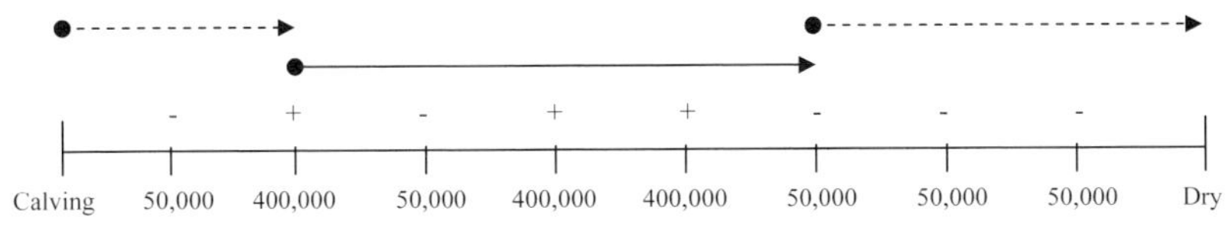

Figure 1. A visualisation of the cow-days at risk in lactation for the definition of subclinical mastitis incidence rate for one individual animal. Straight arrow = infected, dotted arrow = at risk

Results

The dataset for subclinical mastitis compromised 396 dairy herds with 16,571 primiparous and 28,751 multiparous cows, while records on 205 herds with 9,850 primiparous and 16,029 multiparous cows were available for analysis of clinical mastitis. In the total dataset (n=396) the average herd size was 77.4 (SD=25.0) cows and the average bulk milk SCC was 190,000 (SD=78,000) cells/ml. Because animals calved and were culled throughout the study period, the median time primi- and multiparous cows were in the one year study period was 184 (min=1; max=365) and 340 (min=1; max=365) days respectively.

Prevalence of subclinical mastitis

Herd level SCM prevalence at the default threshold (200,000 cells/ml) was estimated to be 13.2% and 27.6% for primi- and multiparous cows (Table 1). SCM prevalence increased with a decreasing threshold for both primi- and multiparous cows, to about 30% and 50% at the threshold of 100,000 cells/ml. SCM prevalence was the highest in August 2004 and the lowest in February 2005 at the default threshold (Figure 2).

Incidence rate of subclinical mastitis

In the default situation (threshold of 200,000 cells/ml), herd level SCM incidence rate is 0.81 (/365 days at risk) in primiparous cows compared to 1.17 (/365 days at risk) in multiparous cows (Table 2). To illustrate SCM incidence rate; if a multiparous cow theoretically would be in lactation for 365 days continuously it would have on average 1.17 new SCM cases during that lactation. From Table 2, an increasing SCM incidence rate can be observed with a decreasing threshold for both primi- and multiparous cows. Similar variation is observed between herds in SCM incidence rates for both primi- and multiparous cows (Figure 3).

Table 1. Estimated herd level subclinical mastitis prevalence with 95%-confidence interval according to four different thresholds from July 1st, 2004 till June 30th 2005 in Dutch primi- and multiparous cows, based on a negative binomial model with a repeated herd effect.

Threshold (cells/ml)	Subclinical mastitis prevalence (%)	
	primiparous cows	multiparous cows
250,000	9.9% [9.3-10.4]	21.9% [21.1-22.7]
200,000	13.2% [12.6-13.9]	27.6% [26.7-28.6]
150,000	19.1% [18.2-19.9]	36.5% [35.3-37.7]
100,000	30.6% [29.6-31.8]	50.5% [49.0-52.0]

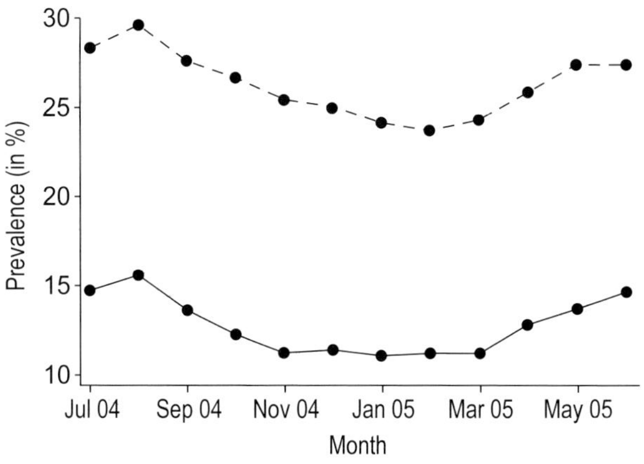

Figure 2. Mean herd level subclinical mastitis prevalence per month at the threshold of 200,000 cells/ml from July 1st, 2004 till June 30th 2005 in Dutch primi- (—) and multiparous (---) cows.

Table 2. Estimated herd level subclinical mastitis incidence rate with 95%-confidence interval, expressed as the number of new cases per 365 days at risk, according to four different thresholds from July 1st, 2004 till June 30th 2005 in Dutch primi- and multiparous cows, based on a negative binomial model.

Threshold (cells/ml)	Subclinical mastitis incidence rate (/365 days at risk)	
	primiparous cows	multiparous cows
250,000	0.58 [0.56-0.62]	0.98 [0.94-1.01]
200,000	0.81 [0.77-0.85]	1.17 [1.13-1.21]
150,000	1.10 [1.05-1.15]	1.45 [1.41-1.50]
100,000	1.75 [1.68-1.83]	1.92 [1.86-1.98]

Incidence rate of clinical mastitis

CM incidence rate was 0.20 [0.18-0.22] and 0.41 [0.39-0.44] (/365 days at risk) for primi- and multiparous cows respectively from July 1st 2004 till 30th June 2004, while overall CM incidence rate was 0.31 [0.29-0.34]. Variation in CM incidence rate, for both primi- and multiparous cows, was seen between herds (Figure 4), although more variation between herds was observed in multiparous cows compared to primiparous cows.

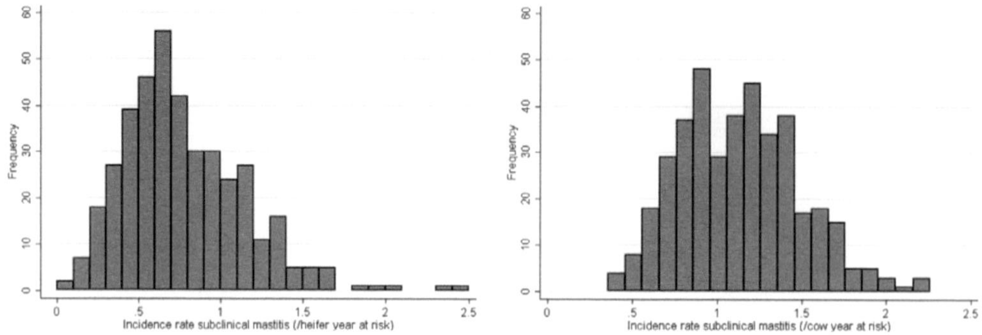

Figure 3. Histograms showing the distribution of herd level subclinical mastitis incidence rate (/365 days at risk) on 396 dairy farms, according to the threshold of 200,000 cells/ml, from July 1st, 2004 till June 30th 2005 in Dutch primi- (left) and multiparous (right) cows.

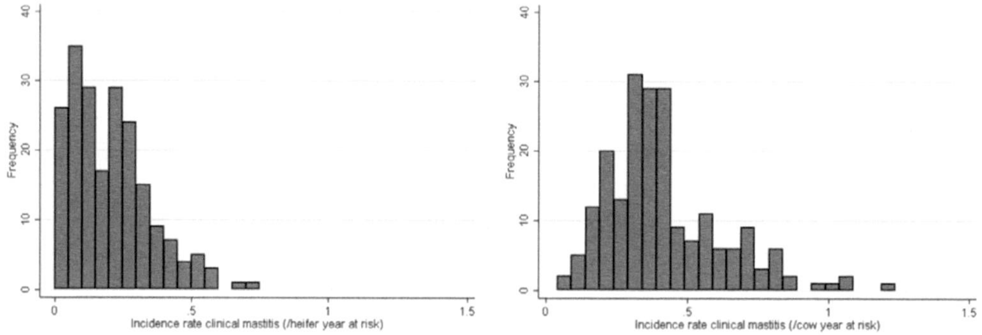

Figure 4. Histograms showing the distribution of herd level clinical mastitis incidence rate (/365 days at risk) on 205 dairy farms, from July 1st, 2004 till June 30th 2005 in Dutch primi- (left) and multiparous (right) cows.

Discussion

CSCC are commonly used as an indication for subclinical mastitis although they may not truly reflect an intramammary infection. Sensitivity and specificity vary between thresholds used, with specificity being high (0.92) for the default threshold (Dohoo and Leslie, 1991), indicating few false positive animals above this threshold. Additionally, CSCC are easily available from the test day recording, making them very suitable for monitoring purposes. To observe the effect of the used thresholds, several were evaluated. An increasing prevalence and incidence rate were observed with a decreasing threshold as expected.

Between herd variation was observed in the incidence rates for SCM and CM, with variation being the highest in multiparous cows for CM. Some herds had a CM or SCM incidence rate twice the average, leaving room for improvement. Mastitis control programs should therefore focus on these herds, as the most gain is to be expected in the age groups of these herds.

Incidence rates of CM in primi- and multiparous cows from this study are comparable with the estimates from Barkema *et al.* (1998), indicating little change in the occurrence of CM in the Netherlands in the last decade. Estimates of CM from this study are higher compared to the number of veterinary-treated clinical cases in Sweden in 2006, being 0.10 (/365 days at risk) in primiparous cows and 0.15 to 0.25 (/365 days at risk) in multiparous cows with an increasing parity (Persson Waller *et al.*, 2007). The Dutch overall (regardless parity) CM incidence rate (0.31/365 days at risk) is in between recent (overall) estimates from other countries worldwide: Olde Riekerink *et al.* (2008) reported 0.23 cases (/365 days at risk) in Canada, Valde *et al.* (2005) observed 0.36 cases (/365 days at risk) in Norway, while Bradley *et al.* (2007) found 0.47 cases (/365 days at risk) in England and Wales. Because no confidence intervals were reported in the other studies, true differences between countries can not be established.

Conclusion

The estimates on prevalence and incidence rates of (sub)clinical mastitis from this study did not seem to differ from the estimates of Barkema and co-workers (1998). Large differences in occurrence of mastitis between farms are observed, leaving room for improvement and therefore justifying a mastitis control program. Using these estimates, focus areas can be identified for research, parity- and herd specific goals can be set for a mastitis control program and the effect of control measures on mastitis can be monitored.

Acknowledgements

This study is part of the five-year udder health program of the Dutch Udder Health Centre and was financially supported by the Dutch Dairy Board.

References

Barkema, H.W., Schukken, Y.H., Lam, T.J.G.M., Beiboer, M.L., Wilmink, H., Benedictus, G. and Brand, A., 1998. Incidence of clinical mastitis in dairy herds grouped in three categories by bulk milk somatic cell counts. J. Dairy Sci. 81: 411-419.

Bradley, A.J., Leach, K.A., Breen, J.E., Green, L.E. and Green, M.J., 2007. Survey of the incidence and aetiology of mastitis on dairy farms in England and Wales. Vet. Rec. 160: 253-258.

Dohoo, I.R. and Leslie, K.E., 1991. Evaluation of changes in somatic cell counts as indicators of new intramammary infections. Prev. Vet. Med. 10: 225-237.

Halasa, T., Huijps, K., Osteras, O. and Hogeveen, H., 2007. Economic effects of bovine mastitis and mastitis management: A review. Vet. Quart. 29: 18-31.

Olde Riekerink, R.G.M., Barkema, H.W., Kelton, D.F. and Scholl, D.T., 2008. Incidence rate of clinical mastitis on Canadian dairy farms. J. Dairy Sci. 91: 1366-1377.

Persson Waller, K., Bengtsson, B., Lindberg, A., Nyman, A. and Unnerstad, H., 2007. Incidence of mastitis and bacterial findings at acute clinical mastitis in Swedish primiparous cows – influence of breed and stage of lactation. Heifer mastitis conference, Gent.

Schukken, Y.H., Wilson, D.J., Welcome, F., Garrison-Tikofsky, L., González, R.N., 2003. Monitoring udder health and milk quality using somatic cell counts. Vet. Res. 34: 579-596.
Valde, J.P., Osteras, O. and Simensen, E., 2005. Description of herd level criteria for good and poor udder health in Norwegian dairy cows. J. Dairy Sci. 88: 86-92.

Prevalence of pathogens in milk samples of dairy cows with clinical mastitis and in heifers at first parturition

B.-A. Tenhagen, I. Hansen, A. Reinecke and W. Heuwieser
Freie Universität Berlin, Tierklinik für Fortpflanzung, Königsweg 65, Hs. 27, 14163 Berlin, Germany
Corresponding author: Bernd-Alois.Tenhagen@Bfr.bund.de

Abstract

Prevalence of mastitis pathogens in milk samples from dairy cows and heifers was studied over a period of one year (Aug 2005 to Aug 2006) in ten dairy herds in Germany. Milk samples (n=8240) were collected from heifers without clinical mastitis at parturition (n=6915), from primiparous cows with clinical mastitis (n=751) and from older cows with clinical mastitis (n=574). Coagulase negative staphylococci (CNS) were the predominant group of bacteria isolated (46.8 % of samples) from clinically healthy quarters of primiparous cows around parturition, followed by streptococci (12.6%), *E. coli* (4.7%) and *S. aureus* (4.0%). 33.0 % of samples were negative on culture (Range on farm level 12.0 to 46.4 %). In cases of clinical mastitis in primiparous and older cows, streptococci were the predominant finding (32.1 and 39.2 %), followed by CNS (27.4 and 16.4%), coliforms (10.3 and 13.1%) and *S. aureus* (10.0 and 11.7%). Negative results were obtained from 21.3 % (range 0.0 to 30.6 %) and 19.5 % (range 0.0 to 32.6 %) of these samples. Results indicated substantial differences in the prevalence of pathogens between herds. There was a positive within herd correlation between the monthly prevalences for *S. dysgalactiae* in the three groups of samples. This correlation was also found between clinical samples of primiparous and older cows for *S. aureus*. Other pathogens were not correlated. Besides herd, prevalence of pathogens was influenced by parity, type of sample and season.

Keywords: heifers, multiparous, prevalence, primiparous

Introduction

A lot of research has been conducted to study risk factors for clinical mastitis and intramammary infection at first parturition, on the prevalence of pathogens in heifers, and on the pathogens associated with clinical mastitis in dairy heifers and primiparous cows (Kalmus *et al.*, 2006; Parker *et al.*, 2007; Compton *et al.*, 2007b). However, the relationsship of intramammary infection, clinical mastitis and the associated pathogens in primiparous and older cows within the same herd has not been studied intensively.

Some studies have reported such a relationsship, without reference to the pathogens involved (Waage *et al.*, 1998; Parker *et al.*, 2007). It was the purpose of this study to analyse patterns of clinical mastitis and intramammary infection in primiparous dairy cows in comparison to their older herdmates.

Material and methods

The study was conducted on 10 commercial dairy farms in north eastern Germany. The herds had on average 700 cows with a milk quota of 6,200 tons per year. All herds used their own replacement exclusively.

Collection of milk samples

Quarter milk samples were collected between August 2005 and August 2006. Farms were advised to sample any case of clinical mastitis during the first month of lactation prior to treatment and a maximum of 5 heifers per week within 48 hours of parturition. Two types of samples were differentiated: (1) 'Clinical samples' were from quarters with clinical mastitis. These were further characterised by the age of the cows (primiparous vs. multiparous) and the time relative to parturition when they were collected. (2) 'Non-clinical samples' were colostrum samples from clinically healthy quarters of primiparous cows.

Samples were collected by trained farm personnel. After cleaning of the teats and discarding the first streaks of milk teats were wiped with commercial towels for teat disinfection as provided together with intramammary drugs by the pharmaceutical companies. Samples were collected in sterile vials and stored in a refrigerator at about 4 °C until transportation to the laboratory and analysis.

Laboratory analysis

In the laboratory 0.01 ml of milk were streaked out on one half of an agar dish (Blood Agar Base Nr. 2, Oxoid, Wesel, supplemented with 5% sheep blood and 0.1% aesculin). After 48 hours of incubation growth was evaluated and preliminary identification by colony morphology and hemolysis was carried out.

Staphylococcus aureus was differentiated from coagulase negative staphylococci (CNS) using a commercial tube coagulase test (BBL Coagulase Plasma, Rabbit; Becton, Dickinson and Company, Heidelberg, Germany). Streptococci were differentiated using the CAMP Test and a commercial test to define Lancefield groups (Streptococcal grouping kit; Oxoid, Wesel, Germany). Streptococci were differentiated into *Streptococcus agalactiae* (positive CAMP test and Lancefield group B), *S. dysgalactiae* (esculin negative, Lancefield C), *S. uberis* (esculin pos., no growth on salt, non Lancefield D) and other streptococci.

Coliforms, yeasts and *Arcanobacterium pyogenes* were identified by colony morphology and gram staining. All other bacteria were summarised as 'others' for the purpose of this study.

Samples with growth of two pathogens were regarded positive for both pathogens. Samples with growth of more than two pathogens were classified as contaminated and withdrawn from the analysis. For *S. aureus* and *A. pyogenes* single colonies (i.e. 100 cfu/ml) were regarded as positive. For all other pathogens a minimum of 300 cfu/ml was required.

Statistical analysis

Analysis was based on quarters. Proportions are given as proportions of samples that could be analysed. Contaminated samples were withdrawn from the analysis. Factors influencing the outcome of the milk sample were studied using separate binary logistic regression for the six most prevalent pathogens. The outcome variable was presence of the respective pathogen. The independent factors were herd, season, location of quarter, type of sample and parity. As location of quarter had no significant effect, it was dropped from the final model.

The relationship between the prevalence of pathogens in the three groups of samples (primiparous colostrum, primiparous mastitis, multiparous mastitis) was analysed using Spearmans correlation coefficient for each pair based on the prevalence of the pathogen stratified by herd and month. All analyses were carried out using SPSS Version. 12.0 (SPSS Inc. München, Germany).

Results

The prevalence of pathogens in the different types of milk samples is presented in Figure 1. Herd influenced the prevalence of all pathogens in the samples. Primiparous cows were more likely to harbour CNS (OR 2.08 95% CI 1.57-2.75) and *Sc. dysgalactiae* (1.74 95% CI 1.14-2.65). On the other hand, their mammary glands were less likely to be infected with *Streptococcus* species other than *Sc. agalactiae, Sc. uberis* and *Sc. dysgalactiae.* (OR 0.60, 95% CI 0.46-0.79). As expected, major pathogens were more often found in clinical samples than in non clinical samples (OR between 2.16 for *S. aureus* and 4.83 for *Sc. uberis*). CNS were more prevalent in non clinical samples than in clinical samples (OR 2.18, 95% CI 1.82-2.60). CNS, *S. aureus* and coliforms were more prevalent in summer while all *Streptococcus* species were more prevalent in winter.

The prevalence of *S. aureus* in mastitis samples from older cows was significantly related to the prevalence in of *S. aureus* in mastitis samples of primiparous cows in the same herd (ρ=0.92, P<0.01). However, both were not related to the prevalence in non-clinical colostral samples. The prevalence of *S. dysgalactiae* in clinical mastitis samples was also correlated between the different age groups (ρ=0.95, P<0.01). For *S. dysgalactiae* there was also a significant correlation of the prevalence in non-clinical samples with the prevalence in clinical mastitis samples from primiparous (ρ=0.67, P<0.05) and multiparous cows (ρ=0.75, P<0.05). All other prevalences were not significantly correlated between the three groups of samples.

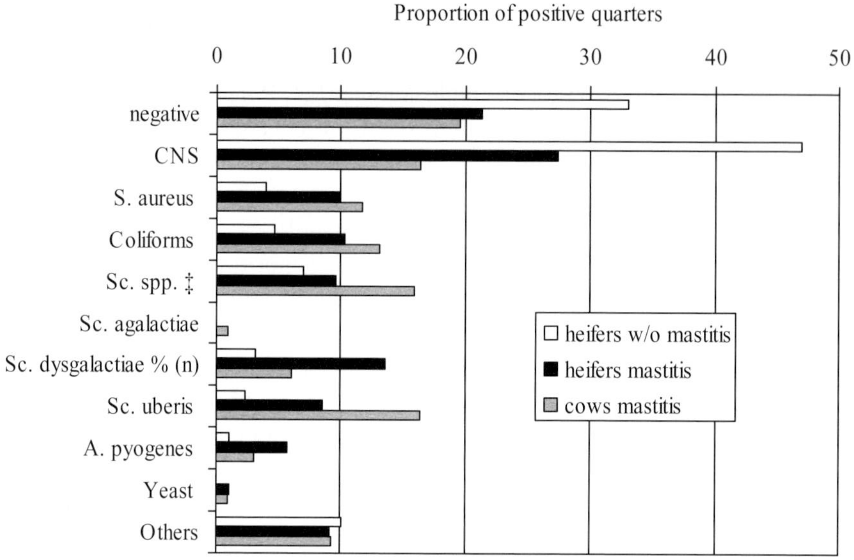

Figure 1. Prevalence of pathogens in quarter milk samples from heifers at parturition without clinical mastitis (n=6,915), and from cases of clinical mastitis in primiparous cows (n=751)[‡] and multiparous cows (n=574). Samples do not add up to 100% because of mixed infections. [‡]*excluding* S. agalactiae, S. dysgalactiae and S. uberis.

Discussion

It was the objective of this study to analyse the relationship of the prevalence of pathogens in milk samples of heifers at parturition, in samples from clinical mastitis quarters in primiparous cows and in samples from clinical mastitis quarters in older cows. Results of the study demonstrate that this relationship differs between pathogens.

Coagulase negative staphylococci are the predominant pathogen isolated from heifers at parturition in countries with intensive milk production(Borm *et al.*, 2006; Tenhagen *et al.*, 2006; Compton *et al.*, 2007a). With respect to udder health in primiparous cows they have received considerable attention. It has been demonstrated that intramammary infection (IMI) at parturition was associated with higher cell counts and lower milk yield in first lactation (Timms und Schultz, 1987). CNS were the group of bacteria with the highest prevalence in non-clinical samples in all of the 10 herds studied. However, their contribution to samples with mastitis was lower than to the non-clinical samples. This is a substantial difference to all other pathogens included in this study. In line with this observation, it has recently been reported that the presence of *S. chromogenes*, one of the most prevalent CNS on the teat apex prior to parturition, was associated with a lower risk of high somatic cell counts post partum (De Vliegher *et al.*, 2003).

Statistically, the lower prevalence in mastitis samples indicates a protective effect of CNS. However, as CNS are part of the normal skin flora, they might also have been derived from colonised streak canals or colonisation of the teat cistern. Colonisation of the streak canal could explain the substantial reduction of CNS in quarters sampled a couple of days into lactation (Aarestrup and Jensen, 1997; Edinger *et al.*, 2000; Calvinho *et al.*, 2007). Such a reduction was also reported for other pathogens (Compton *et al.*, 2007a).

Staphylococcus aureus is still one of the most prevalent major mastitis pathogens in dairy herds (Tenhagen *et al.*, 2006; Osteras *et al.*, 2006). Although it is predominantly spread during the milking process, it has also been isolated from heifers and primiparous cows prior to and at parturition (Roberson *et al.*, 1998; Edinger *et al.*, 2000). In this study the prevalence of *S. aureus* was higher in mastitis samples than in non-clinical samples. While in primiparous cows it was found more often in summer than in winter, the opposite was observed for the older cows with clinical mastitis. In a recent survey from Norway, the prevalence of *S. aureus* was higher in summer (Osteras *et al.*, 2006). The prevalence of *S. aureus* in mastitis samples from older cows did not differ significantly from those of primiparous cows. In contrast, we have reported that the prevalence of *S. aureus* in samples from clinically healthy cows was higher in older than in younger cows in our region (Tenhagen *et al.*, 2006). However, this was observed in later lactation, while early in lactation, the difference was not significant. This is in accordance with the data of this study that focussed on the beginning of lactation. From Norway it was reported that the prevalence of *S. aureus* in primiparous and older cows did not differ significantly (Osteras *et al.*, 2006).

Non-agalactiae streptococci are one of the major groups of environmental pathogens associated with mastitis. As a group, their prevalence in samples from cases of clinical mastitis in cows was highest. Likewise, in heifers streptococci had a high prevalence in clinical mastitis samples. Their prevalence in non-clinical samples was substantially lower. The higher prevalence of environmental streptococci in older cows, compared to heifers, is supported by recent data from large dairy herds in Germany (Tenhagen *et al.*, 2006).

Streptococcus dysgalactiae showed some differences to the other streptococci. The major difference was the strong correlation of the prevalence of *S. dysgalactiae* in non-clinical samples from primiparous cows, clinical samples from primiparous cows and clinical samples from multiparous cows. *S. dysgalactiae* was the only pathogen that showed these strong correlations. The reasons for these correlations are not clear. Besides for *S. dysgalactiae* these correlations were only partly observed for *S. aureus*. The relationship may be a typical feature indicating a contagious nature of a pathogen, because the feature was not observed in other streptococci and in coliforms. *Streptococcus dysgalactiae* has been reported to invade into epithelial cells and survive there for a longer period without damaging the cells (Calvinho und Oliver, 1998). This may explain the comparatively high proportion of positive colostral samples.

Furthermore, *S. dysgalactiae* was more prevalent in primiparous than in older cows, which is in contrast to two other recently published studies (Tenhagen *et al.*, 2006; Osteras *et al.*, 2006). However, these studies dealt with non-clinical samples. This indicates that pathogenicity of *S. dysgalactiae* may be higher for primiparous cows than for older cows. In line with this, S. dysgalactiae has been associated with cases of summer mastitis in heifers, a condition that is commonly attributed to *A. pyogenes* (Madsen *et al.*, 1992).

Strains of *S. dysgalactiae* that were isolated from heifers in the week prior to parturition were observed in the same quarter after parturition (Aarestrup und Jensen, 1997). The prevalence of *S. dysgalactiae* in Scandinavian studies on heifers was higher than that of other streptococci (Aarestrup und Jensen, 1997; Waage *et al.*, 1999).

In contrast to the Norwegian investigation, in our study *S. dysgalactiae* was more prevalent in winter than in summer, just like the other streptococci. In the Norwegian survey, *S. dysgalactiae* and *S. uberis*, were more prevalent in summer than in winter. The reason for the difference is not clear. However, there are substantial differences in herd sizes and climatic conditions between the Norwegian herds (15 cows) and the herds that we included in the study (700 cows).

As expected, *Streptococcus uberis* was far more prevalent in clinical than in non-clinical samples (Compton *et al.*, 2007a). Unlike in studies from North America (Todhunter *et al.*, 1995), *S. uberis* was more prevalent in winter than in summer.

In our study herds, coliforms were isolated from 10% of mastitis samples from primiparous cows and from 13% of mastitis samples from older cows. However, as with all pathogens, the contribution of coliforms varied substantially between herds ranging from 5 to 25% in primiparous and from 7 to 43% in older cows. As in other studies, coliforms were found more often in summer than in winter. In non-clinical samples the prevalence of coliforms was significantly lower.

Conclusion

Our data indicate that mastitis in primiparous and older cows differs with respect to pathogen pattern. Furthermore, pathogens isolated from clinically healthy quarters of primiparous cows at parturition differ from those isolated from clinical mastitis. Reports on the reduction of peripartum intrammammary infections in heifers by management have to differentiate between the various pathogens. Further research will be needed to increase our understanding of the role of the different CNS in heifer mastitis and to understand the mechanisms of spontaneous elimination of bacteria from the mammary gland early postpartum.

References

Aarestrup, F.M. and Jensen, N.E., 1997. Prevalence and duration of intramammary infection in Danish heifers during the peripartum period. J. Dairy Sci. 80: 307-312.

Borm, A.A., Fox, L.K., Leslie, K.E., Hogan, J.S., Andrew, S.M., Moyes, K.M., Oliver, S.P., Schukken, Y.H., Hancock, D.D., Gaskins, C.T., Owens, W.E. and Norman, C., 2006. Effects of prepartum intramammary antibiotic therapy on udder health, milk production, and reproductive performance in dairy heifers. J. Dairy Sci. 89: 2090-2098.

Calvinho, L.F., Canavesio, V.R., Iguzquiza, I.A., Marioni, I., Puricelli, F.G., Neder, V.E., Tarabla, H.D. and Aubagna, M.D., 2007. Intramammary infections during the periparturient period in Argentine dairy heifers. Rev. Argent. Microbiol. 39: 84-89.

Calvinho, L.F. and Oliver, S.P., 1998. Invasion and persistence of Streptococcus dysgalactiae within bovine mammary epithelial cells. J. Dairy Sci. 81: 678-686.

Compton, C.W., Heuer, C., Parker, K. and McDougall, S., 2007a. Epidemiology of mastitis in pasture-grazed peripartum dairy heifers and its effects on productivity. J. Dairy Sci. 90: 4157-4170.

Compton, C.W., Heuer, C., Parker, K. and McDougall, S., 2007b. Risk factors for peripartum mastitis in pasture-grazed dairy heifers. J. Dairy Sci. 90: 4171-4180.

De Vliegher, S., Laevens, H., Devriese, L.A., Opsomer, G., Leroy, J.L., Barkema, H.W. and De Kruif, A., 2003. Prepartum teat apex colonization with Staphylococcus chromogenes in dairy heifers is associated with low somatic cell count in early lactation. Vet. Microbiol. 92: 245-252.

Edinger, D., Tenhagen, B.A., Kalbe, P., Klunder, G., Baumgartner, B. and Heuwieser, W., 2000. Effect of teat dipping with a germicide barrier teat dip in late gestation on intramammary infection and clinical mastitis during the first 5 days post-partum in primiparous cows. J. Vet. Med. A 47: 463-468.

Kalmus, P., Viltrop, A., Aasmae, B. and Kask, K., 2006. Occurrence of clinical mastitis in primiparous Estonian dairy cows in different housing conditions. Acta Vet. Scand. 48: 21-26.

Madsen, M., Aalbaek, B. and Hansen, J.W., 1992. Comparative bacteriological studies on summer mastitis in grazing cattle and pyogenes mastitis in stabled cattle in Denmark. Vet. Microbiol. 32: 81-88.

Osteras, O., Solverod, L. and Reksen, O., 2006. Milk culture results in a large Norwegian survey--effects of season, parity, days in milk, resistance, and clustering. J. Dairy Sci. 89: 1010-1023.

Parker, K.I., Compton, C.W., Anniss, F.M., Weir, A.M. and McDougal, S., 2007. Management of dairy heifers and its relationships with the incidence of clinical mastitis. N.Z. Vet. J. 55: 208-216.

Roberson, J.R., Fox L.K., Hancock, D.D., Gay, J.M. and Besser, T.E., 1998. Sources of intramammary infections from Staphylococcus aureus in dairy heifers at first parturition. J. Dairy Sci. 81: 687-693.

Tenhagen, B.A., Koster, G., Wallmann, J. and Heuwieser, W., 2006. Prevalence of mastitis pathogens and their resistance against antimicrobial agents in dairy cows in Brandenburg, Germany. J. Dairy Sci. 89: 2542-2551.

Timms, L. L., and Schultz, L. H., 1987. Dynamics and significance of coagulase-negative staphylococcal intramammary infections. Journal of Dairy Science 70: 2648-2657.

Todhunter, D.A., Smith, K.L. and Hogan, J.S., 1995. Environmental streptococcal intramammary infections of the bovine mammary gland. J. Dairy Sci. 78: 2366-2374.

Waage, S., Mork, T., Roros, A., Aasland, D., Hunshamar, A. and Odegaard, S.A., 1999. Bacteria associated with clinical mastitis in dairy heifers. J. Dairy Sci. 82: 712-719.

Waage, S., Sviland, S. and Odegaard, S.A., 1998. Identification of risk factors for clinical mastitis in dairy heifers. J. Dairy Sci. 81: 1275-1284.

'animal associated MRSA' (AA-MRSA) were shown to be able to colonise also humans. An increase in detection of these strains in humans from 0% in 2002 to 21% in 2007 was reported (Van Loo *et al.*, 2007, Van Rijen *et al.*, 2008). It should be noted that meanwhile the detection methodology has changed and this might have influenced the increase substantially. This AA-MRSA clone is typically non-typable MRSA by use of PFGE with *Sma*I, the international standard for MRSA typing (Bens *et al.*, 2006). All AA-MRSA belong to one clonal complex, being the multilocus sequence type 398 (ST398) (Van Loo *et al.*, 2007). However, different spa types were recovered.

Meanwhile ST398 has been recovered in several European countries, e.g. Belgium, the Netherlands, Germany, Italy, Spain and Denmark and also in Canada and Singapore (Wulf and Voss, 2008). It appears to be an international spreading of the strain, as has been demonstrated for other MRSA (both hospital and community acquired MRSA). MRSA ST398 is unfortunately capable of colonising several animal species, such as pigs, cattle, sheep, horses, dogs, cats and chicken (Middleton *et al.*, 2005; Leonard and Markey, 2008). In horses, it has been shown to be pathogenic (Van den Eede *et al.*, 2007). First isolations of MRSA in animals were from a mastitic cow. However, this strain was supposed to be human contamination since it had the typical human biotype profile (Devriese *et al.*, 1972; Devrieze and Hommez, 1975). Recently MRSA ST 398 has been shown to be implicated in clinical and subclinical mastitis (P. Butaye, unpublished data).

Staphylococcus aureus is frequently isolated from dairy cows with clinical and subclinical mastitis. These infections have high economic consequences due to difficulties in the treatment (Nickerson *et al.*, 1995; Akineden *et al.*, 2001; Zschock *et al.*, 2005; Piepers *et al.*, 2007). MRSA has been previously associated with mastitis in dairy (P. Butaye, unpublished data; Kwon *et al.*, 2005; Middleton *et al.*, 2005; Monecke *et al.*, 2007), but there is a lack in data describing the prevalence of MRSA within herds. Therefore, the present study aimed to estimate the spread of MRSA strains within dairy herds previously proven to be MRSA-positive.

Material and methods

Herd selection and sampling

In a previous research, conducted in 2006, control milk samples from clinical and subclinical mastitis were found to be MRSA positive. The related herds were contacted and consecutively, all lactating cows were sampled at quarter level using a standardised method of cleaning, disinfecting and milking the udder quarters.

Bacteriology and MRSA typing

The same day, milk samples were inoculated on agar plates with 5% sheep's blood (CSA-plates) and MRSA-ID plates. Typical colonies from MRSA-ID were purified on CSA-plates for control on the typical morphology. Strains compiling with the typical *S. aureus* morphology were subsequently confirmed by 16S rRNA-mecA-nuc triplex PCR as previously described (Maes *et al.*, 2002). Determination of the Staphylococcal Chromosome Cassette (SCCmec) type was performed by multiplex PCR (Oliveira and De Lencastre, 2002). A subset of MRSA strains were subjected to Multi-Locus Sequence Typing (MLST) (Enright *et al.*, 2000). Spa-types were determined as previously described (n=112) (Harmsen *et al.*, 2003).

Results and discussion

Intra-herd prevalence of MRSA positive cows did differ considerably, 0-14.3% (Table 1). The reason for this variation between dairy herds remains unclear. Milking techniques have been shown to influence prevalence of *S. aureus* in herds, as did some housing aspects (Barkema *et al.*, 1999). Pigs were kept at herds 1 and 4 of our study. These herds vary considerably in MRSA prevalence, 9.5 and 3.9%, respectively. It is unclear what the role of this mixed farms is in the prevalence of MRSA in bovines. Further studies analysing the risk factors are necessary.

Hygienic measures taken by the farmer when visiting one groups of animals after the other will play a primordial role in the possible spread of MRSA. The infection pressure of *Staphylococcus aureus* on the herd and the antibiotic use in general, specifically to treat mastitis, and as prevention in dry cows, will strongly influence the prevalence of MRSA at the herd.

MRSA strains from farm 1, 3 and 4 were further analysed by spa typing, strains from farm 1 and 4 by MLST, and strains from farm 4 were analysed by SCCmec typing. Strains from farm 2 could not be further analysed due to laboratory circumstances. Typing showed that the strains isolated in this study were ST398 associated with animals, and were of spa type t011, the type most prevalent in pigs in Belgium (Willems *et al.*, 2007). This type has also been found in the previous study in bovines (P. Butaye, unpublished data). The strains of farm 4 were all

Table 1. Overview of number of lactating cows per sampled herd, percentage of MRSA positive cows and typing of the isolated bacteria.

Herd	Number of lactating cows	% of MRSA positive cows	MLST[1]	*spa*-typing
1	63	9.5	ST398	t011
2	77	14.3	ND	ND
3	68	7.4	ND	t011
4	77	3.9	ST398	t011
5	51	0	NA	NA

[1] Multi Locus Sequence Typing.

of SCCmec type IV, a type also found back in other ST398 strains. Since only few data are available, further investigations on the prevalence of the SCCmec types are necessary.

It is important to have an idea of MRSA prevalence in cattle in order to estimate the risk for the animals and also for persons in close contact with the animals. As has been demonstrated previously, farmers, veterinarians and slaughterhouse personnel are at higher risk to get colonised with MRSA (Vandenbroucke-Grauls and Beaujean, 2006; Moodley *et al.*, 2008). Since the spread of MRSA in positive farms is limited to less than 15% of the cows in the herd, it is reasonable to consider culling of the infected animals. This is rectifiable seen the thread of MRSA strains and the problematic treatment due to multiple resistances.

In conclusion, MRSA has been shown to be at dairy farms. The spread within the farms is rather limited with a large variation between farms. The types found were all types previously described in pigs in Belgium and also in other animal species in other countries.

References

Akineden, O., Annemuller, C., Hassan, A.A., Lammler, C., Wolter, W. and Zschock, M., 2001. Toxin genes and other characteristics of *Staphylococcus aureus* isolates from milk of cows with mastitis. Clin. Diagn. Lab. Imm. 8: 959-964.

Barkema, H.W., Schukken, Y.H., Lam, T.J.G.M., Beiboer, M.L., Benedictus, G. and Brand, A., 1999. Management practices associated with the incidence rate of clinical mastitis. J. Dairy Sci. 82: 1643-1654.

Bens, C.C., Voss, A. and Klaassen, C.H., 2006. Presence of a novel DNA methylation enzyme in methicillin-resistant *Staphylococcus aureus* isolates associated with pig farming leads to uninterpretable results in standard pulsed-field gel electrophoresis anaylsis. J. Clin. Microb. 44: 1875-1876.

Deresinski, S., 2005. Methicillin-resistant *Staphylococcus aureus*: an evolutionary, epidemiologic and therapeutic odyssey. Clin. Inf. Dis. 40: 562-573.

Devriese, L.A. and Hommez, J., 1975. Epidemiology of methicillin-resistant *Staphylococcus aureus* in dairy herds. Res. Vet. Sci. 19: 23-27.

Devriese, L.A., Vandamme, L.R. and Fameree, L., 1972. Methicillin (cloxacillin)-resistant *Staphylococcus aureus* strains isolated from bovine mastitis cases. Zentralblatt fur Veterinarmedizin B 19: 598-605.

Enright, M.C., Day, N.P.J., Davies, C.E., Peacock, S.J. and Spratt, B.G., 2000. Multilocus sequence typing for characterization of methicillin-resistant and methicillin-susceptible clones of *Staphylococcus aureus.* J. Clin. Microb. 38: 1008-1015.

Harmsen, D., Claus, H., Witte, W., Rothgänger, J., Claus, H., Turnwald, D. and Vogel., U., 2003. Typing of methicillin-resistant *Staphylococcus aureus* in a university hospital setting by using novel software for spa repeat determination and database management. J. Clin. Microb. 41: 5442-5448.

Kwon, N.H., Park, K.T., Moon J.S., Jung, W.K., Kim, S.H., Kim, J.M., Hong, S.K., Koo, H.C., Joo, Y.S. and Park, Y.H., 2005. Staphylococcal cassette chromosome mec (SCCmec) characterization and molecular analysis for methicillin-resistant *Staphylococcus aureus* and novel SCCmec subtype IVg isolated from bovine milk in Korea. J. Antimicr. Chem. 56: 624-632.

Leonard, F.C. and Markey, B.K., 2008. Methicillin-resistant *Staphylococcus aureus* in animals: A review. Vet. J. 175: 27-36.

Maes, N., Magdalena, J., Rottiers, S., De Gheldre, Y. and Struelens, M.J., 2002. Evaluation of a triplex PCR assay to discriminate *Staphylococcus aureus* from coagulase-negative Staphylococci and determine methicillin resistance from blood cultures. J. Clin. Microb. 40: 1514-1517.

Middleton, J.R., Fales, W.H., Luby, C.D., Oaks, J.L., Sanchez, S., Kinyon, J.M., Wu, C.C., Maddox, C.W., Welsh, R.D. and Hartmann, F., 2005. Surveillance of *Staphylococcus aureus* in veterinary teaching hospitals. J. Clin. Microb. 43: 2916-2919.

Monecke, S., Kuhnert, P., Hotzel, H., Slickers, P. and Ehricht, R., 2007. Microarray based study on virulence-associated genes and resistance determinants of *Staphylococcus aureus* isolates from cattle. Vet. Microb. 125: 128-140.

Moodley, A., Nightingale, E.C., Stegger, M., Nielsen, S.S., Skov, R.L. and Guardabassi, L., 2008. High risk for nasal carriage of methicillin-resistant Staphylococcus aureus among Danish veterinary practitioners. Scand. J. Work Environ. Health 34: 151-157.

Nickerson, S.C., Owens, W.E. and Boddie, R.L., 1995. Mastitis in dairy heifers: initial studies on prevalence and control. J. Dairy Sci. 78: 1607-1618.

Oliveira, D. C., and H. de Lencastre. 2002. Multiplex PCR strategy for rapid identification of structural types and variants of the mec element in methicillin-resistant *Staphylococcus aureus*. Antimicrobial Agents and Chemotherapy 46: 2155-2161.

Piepers, S., De Meulemeester, L., De Kruif, A., Opsomer, G., Barkema, H.W. and De Vliegher, S., 2007. Prevalence and distribution of mastitis pathogens in subclinically infected dairy cows in Flanders, Belgium. J. Dairy Res. 74: 478-483.

Vandenbroucke-Grauls, C.M.J.E. and Beaujean, D.J.M.A., 2006. Methicillin-resistant *Staphylococcus aureus* in pig breeders and cattle breeders. Ned. Tijdschr. Diergen. 150: 1710-1712.

Van den Eede, A., Hermans, K., Lipinska, U., Struelens, M., Deplano, A., Denis, O., Gasthuys, F., Haesebrouck, F. and Martens A., 2007. Nasal carriage of methicillin-resistant *Staphylococcus aureus* in the equine population: prevalence, typing and antimicrobial resistance. 2nd Symposium on Antimicrobial Resistance in Animals and the Environment, 17-19 December 2007, Tours, France.

Van Loo, I., Huijsdens, X., Tiemersma, E., de Neeling, A., Van de Sande-Bruinsma, M., Beaujean, D., Voss, A. and Kluytmans, J., 2007. Emerence of methicillin-resistant *Staphylococcus aureus* of animal origin in humans. Emerg. Infect. Dis. 13: 1834-1839.

Van Rijen, M.M.L., Van Keulen, P.H. and Kluytmans, J.A., 2008. Increase in a Dutch hospital of Methicillin-Resistant *Staphylococcus aureus* related to animal farming. Clin. Infect. Dis. 46: 261-263.

Willems, G., Dispas, M., Denis, O., Hallin, M., Suetens, C., Gordts, B., Streulens, M. and Butaye, P., 2007. Characterisation of MRSA from pigs in Belgium. 2nd Symposium on Antimicrobial Resistance in Animals and the Environment, 17-19 December 2007, Tours, France.

Wulf, M. and Voss, A., 2008. MRSA in livestock animals – an epidemic waiting to happen? Clin. Microb. Inf. 14: 519-521.

Zschock, M., Kloppert, B., Wolter, W., Hamann, H.P. and Lammler, C., 2005. Pattern of enterotoxin genes seg, seh, sei and sej positive *Staphylococcus aureus* isolated from bovine mastitis. Vet. Microb. 108: 243-249.

Comparing bacterial counts on bare hands with gloved hands during milking

R.G.M. Olde Riekerink[1], O.C. Sampimon[1], V.J. Eerland[1], M.J. Swarts[1] and T.J.G.M. Lam[1,2]
[1]GD Animal Health Service, P.O. Box 9, 7400 AA, Deventer, the Netherlands
[2]Dutch Udder Health Center, P.O. Box 2030, 7420 AA, Deventer, the Netherlands
Corresponding author: r.olderiekerink@gddeventer.com

Abstract

Milking parlor hygiene has been propagated by many veterinarians, extension specialists, and researchers. Research has shown that producers that work clean and precise have in general lower incidence rates of clinical mastitis and lower bulk milk somatic cell counts. Part of the recommended milking procedures is wearing milkers gloves during milking. Some studies have shown that similar strains of mastitis pathogens can be found in milk samples, udder skin, and on milkers' hands, suggesting that mastitis pathogens can be transmitted from cow to cow via hands. The goal of the present study was to conduct a quantitative comparison of bacterial counts on bare hands, disinfected hands, gloves, and disinfected gloves. The glove-juice method (50 ml 0.9% NaCl) was used to quantify bacterial presence on 27 milkers' hands. The milkers were asked, after milking a full parlor of cows (8 to 36 stalls), to rinse off his hands and wipe them dry using a cloth or paper towel before the bare or gloved hand was sampled. After sampling the bare or gloved hand, the milker was asked to disinfect his hand or glove with alcohol-impregnated udder wipes (TeaterClean®) before sampling the disinfected hand or glove again. Disinfecting bare hands reduced bacterial load with 85%. Wearing gloves and disinfected gloves reduced bacterial loads compared with bare hands with 75% and 98%, respectively. This method only evaluated the total bacterial load on milkers' hands. The vast majority of the isolated bacteria are most likely harmless. This study showed, however, that using gloves during milking will reduce the exposure of teats to bacteria through milkers' hands.

Keywords: disinfection gloves, hands, milking

Introduction

Mastitis still is an important disease to the dairy industry. Infected cow's udders are an important reservoir of mastitis pathogens. Transmission from cow to cow mostly occurs during milking. Prior to causing an intramammary infection (IMI), contagious bacteria will most likely colonise the teat canal or teat skin (Fox and Gay, 1993). Milking time hygiene and prevention of cow-to-cow transmission is effective in reducing new IMI (Neave *et al.*, 1969). Post-milking teat disinfection has been shown to be an effective measure to reduce new IMI since it reduces bacterial loads on teat skin (Pankey *et al.*, 1984; Lam *et al.*, 1996). It seems logical that reducing bacterial loads on teat skin reduces the probability of IMI (Fox and Gay, 1993).

Because many IMI are established during milking, fomites that contact the teat skin during milking are most likely an important vector in transmitting bacteria from cow to cow. Liners, udder cloths, and milkers' hands do come in contact with teat skin. Early studies suggest that humans can be the source of IMI caused by methicillin-resistant *Staphylococcus aureus* (Devriese and Hommez, 1975) or a possible mutual human-animal transfer of Staphylococcus strains (Swartz *et al.*, 1985). Thorberg *et al.* (2006) suggested in a more recent study that IMI caused by *Staph. epidermidis* might be a zoonosis emanating from man.

Wearing milkers' gloves is recommended by many dairy extension specialists and is often part of a mastitis control programme. It is general accepted that milkers' hands often have many cracks that can harbor plenty of bacteria. Gloves, either made from nitrile or latex, have a smooth surface which is easy to clean and will harbor less dirt and bacteria.

The Dutch Udder Health Center, planned a national campaign to raise farmers' awareness of the importance of wearing milkers' gloves. However, to-date, there is no scientific support that wearing gloves will reduce incidence of mastitis. The objective of this study was to compare bacterial loads on bare hands with bacterial loads on disinfected hands, gloved hands, and disinfected gloved hands during milking.

Materials and methods

Farm selection

In total, 27 farms were selected by convenience, some were participating in other research, some were selected because of their proximity to GD Animal Health Service. Farmers were asked to have their dominating hand tested 4 times during milking. The dominating hand was the right hand for right-handed farmers and the left for left-handed farmers.

Sampling strategy

At the beginning of milking time, farmers were asked to routinely milk 1 round of cows with bare hands. The sampling hand was wiped off with an available udder paper or cloth to remove excess manure if present. The hand was sampled using the method described below. After the bare hand was sampled, the farmer was asked to disinfect the hand with disposable pre-moistened teat wipes (Teater Clean®, Ingenieursbureau Heemskerk b.v., Hilvarenbeek, the Netherlands). These wipes were chosen for disinfection to mimic a realistic and practical method in the milking parlor. The disinfected bare hand was sampled using the same method and immediately after sampling the farmer put on clean nitrile gloves. The farmer would continue milking with gloves on. After 1 round of milking the sampling strategy was repeated with the milkers' gloves on.

Sampling method

The glove juice method was used for sampling. This method was selected because it is a quantitative method and is least sensitive for contamination under milking parlor circumstances. The glove juice technique (Michaud *et al.*, 1976) has become widely accepted by industry and the American Society for Testing Materials in the development and testing of antimicrobial hand wash products (Mahl, 1989). In short, the tested hand was gloved with a new, clean (non-sterile) latex glove containing 50 ml of a sterile 0.9% saline solution. The gloved hand with solution was massaged for 60 seconds. The solution was consequently poured into a sample bottle. Standard plate counts were determined in serial dilutions of the sampling fluids.

Statistical analyses

A linear mixed model with herd as a random effect was used to estimate the effect of wearing gloves and disinfection. Effects of parlor size, herd size, previous glove use, stripping, and all possible and epidemiological reasonable interactions, such as the interaction between glove use and disinfection, were checked and removed if their effect was not significant ($P<0.05$) or had a tendency of significance ($0.05<P\leq 0.10$). To approximate a normal distribution a natural logarithm transformation of colony counts (cfu/ml) was used. The resulting model for the natural logarithm of colony count was as follows:

$$\log(\text{cfu/ml}) = \beta_0 + \beta_1\text{disinfect} + \beta_2\text{glove} + \beta_3\text{strip} + \beta_4\text{glove*strip} + u + \varepsilon$$

where β_0 is the intercept, $\beta_{1\text{-}4}$ the regressions coefficients for disinfection, wearing gloves, stripping, and the interaction between wearing gloves and stripping, respectively, u is the herd random effect, and ε the error term. All statistical calculations were carried out using Stata software (Stata SE for Windows, version 10; Stata Corporation, College Station, Texas, USA).

Results

In total, 27 herds were involved, all located in the eastern part of the Netherlands. Mean herd size was 80 milking cows, ranging from 25 to 158 cows. A herringbone milking parlor was used on 21 farms, followed by a rapid exit (2), tie-stall barn (2), open tandem (1), and a rotary parlor (1). Mean parlor size was 14 milking stalls, ranging from 8 to 36 milking stalls. Wearing gloves during milking and stripping teats before cluster attachment was carried out on 16 (59%) and 15 (56%) farms, respectively. In total, 107 samples were examined, 1 bottle was lost during transport.

Farmers that stripped teats had larger bacterial loads on their hands and gloves than farmers that did not strip, 447,000 cfu/ml and 178,000 cfu/ml on bare hands and 62,000 and 52,000 cfu/ml on gloves, respectively (Table 1; Figure 1).The difference in bacterial load between

Table 1. Linear mixed model of the natural logarithm of colony forming units per ml.

	Coefficient β	SE	*P*-value
Intercept	12.09	0.31	< 0.01
Gloves	-1.23	0.31	< 0.01
Disinfected	-2.14	0.20	< 0.01
Strip	0.92	0.39	0.02
Gloves*Strip	-0.75	0.41	0.06

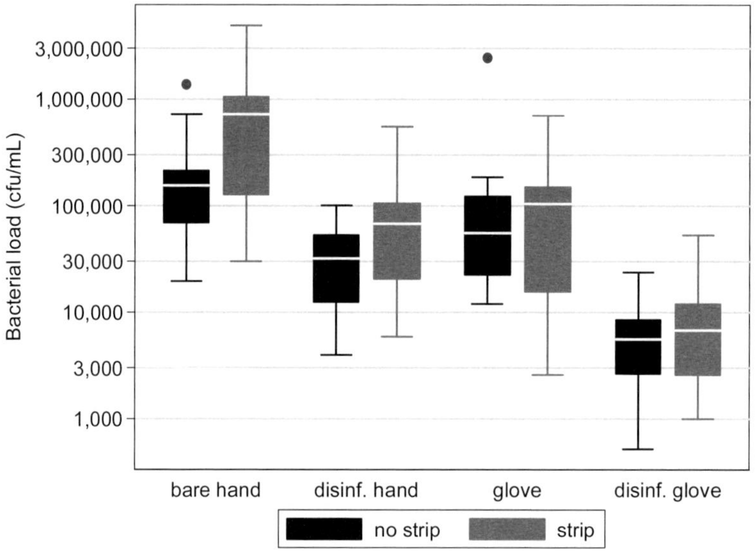

Figure 1. Bacterial load on bare hands, disinfected hands, gloves, and disinfected gloves by practice of stripping.

stripping and not stripping on a gloved hand tended (*P*=0.06) to be smaller than on a bare hand (Table 1; Figure 1). Disinfecting bare hands reduced bacterial load with 85%. Wearing gloves and disinfected gloves reduced bacterial loads compared with bare hands with 75% and 98%, respectively.

Discussion

This study showed that using gloves and disinfecting hands and gloves during milking will reduce the exposure of teats to bacteria through milkers' hands. However, we counted the total bacterial loads on hands and gloves. We did not make the distinction between pathogenic and non-pathogenic bacteria, but assumed that the effect of wearing gloves and disinfecting hands and gloves would be the same for pathogenic and non-pathogenic bacteria. Reducing bacterial loads on hands will reduce the exposure of teats to bacteria on hands. An association between bacterial loads on teat skin and incidence rate of new IMI (Galton *et al.*, 1988) is the basis for the success of reducing new IMI by application of teat disinfectants. In more recent epidemiologic studies in the UK wearing gloves during milking was associated with an increased incidence rate of clinical mastitis (Peeler *et al.*, 2000; O'Reilly *et al.*, 2006). However, the latter two studies did not show a causal relation between wearing gloves and incidence of clinical mastitis. A higher incidence of clinical mastitis could have motivated the farmer to wear gloves, or farmers that wear gloves more frequently strip and detect more clinical mastitis. On the other hand, farmers that work clean and accurate will have more likely a lower bulk milk SCC (Barkema *et al.*, 1999). Although this study did not include wearing milkers' gloves in the analyses it did find an association with cleanliness of farmers' hands.

Bare hands of farmers that checked foremilk before attaching the milking cluster (stripping) had larger bacterial loads on their hands than farmers that did not practice this. Bacterial loads could increase because of the frequent touching of dirty teats. The difference in bacterial loads of gloved hands was not as large as on bare hands. This finding supports the suggestion that if a farmer strips teats before attachment, he should wear gloves.

The glove juice method seemed to be a practical and reliable method to measure bacterial loads on milkers' hands. The gloves that were used were not sterile gloves and contained cornstarch powder. We assumed that because we used new, clean gloves every test, non-sterility and powder would not affect the effect of wearing gloves and disinfecting hands.

Hands and gloves were disinfected and measured immediately after the hands and gloves had contact with the testing juice. Bacterial counts could be reduced by contact with the juice alone. This would reduce the effect of the disinfection. However, the glove juice method is an approved method for testing disinfecting soaps and solutions (Michaud *et al.*, 1976).

Conclusion

Wearing gloves and regularly disinfecting hands or gloves result in considerable smaller bacterial loads on hands or gloves. This reduction is larger for farmers that strip the teats before they attach the milking cluster. Thus, wearing gloves and regularly disinfect them, especially if stripping is practiced, will attribute to reduction of IMI by reduction of exposure to potential pathogenic bacteria.

Acknowledgements

This study was part of the five-year udder health program of the Dutch Udder Health Centre and was financially supported by the Dutch Dairy Board, Ingenieursbureau Heemskerk, and

CA-FNZ Agri. We thank the participating farmers for their time and special thanks to Ms. Sarienke Barneveld for the sampling work.

References

Barkema, H.W., Van der Ploeg, J.D., Schukken, Y.H., Lam, T.J.G.M., Benedictus, G. and Brand, A., 1999. Management style and its association with bulk milk somatic cell count and incidence rate of clinical mastitis. J. Dairy Sci. 82: 1655-1663.

Devriese, L.A. and Hommez, J., 1975. Epidemiology of methicillin-resistant *Staphylococcus aureus* in dairy herds. Res. Vet. Sci. 19: 23-27.

Fox, L.K. and Gay, J.M., 1993. Contagious mastitis. Vet. Clin. N. Am. – Food Anim. Pract. 9: 475-487.

Galton, D.M., Peterson, L.G. and Merrill, W.G., 1988. Evaluation of udder preparations on intramammary infections. J. Dairy Sci. 71: 1417-1421.

Lam, T.J.G.M., De Jong, M.C., Schukken, Y.H. and Brand, A., 1996. Mathematical modeling to estimate efficacy of postmilking teat disinfection in split-udder trials of dairy cows. J. Dairy Sci. 79: 62-70.

Mahl, M.C., 1989. New method for determination of efficacy of health care personnel hand wash products. J. Clin. Microbiol. 27: 2295-2299.

Michaud, R.N., McGrath, M.B. and Goss, W.A., 1976. Application of a gloved-hand model for multiparameter measurements of skin-degerming activity. J. Clin. Microbiol. 3: 406-413.

Neave, F.K., Dodd, F.H., Kingwill, R.G. and Westgarth, D.R., 1969. Control of mastitis in the dairy herd by hygiene and management. J. Dairy Sci. 52: 696-707.

O'Reilly, K.M., Green, M.J., Peeler, M.J., Fitzpatrick, J.L. and Green, L.E., 2006. Investigation of risk factors for clinical mastitis in British dairy herds with bulk milk somatic cell counts less than 150,000 cells/ml. Vet. Rec. 158: 649-653.

Pankey, J.W., Eberhart, R.J., Cuming, A.L., Daggett, R.D., Farnsworth, R.J. and McDuff, C.K., 1984. Uptake on postmilking teat antisepsis. J. Dairy Sci. 67: 1336-1353.

Peeler, E.J., Green, M.J., Fitzpatrick, J.L., Morgan, K.L. and Green, L.E., 2000. Risk factors associated with clinical mastitis in low somatic cell count British dairy herds. J. Dairy Sci. 83: 2464-2472.

Swartz, R., Jooste, P.J. and Novello, J.C., 1985. Bacteriophage typing of *Staphylococcus aureus* strains isolated from Bloemfontein dairy herds. J. South Afr. Vet. Ass. 56: 69-73.

Thorberg, B.M., Kuhn, I., Aarestrup, F.M., Brandstrom, B., Jonsson, P. and Danielsson-Tham, M.L., 2006. Pheno- and genotyping of *Staphylococcus epidermidis* isolated from bovine milk and human skin. Vet. Microbiol. 115: 163-172

Changes of mastitis pathogen spectrum in dairy herds of Latvia

A. Jemeljanovs, I.H. Konosonoka, J. Bluzmanis and D. Ikauniece
Latvia University of Agriculture, Research Institute of Biotechnology and Veterinary Medicine Sigra, Instituta street no 1, Sigulda, LV2150, Latvia
Corresponding author: biolab.sigra@lis.lv

The objective of the current study was to investigate spectrum of the mastitis pathogens in the dairy farms in Latvia of the last years compared with those 25-30 years backwards. In total, 577 subclinical and clinical mastitis secretion samples from the different dairy farms in Latvia were analysed. Samples were inoculated on 5% sheep blood agar and different selective culture media. Isolated microorganisms were further identified to species level using gram-positive and gram-negative kits of BBL Crystal Identification System. *Staphylococcus aureus* and coagulase negative staphylococci prevail in subclinically (72.7%; n=440) and clinically (46.7%; n=137) diseased cows' udder secretion samples. *Staphylococcus aureus* were isolated from 41.1% of subclinically and 24.1% of clinically diseased cows' udder secretion samples, but coagulase negative staphylococci from 27.0% and 20.4%, respectively. The most frequently isolated coagulase negative staphylococci were *Staphylococcus haemolyticus* in both cases of mastitis. *Streptococcus* spp. were isolated from 5.9% of subclinically and 33.6% of clinically diseased cows' udder secretion samples. The genus *Streptococcus* species were mastitis agents in 65.5% of subclinical and 64.8% of clinical mastitis cases in the 1980s. Our studies revealed that replacement of predominating agents of mastitis from the genus *Streptococcus* to the genus *Staphylococcus* has been occurred in Latvia. *Staphylococcus aureus* antigen is developed and experimentally tested at the research Institute of Biotechnology and Veterinary Medicine 'Sigra'. The results established that the number of cows, the milk of which contains *Staphylococcus aureus*, after the 1st vaccination diminished 1.5 times.

Molecular testing, epidemiological aspects, prevalence and distribution of mastitis pathogens in dairy bovine, caprine and ovine herds

P. Cremonesi[1], B. Castiglioni[1], P. Moroni[2] and G. Pisoni[2]
[1]IBBA, CNR, Via Bassini 15, 20133 Milano, Italy
[2]DIPAV, UNIMI, Via Celoria 10, 20133 Milano, Italy
Corresponding author: paola.cremonesi@unimi.it

Mastitis is a disease of major economic importance in dairy herds resulting in reduced milk yield and loss of income. The objective of this study was to investigate the prevalence and the distribution of mastitis pathogens in different dairy bovine, caprine and ovine herds, located in Italy. Milk samples from 355 cows, 296 goats, and 63 ewes were collected for bacteriological examination and molecular testing (PCR, multiplex-PCR, array diagnostic kit) for the detection of the main pathogens involved in mastitis. The prevalence of infection in bovine herds was 41.9% with isolation of *Staphylococcus aureus* (7.6%), *Streptococcus* spp. (1.4%), other *Staphylococcus* spp. (30.4%), and *Mycoplasma bovis* (1.1%), *Escherichia coli* (0.8%); the prevalence of infection in goat herds was 52.0% with isolation of *Staphylococcus aureus* (33.4%), *Streptococcus* spp. (0.3%), other *Staphylococcus* spp. (18.2%); the prevalence of infection in ovine herds was 96.8% with isolation of *Staphylococcus aureus* (77.7%), *Streptococcus* spp. (7.9%), other *Staphylococcus* spp. (4.7%), and *Mycoplasma agalactiae* (1.3%). We conclude that rapid, sensitive and specific diagnostic method can be performed within hours and represents an innovative diagnostic tool for the detection and analysis of epidemiological distribution of milk pathogens in dairy herds.

Prevalence of bovine mastitis and causal agents in the state of Jalisco, Mexico

H. Castañeda[1], W. Wolter[2], S.P. Jäger[2], M. Szchöck[2], M.A. Castañeda[1], G. Perez[1] and C. Bedolla[1]
[1]University of Guadalajara, Km. 15.5 Carretera Guad.-Nogales, 45150, Zapopan, Mexico
[2]Landesbetrieb Hessisches Landeslabor, Marburgerstrasse 54, 35396 Giessen, Germany
Corresponding author: hcastane@cucba.udg.mx

Aim of the present work was to prove the occurrence of subclinic and clinic disturbances of udder health in 33 herds of dairy cattle in Jalisco, Mexico. 1996 (66.9%) out of 2937 udder quarters examined by CMT showed a positive reaction. 1087 (37%) of these reactions were from clearly up to significantly positive reactions. Compared to the bacteriological examinations the prevalence of subclinical mastitis came up to 43.7%. On the other hand clinical mastitis could be proven in 2.5 %. In 53.8% of the examined quarter milk samples there was not bacteriological pathogen content. From the rest of the samples we could isolate CNS (15.4%), *Corynebacterium* spp. (13.9%) S. *agalactiae* (6.6%), *S. aureus* (5.8%) coliform pathogens (3.6%) and others (*Bacillus* spp., *Nocardia* spp, *Candida* spp.) (1.7%). These results demonstrate a significant share of minor pathogens beside contagious mastitis pathogens as *S. aureus* and *S. agalactiae* in mastitis incidents in Jalisco. By means of pulse field gel electrophoresis we proved that in each of those farms where *S. aureus* had been isolated, only one genotype was responsible for mastitis incidents. The farm specific genotypes mostly showed a close relationship to the genotypes of other farms. Therefore the contagious character of mastitis pathogens and the dominating occurrence of certain *S. aureus* clones could be proved.

Etiology of subclinic mastitis in Patzcuaro Michoacan

L.C. Bedolla[1], R. Mejia[1], I. Renteria[1], E. Bedolla[1], E. Garcia[1], H. Castañeda[2], M.A. Castañeda[2], J.C. Serratos[2] and W. Wolter[3]
[1]Universidad de Michoacan, Veterinaria, Av. Acueducto y Tzintzuntzan s/n C.P. 58000, Morelia, Michoacan, Mexico
[2]Universidad de Guadalajara, Veterinary Medicina, Km. 15.5 Carretera Guadalajara-Nogales., 45159, Zapopan, Mexico
[3]Landesbetrieb Hessisches Landeslabor, Marburgerstrasse 54, 35396 Giessen, Germany
Corresponding author: hcastane@cucba.udg.mx

The objective of this study was to determine the etiology of subclinic mastitis in Patzcuaro, Michoacan, Mexico. The study was conducted from September to November of 2007. Eight barns with dairy cattle of the race Holstein Friesian were sampled, which had 10 cows in average raised under the system of production in small scale cattle barns. A total of 347 milk samples was collected aseptically in disposable tubes of single udder quarters of the mammary gland of 88 cows in lactation and transported to the laboratory at low temperatures (4 °C). The samples were inoculated in both blood agar with esculin and McConkey agar, and incubated at 37 °C, and observed 24 h and 48 h after inoculation to assess colony growth. The staphylococci isolations were again inoculated in agar with lamb blood, isolated, in order to observe colonial morphology, haemolysis as well as Gram stain, catalase tests, coagulase, manitol and gelatinase. The negative pathogens were identified according to colonial morphology, and biochemical tests. The results of the bacteriological examination of the milk samples were that 64 (18.44%) corresponded to *Staphylococcus aureus*, 85 (24.49%) to coagulase negative staphylococci, 24 (6.91%) to esculin positive streptococci, 2 (0.57%) to *Escherichia coli*, whereas the rest 122 (35.46%) corresponded to other pathogenic causes of mastitis. We concluded that coagulase negative staphylococci were the main pathogen agents found in the subclinic mastitis, and that *Staphylococcus aureus* was the main causal agent of contagious bovine mastitis in this study.

If ten points are no longer sufficient: an observational study on factors related to udder health and milk quality in Flanders, Belgium

B. Verbist[1], B. Sonck[2], V. Piessens[1], G. Braem[3], L. Herman[1] and S. de Vliegher[4]
[1]Min. of Flemish Community, Inst. for Agric. and Fish. Research; Techn. and Food, Van Gansberghelaan 115 bus 1, 9820 Merelbeke, Belgium
[2]Inst. for Agric. and Fisheries Research, Animal Science Unit, Merelbeke, Belgium
[3]Res. Group Industr. Microb. and Food Biotechnology, VUB, Brussels, Belgium
[4]Ghent University, Fac. Vet. Med., Dept. of Reprod., Obstet. and Herd Health, Merelbeke, Belgium
Corresponding author: bart.verbist@ilvo.vlaanderen.be

In Flanders, a shift of the distribution of mastitis pathogens towards coagulase-negative staphylococci (CNS) and coliforms has been observed and this may be the cause of the recent problems of increasing bulk milk somatic cell counts and/or decreasing milk quality. Ten randomly selected cows are monitored during one year on 6 Flemish dairy herds. For comparison, three farms with and three without specific coliform problems are included in the study. Milk samples are cultured for presence of mastitis bacteria and somatic cell counts are measured. Monthly climate variations (temperature, humidity, gas concentrations, dust) are investigated with innovative techniques. At the cow level, zootechnical information is complemented with recording of cleanliness, body condition, gait and milking characteristics, and at the quarter level teat conformation, teat apex condition and teat cleanliness are observed with recently developed digital image-analysis technology. These monthly observations will contribute to the clarification of the complex relationships between different factors explaining the mastitis status of cows and quarters and its evolution over time.

Protocol for evaluation of teat dips efficacy on mastitis prevention

H. Charier and R. Alasri
Cid Lines NV, Waterpoostraat 2, 8900 Ieper, Belgium
Corresponding author: helene.charier@cidlines.com

Teat dips are now recognised in Europe as veterinary medicinal products for mastitis prevention. The efficacy of those products is evaluated in farm, in real conditions. The only recognised protocol allowing the efficacy evaluation of teat dips has been published by the NMC on the US referential. In Europe, such protocol doesn't exist. This void is partly filled by a general guideline on clinical trials 'Good Clinical Guidelines' published by the EMEA. The aim of this article is to propose a protocol for European evaluation of teat dips as part of mastitis prevention hygiene program, combining NMC and GCP guidelines. A clinical teat dip trial is preferably a multicentric trial with randomised blocked design versus a positive control, with blinding. The treatment is compared to a positive control: a registered veterinary medicinal product in the test country. At least 2 farms, preferably in different countries if a mutual recognition procedure is intended to be followed, must be involved in the study and each product must be tested on at least 60 cows each. The trial must last at least 12 months in order to test the efficacy of the treatment during all seasons. The teat dip is applied with a dip cup or a sprayer after each milking. Teat condition and mastitis results must be collected once a month during all trial period; teat condition results are analysed by ANOVA (analysis of variance) and mastitis results of the tested treatment is compared to the positive control results by Student test. If there is no significant difference or if the number of mastitis per cow per time unit, is significantly lower for the tested treatment, the tested teat dip can be considered efficient for mastitis prevention. This is the basis of the efficacy protocol. If necessary, others parameters can be analysed, as cell count, to support and/or to enlarge the medicinal indication.

Good hygiene practice on dairy farms

J. Verhaeghe and R. Alasri
Cid Lines NV, Waterpoortstraat 2, 8900 Ieper, Belgium
Corresponding author: josephine.verhaeghe@cidlines.com

Good hygiene practice on dairy farms is essential to obtain good quality milk with low bulk bacteria count (BBC) and somatic cell counts (SCC). The FAO (Food and Agriculture Organisation) writes guideline on: Milking, milk production hygiene and udder health. The aim of our study is to make a critical understanding of the FAO's guideline and to lay the emphasis on the best way to apply it in order to be cost effective. General preventive measures should be established for feeding, housing, milking and managing cattle. The farmer must be aware of the importance of management and hygiene prevention. Equipment must be correctly tested, maintained, cleaned and renewed if necessary in order to avoid contamination of milk and teats. Housing is a reservoir of pathogens potentially responsible of mastitis. Clean and disinfect the sleeping area, control the area available per cow. Use insecticide. Teats must be in good condition. Several teat dips with varied qualities are available on the market. Choose teat dips with field trials led with a recognised protocol. Several parameters should be tested: teat condition improvement, bulk somatic cell count and of course the number of new infection cases. In Europe these parameters are usually controlled during the medicinal registration process. Therefore Registered Medicinal teat dips for mastitis prevention should be preferred for their certified efficacy. A method of detection of clinical mastitis must be established. The treatment must be done in a reasoned way: treat with antibiotic preparation under veterinary supervision and use hygienic measures before application. Preventive or curative habits must be taken during drying off. The poster gives figures, norms and limits to choose the best scheme of mastitis prevention and all the steps are detailed. Good preventative habits are useful if they are well understood and in that case, users can reap the benefits of their application.

Coagulase-negative staphylococci: a matter of lesser concern?

K. Supré[1], S. de Vliegher[1], R.N. Zadoks[2] and F. Haesebrouck[3]
[1]Ghent University Fac. Vet. Med., Dept. Reprod. Obstetrics, Herd Health, Salisburylaan 133, 9820 Merelbeke, Belgium
[2]Moredun Research Institute, Penicuik, Scotland, United Kingdom
[3]Ghent University Fac. Vet. Med., Dept. Pathology, Bact. and Poultry Diseases, Salisburylaan 133, 9820 Merelbeke, Belgium
Corresponding author: karlien.supre@UGent.be

In many European dairy farms that have adopted the 10-point mastitis prevention program, coagulase-negative staphylococci (CNS) have become the predominant pathogens found in milk samples. The fact that CNS are found as protective commensals on teat apices but also in milk samples from cows with or without elevated somatic cell counts (SCC) or clinical mastitis, emphasises that it is a heterogeneous group of bacteria, of which some are presumably clinically important and others are not. Epidemiological studies to elucidate the importance of CNS have already been conducted using phenotypic identification methods which lack accuracy. In order to clarify the epidemiology and importance of different CNS species as cause of rise in SCC or of clinical mastitis, or as protective organisms we conduct a longitudinal study on 3 Flemish dairy herds. Milk samples are collected monthly during an 18 month period for bacteriological culture and SCC determination at the quarter level. Relevant information on body condition score, parity, teat skin and apex condition, and presence of teat lesions is gathered in order to determine risk factors at the cow and quarter level for infection with the biologically most relevant species. Additional milk samples are taken at special events (clinical mastitis, drying-off, calving, culling). CNS species are differentiated by tDNAintergenic spacer PCR. Identification of cow and quarter level risk factors of the biologically most relevant species will give insight in the epidemiology of CNS and will help to formulate preventive strategies against CNS-infections, if, at all, necessary.

Molecular typing of microflora on teat apices using culture-dependent and culture-independent methodologies

G. Braem[1], S. de vliegher[2], B. Verbist[3], V. Piessens[3], F. Leroy[1] and L. de vuyst[1]
[1]Res. group of Industr. Microbiol. and Food Biotechnol. (IMDO), Dept. of Applied Biol. Sci. and Engin., Vrije Universiteit, Pleinlaan 2, 1050 Brussels, Belgium
[2]Ghent University, Fac. Vet. Med., Dept. Reprod., Obstetr. and Herd Health, B 9820 Merelbeke, Belgium
[3]Ministry of the Flemish Community, Inst. for Agric. and Fisheries Res., Unit Technology and Food, 9090 Melle, Belgium
Corresponding author: gorik.braem@vub.ac.be

In Flanders, a shift of the distribution of mastitis pathogens towards coagulase-negative staphylococci (CNS) and coliforms has been observed and this may be the cause of the recent problems of increasing bulk milk somatic cell counts and/or decreasing milk quality. An observational study is being conducted to study different aspects of the observed phenomena. Therefore, the diversity of microorganisms from teat apices of lactating cows will be pictured. For comparison, three farms with and three without specific coliform problems are included in the study and on each farm, ten randomly selected cows are monitored during one year. Identification of microorganism from teats consists of both culture-dependent and -independent methodologies. Culture-dependent identification uses rep-PCR, based on a (GTG) 5 primer. For typing of CNS, identification is done using a reference library (isolates originating from culture collections, milk and teat apices, which have been identified using rpoB sequencing). The culture-independent method is based on Denaturing Gradient Gel Electrophoresis (DGGE) profiles of PCR amplicons targeting the V3 region of 16S rRNA. Preliminary results show presence of Aerococcus, Lactobacillus and Staphylococcus spp. Results from the current project will help to elucidate the actual role of microorganisms present on teats from dairy cows.

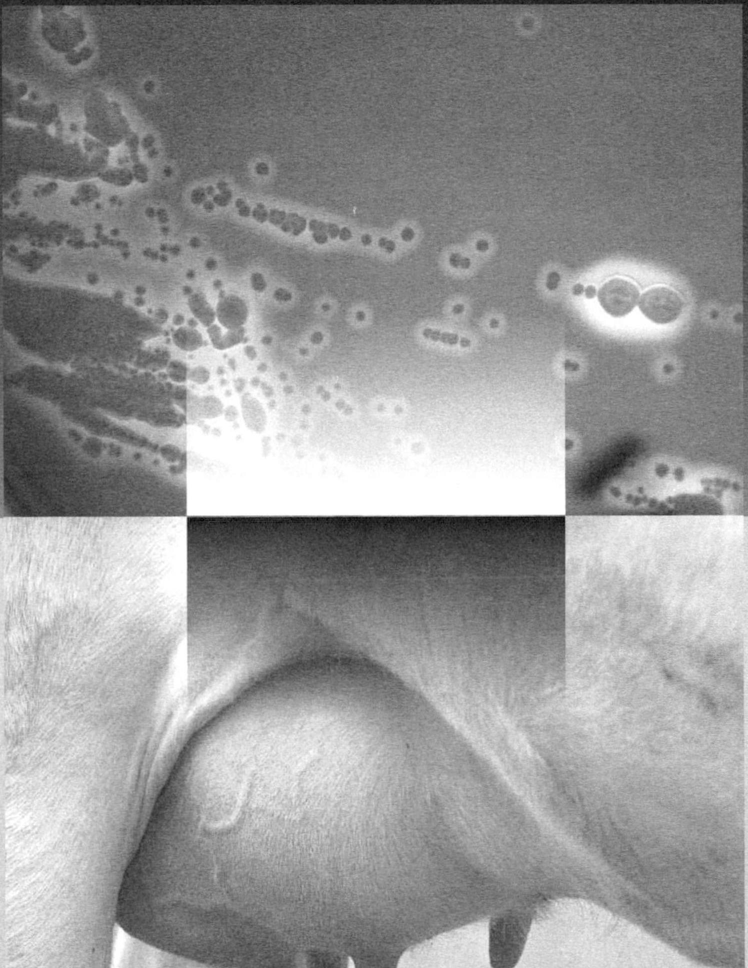

Heifer and quarter characteristics associated with periparturient blood and milk neutrophilic viability

S. Piepers[1], G. Opsomer[1], K. Demeyere[2], A. de Kruif[1], E. Meyer[2] and S. de Vliegher[1]
[1]Department of Reproduction, Obstetrics and Herd Health, Faculty of Veterinary Medicine, Ghent University, Merelbeke, Belgium
[2]Laboratory of Biochemistry, Faculty of Veterinary Medicine, Ghent University, Belgium
Corresponding author: Sofie.Piepers@UGent.be

Abstract

Polymorphonuclear neutrophilic leukocytes (PMN) play an important role in the first line immune defence of the mammary gland. Reduced blood and/or milk PMN viability around parturition may therefore at least partly explain the high prevalence of intramammary infections (IMI) in fresh dairy heifers. The present study is the first to identify both heifer and quarter characteristics associated with the viability of blood and milk PMN in periparturient dairy heifers. A total of 82 heifers from 19 dairy herds were included in the study. Polymorphonuclear neutrophilic leukocyte viability in blood (at 1 week before calving and at 1 to 4 days in milk (DIM)) and in milk (at 1 to 4 DIM) was estimated by determining the proportion of apoptotic cells using flow cytometry. Information on heifer and quarter characteristics was collected in early lactation. Data were analysed using multivariable, multilevel regression analysis. Supplementation of minerals/vitamins was associated with a higher blood and milk PMN viability (less apoptosis) around calving. Both blood and milk PMN viability showed a seasonal variation with the highest proportion of apoptotic cells between April and June. Heifers losing condition (>0.5 points on a 5 point scale) between one week before expected calving date and 1 to 4 DIM had a higher proportion of apoptotic blood PMN in early lactation. The variation in PMN viability mainly resided at the heifer and quarter level rather than at the herd level, indicating that measures to optimise the non-specific immunity around calving should focus at these levels. Knowledge of the here described risk factors can be helpful in improving the innate immunity of the mammary gland around calving in dairy heifers, and so in the resistance against IMI and/or in their clearance.

Keywords: periparturient, flow cytometry, heifers, immunology, leukocytes, risk factors

Introduction

A high proportion of heifers freshens with one or more subclinically infected quarters (Fox *et al.*, 1995). Clinical mastitis in dairy heifers is not uncommon either (Barkema *et al.*, 1998). The impact of subclinical intramammary infections (IMI) on the heifers' future performances is most likely related to the persistence of the infection when milk production has started (De Vliegher *et al.*, 2005). Some heifers eliminate IMI at calving within a short time span whereas others do not. This difference is most likely due to variation in the pathogen virulence and its capability of persisting, but also due to the immune status of the host (Taponen *et al.*, 2007).

The available number of polymorphonuclear neutrophilic leukocytes (PMN) and their functionality contribute to a considerable extent to the first line of immune defence of the mammary gland (Rainard *et al.*, 2006). Differences in the number and viability of PMN at the heifer and quarter level could therefore, at least partly, explain why an IMI occurs and why it persists or not in a specific heifer/quarter rather than in others. After all, apoptosis of bovine PMN is closely related to their activity (Mehrzad *et al.*, 2004).

Genetic variation in the innate immunity of the mammary gland has been demonstrated (Detilleux, 2002), but very little is known about other potential risk factors affecting the immunity of the heifers in early lactation. Moreover, most epidemiological studies identifying risk factors associated with bovine PMN viability focussed on blood PMN features, and only to a very limited extent on milk PMN activity. Compared to blood, milk is a difficult matrix to analyse and because an accurate technique allowing the quantification of milk PMN viability on a larger number of milk samples was lacking until now. Knowledge of factors associated with the viability of both heifers' blood and milk PMN around calving could be helpful to open up new perspectives in how to prevent and control heifer mastitis.

The aims of the present study were (1) to identify heifer and quarter characteristics associated with periparturient blood and milk PMN viability, and (2) to determine the contribution of herd, heifer and quarter to the total variance of blood and milk PMN viability.

Materials and methods

Herds, animals and data

Nineteen dairy herds were randomly selected from a database (n=241) of the Flemish Cattle Breeding Association (Oosterzele, Belgium) including all dairy herds within the vicinity (30 km radius) of the Faculty of Veterinary Medicine. The selected herds were not allowed to treat their heifers with antibiotics before calving. Teat apex swabs were collected at one week before expected calving date. Blood PMN viability from 82 clinically healthy dairy heifers belonging to the 19 dairy herds (on average 4 heifers per herd, ranging from 1 to 7) was determined twice, at one week before expected calving date, and at 1 to 4 DIM. Milk PMN viability, quarter milk somatic cell count SCC (qSCC), and bacteriological status were determined by collecting quarter foremilk samples (n=328) between 1 and 4 DIM. Heifer and quarter characteristics were recorded at sampling (Table 1) and were included as independent variables in the modelling process.

Table 1. Multivariable associations between heifer and quarter level characteristics and blood and milk PMN[1] apoptosis of 82 dairy heifers from 19 dairy herds.

Independent variables	Proportion of apoptotic PMN[1]		
	milk after calving	blood before calving	blood after calving
Heifer characteristics			
Admittance to pasture before calving	ns[2]	ns	ns
Age at calving	ns	ns	ns
Body condition loss[3]	ns	ns	+++
Breed[4]	ns	ns	ns
Heifer dirty before calving[5]	ns	nt	nt
Contact with lactating cows before calving	ns	ns	ns
Excessive udder oedema between 1 and 4 DIM	ns	nt	nt
Calving in April to June	+++	++	++
Supplementation with minerals/vitamins	-	-	ns
Quarter characteristics			
Infection status between 1 and 4 DIM[6]	ns	nt	nt
Front quarter	ns	nt	nt
Teat apex colonisation with non-*aureus* staphylococci	--	nt	nt
Teat end lesions	ns	nt	nt
Teat skin lesions	ns	nt	nt

[1] Polymorphonuclear neutrophilic leukocytes.
[2] Multivariable model: +(-) = more (less) apoptosis if factor is present (P<0.05); ++ (--) = P<0.01; +++ (---) = P<0.001; ns = not significant; nt = not tested.
[3] Body condition loss of at least 0.5 point from 1 week before expected calving date to 1-4 days after calving. Based on the visual body condition scoring system of Edmondson *et al.* (1989).
[4] Holstein-Friesian, Red Holstein and Red Holstein crossbreds.
[5] Based on the visual cleanliness scoring system of Hughes (2001).
[6] (1) culture-negative, (2) non-*aureus* staphylococci, *Corynebacterium bovis,* (3) *Staphylococcus aureus, aesculin*-positive cocci, *aesculin*-negative cocci.

Laboratory procedures

Bacteriological culturing of both milk (Animal Health Service Flanders, Torhout, Belgium) and swabs (Faculty of Veterinary Medicine, Merelbeke, Belgium) were done as previously described (De Vliegher *et al.*, 2003; Piepers *et al.*, 2007). A teat apex was classified as colonised with non-*aureus* staphylococci (NAS) when at least 50 CFU were isolated on a blood agar plate. Additional quarter milk samples for somatic cell counting were stored at 4 °C and were immediately transported to the laboratory of the Milk Control Centre Flanders (Lier, Belgium) for electronic counting (Fossomatic 5000™, Foss Electric, Hillerød, Denmark).

Isolation of the blood leukocytes was performed by centrifugation (300×g), removal of plasma and buffy coat, hypotonic lyses of erythrocytes, and two washing steps. For milk, the initial volume of quarter foremilk was divided equally over two 50-ml Falcon-tubes, diluted 50% vol/vol with cold Phosphate Buffered Saline (PBS), and centrifuged (300×g) during 15 minutes. After carefully removing the cream layer, the pellet was suspended into 10 ml PBS, centrifuged at 200×g for 10 min, and washed two more times. Blood PMN were discriminated from other blood cells based on their size and internal complexity in a forward-side scatter dot plot. As this approach is not feasible for milk, differentiation between milk PMN and other milk cells was done as described previously (Piepers, unpublished data). The proportion of apoptotic blood and milk PMN were identified and differentiated from the necrotic subpopulation using a double fluorescein isothiocyanate (FITC)-annexin-V and propidium iodide (PI) staining. As apoptosis does not occur in circulation, the blood cell pellet was first incubated for 18h at 37 °C before PMN viability was determined. All analyses were performed on a double-laser, bench-top flow cytometer (BD FACSCanto II). Data were acquired and processed using FacsDiva Software (Becton Dickinson, Belgium).

Data handling and statistical analysis

The PMN viability was represented by the proportion of apopotic PMN. A square-root transformation was used to normalise the data. The regression-model building process involved several steps as described by De Vliegher *et al.* (2004) using MlwiN 2.02 (Centre for Multilevel Modelling, Bristol, UK). The difference in the Ln-transformed qSCC between the quarters of which the teat apex was colonised with non-*aureus* staphylococci and those which were not, was analysed by an independent samples t-test using SPSS 16.0 (Chicago, USA).

Results

Descriptive analysis

Average bulk milk SCC on the 19 dairy herds was 278,736 cells/ml [Interquartile Range (IQR) 192,500-343,500 cells/ml]. The average yearly milk production was 8,368 kg milk per year (±1469 kg milk/year), and the herd size consisted on average of 48 cows (±16 cows) (range 24 to 77 cows).

Thirty-three percent (n=27) of the heifers were Holstein Friesian, 40% were Red-Holstein (n=33), and 27% were Red Holstein crossbreds (n=22). The average milk yield at the first test-day after calving i.e. within 35 DIM, was 24.9 kg (SD ±5.21 kg). Nearly eighty-eight percent of the heifers had at least one culture-positive quarter. Geometric mean SCC of the 328 quarter milk samples was 315,422 cells/ml (IQR 97,250-935,000 cells/ml). Sixty-three percent of the teat apices were colonised with NAS. The qLnSCC in early lactation was significantly higher if the teat apex was colonised with NAS before calving ($P<0.05$). Just over fifty percent of the milk samples were culture-positive. Non-*aureus* staphylococci and *C. bovis* were isolated from 84.4% of the culture-positive quarters, whereas *S. aureus* and *aesculin*-positive cocci were isolated from 15.6% of the culture-positive quarters.

The proportion of apoptotic blood and milk PMN at the herd, heifer and quarter level is presented in Table 2. Only taking into consideration the culture-negative quarters per heifer, the difference in the proportion of apoptotic milk PMN varied between 0.1 and 36.4%.

Multivariable, multilevel analysis

Overall, blood and milk PMN apoptosis around calving showed a seasonal variation with the highest number of apoptotic PMN occurring in April to June (Table 1; Figure 1). Apoptosis of blood PMN in the first days after calving was more pronounced in heifers losing condition (threshold of 0.5 points on a 5-points scale) around calving compared to heifers not losing condition during that period. Supplementation of minerals/vitamins before calving was

Table 2. Descriptive statistics of the proportion of apoptotic blood and milk PMN[1] around calving of 82 dairy heifers from 19 dairy herds in Flanders (Belgium).

Data	N	Mean	Median	IQR[2]
Apoptotic blood PMN[1] before calving (%)				
Herd	19	20.3	18.2	11.4-26.7
Heifer	82	20.7	16.7	7.7-30.3
Quarter	328			
Apoptotic blood PMN after calving (%)				
Herd	19	19.7	19.8	13.4-24.6
Heifer	82	19.8	14.8	8.3-26.0
Quarter	328			
Apoptotic milk PMN (%)				
Herd	19	22.6	20.9	18.2-25.0
Heifer	82	23.4	21.0	13.9-31.6
Quarter	328	24.9	21.9	14.1-34.4

[1] Polymorphonuclear neutrophilic leukocytes.
[2] Interquartile range.

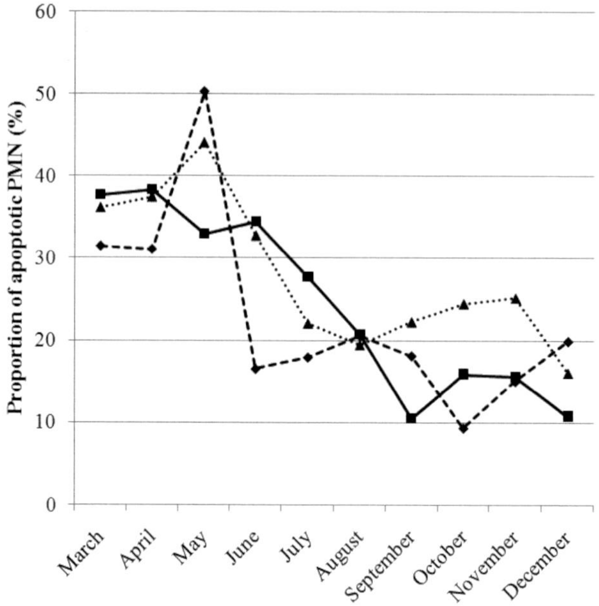

Figure 1. Seasonal variation in the proportion of apoptotic blood polymorphonuclear neutrophilic leukocytes (PMN) before (—■—) and after calving (--◆--), and in the proportion of apoptotic milk PMN after calving (·· ▲··).

significantly related with a lower proportion of apoptotic blood PMN before calving and a lower proportion of apoptotic milk PMN (Table 1). Overall, 71.4% and 98.4% of the variation in the proportion of apoptotic blood PMN before and after calving, respectively, occurred at the heifer level. For the proportion of apoptotic milk PMN, 8.8%, 45.7% and 45.5% of the variation resided at the herd, heifer and quarter level, respectively.

Discussion and conclusions

The present study is, to the best of our knowledge, the first one that deals with heifer and quarter level characteristics related to the viability of both blood and milk PMN in recently freshened heifers. The variation in PMN viability mainly resides at the heifer and quarter level indicating that measures to optimise the innate immunity around calving should focus at these levels rather than at the herd level. Heifers freshening in April to June may have a less optimised systemic and/or local immune system. In Flanders, heifers calving during these months were indeed at a higher risk to suffer from an elevated SCC in early lactation (De Vliegher *et al.*, 2004).

The beneficial impact of supplementing minerals and vitamins on the udder health and immune cell activity has been previously demonstrated in multiparous cows (Persson-Waller, 2000).

Supplementation with vitamins and minerals and other risk factors related to the feeding and management of dairy heifers around calving should be evaluated more in depth as they could be valuable in optimising the first line of defence of the mammary gland around calving, and in enhancing the natural resistance or the bacterial clearance during this period of immune suppression.

A slightly increased quarter milk SCC due to IMI with non-*aureus* staphylococci may contribute to the protective effect of those pathogens against IMI with major pathogens (Green *et al.*, 2004). In the present study, quarters from which the teat apex was colonised with NAS had a substantially higher SCC and significantly less apoptotic milk PMN compared to those from which the teat apex was not colonised. Delayed apoptosis of PMN is known as an important mechanism for PMN accumulation in many bacterial inflammatory diseases (Dibbert *et al.*, 1999). Teat apex colonisation with NAS may therefore generate new hypotheses in protecting the mammary gland against IMI. Overall, only a small amount of the total variation in the blood PMN viability before and after calving (19.1 and 25.0, respectively) and milk PMN viability (22.1%) was explained by the examined factors. Still, some potentially important risk factors, e.g. the genetic background of the heifers, were not included in the study, but definitely warrant further research.

References

Barkema, H.W., Schukken, Y.H., Lam, T.G.J.M., Beiboer, M.L., Benedictus, G. and Brand, A., 1998. Management practices associated with low, medium, and high somatic cell counts in bulk milk. J. Dairy Sci. 81: 1917-1927.

Detilleux, J.C., 2002. Genetic factors affecting susceptibility of dairy cows to udder pathogens. Vet. Immun. Immunopath. 88: 103-110.

De Vliegher, S., Laevens, H., Devriese, L.A., Opsomer, G., Leroy, J.L., Barkema, H.W. and de Kruif, A., 2003. Prepartum teat apex colonization with *Staphylococcus chromogenes* in dairy heifers is associated with low somatic cell count in early lactation. Vet. Microbiol. 92: 245-252.

De Vliegher, S., Laevens, H., Barkema, H.W., Dohoo, I.R., Stryhn, H., Opsomer, G. and de Kruif, A., 2004. Management practices and heifer characteristics associated with early lactation somatic cell count of Belgian dairy heifers. J. Dairy Sci. 87: 937-947.

De Vliegher, S., Barkema, H.W., Stryhn, H., Opsomer, G. and de Kruif, A., 2005. Impact of early somatic cell count in heifers on milk yield over the first lactation. J. Dairy Sci. 88: 938-947.

Dibbert, B., Weber, M., Nikolaizik, W.H., Vogt, P., Schoni, M.H., Blaser, K. and Simon, H.U., 1999. Cytokine-mediated Bax deficiency and consequent delayed neutrophil apoptosis: A general mechanism to accumulate effector cells in inflammation. PNAS 96: 13330-13335.

Edmondson, A.J., Lean, I.L., Weaver, L.D., Farver, T. and Webster, G., 1989. A body condition scoring chart for Holstein dairy cows. J. Dairy Sci. 72: 68-78.

Fox, L.K., Chester, S.T., Hallberg, J.W., Nickerson, S.C., Pankey, J.W. and Weaver, L.D., 1995. Survey of intramammary infections in dairy heifers at breeding age and first parturition. J. Dairy Sci. 78: 1619-1628.

Green, M.J., Burton, P.R., Green, L.E., Schukken, Y.H., Bradley, A.J., Peeler, E.J. and Medley, G.F., 2004. The use of Markov chain Monte Carlo for analysis of correlated binary data: patterns of somatic cells in milk and the risk of clinical mastitis in dairy cows. Prev. Vet. Med. 64: 157-174.

Hughes, J., 2001. A system for assessing cow cleanliness. In Practice 23: 517-524.

Mehrzad, J., Duchateau, L. and Burvenich, C., 2004. Viability of milk neutrophils and severity of bovine coliform mastitis. J. Dairy Sci. 87: 4150-4162.

Persson-Waller, K., 2000. Mammary gland immunology around parturition – influence of stress, nutrition and genetics. Adv. Exp. Med. Biol. 480: 231-245.

Piepers, S., De Meulemeester, L., de Kruif, A., Opsomer, G., Barkema, H.W. and De Vliegher, S., 2007. Prevalence and distribution of mastitis pathogens in subclinically infected dairy cows in Flanders, Belgium. J. Dairy Res. 74: 478-483.

Rainard, P. and Riollet, C., 2006. Innate immunity of the bovine mammary gland. Vet. Res. 37: 369-400.

Taponen, S., Koort, J., Björkroth, J., Saloniemi, H. and Pyörälä, S., 2007. Bovine intramammary infections caused by coagulase-negative staphylococci may persist throughout lactation according to amplified fragment length polymorphism-based analysis. J. Dairy Sci. 90: 3301-3307.

Parameters for natural resistance in bovine milk

T.C.W. Ploegaert[1], E.J. Tijhaar[1], H.K. Parmentier[2], J.J. van der Poel[3], J.A.M. van Arendonk[3] and H.F.J. Savelkoul[1]
[1]Cell Biology and Immunology Group, Department of Animal Sciences, Wageningen University, Marijkeweg 40, 6709 PG Wageningen, the Netherlands
[2]Section of Immunology, Adaptation Physiology Group, Department of Animal Sciences, Wageningen University, Marijkeweg 40, 6709 PG Wageningen, the Netherlands
[3]Animal Breeding and Genetics Group, Department of Animal Sciences, Wageningen University, Marijkeweg 40, 6709 PG Wageningen, the Netherlands
Corresponding author: Tosca.ploegaert@wur.nl

Abstract

Natural disease resistance of the cow is one of the factors that can play a role in preventing and combating mastitis. It is well documented how immune parameters change following an experimental mammary infection with different pathogens. However, knowledge of the role of natural resistance to infection and parameters to best measure natural resistance in an uninfected animal, is scarce. The hypothesis of this project is that such parameters of natural resistance in milk do correlate with the cow's capacity to resist mastitis. Identification of such parameters can enable the development of tests to monitor the level of natural resistance to mastitis on the dairy farm in a non-invasive way. Monitoring of natural resistance supports the farmer in managing the herd. For this project milk and blood samples were taken from cows without clinical signs of diseases to study: (1) the repeatability of the selected parameters within cows; (2) variation of these parameters between cows; and (3) the relation between these parameters in milk and blood. The humoral parameters that were measured included cytokines, like TNFα (pro-inflammatory) and IFNγ (cell mediated immunity), and (naturally occurring) antibodies against different pathogen associated molecular patterns (PAMPs). The (natural) antibody titres and to a lesser extend the cytokine levels, showed repeatability within and variation between cows. These selected parameters are being measured in milk samples of nearly 2000 heifers of the Dutch Milk Genomics project with known mastitis history to study their relation with natural resistance to mastitis and heritability of measured parameters.

Keywords: genomics, immunology, natural resistance

Introduction

The natural disease resistance of the cow can, among many other factors, play a role in preventing and fighting mastitis. Several immune parameters have been investigated following experimental infection of the mammary gland with different pathogens. Among others, several cytokines like TNFα and IFNγ (expression) were measured following experimental infection with *Staphylococcus aureus* and/or *Escherichia coli* (Bannerman *et al.*, 2004; Lee *et al.*, 2006;

Shuster *et al.*, 1997). However, knowledge about the relationship between different immune parameters in an uninfected animal and its natural resistance to infection, is scarce. Natural antibodies of cows are mentioned (Rainard and Riollet, 2006), but not much studied in relation to natural resistance. Van Knegsel *et al.* (2007) measured antibodies against lipopolysaccharide (LPS) from *E. coli* and hemocyanin from Keyhole Limpet (KLH, from *Megathura crenulata*), but did not fully relate them to resistance yet. The hypothesis of this project is that certain immune parameters in milk do correlate with the cow's ability to resist mastitis. Identification of such parameters can enable the development of tests to monitor objectively in a non-invasive way the level of natural resistance to mastitis. Monitoring of natural resistance supports the farmer in managing the herd. Based on literature, parameters were selected that might be correlated with resistance to bacterial infections.

Before testing these parameters on a large number of samples, the levels were first determined in milk and blood plasma samples taken during the course of nearly 3 weeks on 20 cows without clinical signs of diseases. This was done to study: (1) variation of these parameters between cows; (2) the repeatability of the selected parameters within cows; and (3) the relation between these parameters in milk and blood plasma. The relation between milk and blood is of interest because the goal is to measure parameters in milk, and it is useful to know to what extend (local) levels in the milk correlate with (systemic) levels in the blood. The (humoral) parameters that were measured included cytokines, like TNFα (induction of inflammation) and IFNγ (cell mediated immunity), and (naturally occurring) antibodies against several pathogen associated molecular patterns (PAMPs), like lipoteichoic acid (LTA) and peptidoglycan (PGN) from *S. aureus*, and LPS from *E. coli.* Furthermore, natural antibody titres against a naïve antigen, KLH from *Megathura crenulata*, were determined. A parameter needs to show variability between different animals, otherwise it can never be related to variations in or mastitis susceptibility. Furthermore, a parameter has to show good repeatability when measured a number of times during a relatively short time-span (nearly three weeks). If this is not the case a single measurement of the parameter will most likely not be a good indicator for the cow's natural resistance. In this study it is shown that all the tested parameters showed enough variation between cows and repeatability within a cow to warrant further testing on milk samples of nearly 2000 heifers with known mastitis history. In this way the relation of the parameters with mastitis incidence can be determined. The design of that study enables us to study the heritability of the parameters. This is of interest to evaluate the opportunities to select dairy cows with improved natural resistance to mastitis.

Materials and methods

The observational experiment, mentioned in the introduction, was performed at one farm, using 20 Holstein Friesian dairy cows. Milk and blood samples were obtained from these cows during a period of nearly 3 weeks. At days 1 and 3 samples were taken in the morning only, and at days 8, 10, 15 and 17 in the morning and the afternoon. In total 10 milk and 10 blood samples were collected from each cow, which received no other treatments.

Milk was sampled during routine milking. Just after milking blood samples were taken using vacutainers with K2EDTA (BD, Plymouth, PL67BP, United Kingdom). Milk and plasma samples were aliquoted at the day of collection and stored at -20 °C. In milk and plasma samples of all 20 cows, the cytokines TNFα and IFNγ and total (natural) antibody titres against *E. coli*-derived LPS (L2880, serotype O55:B5) and *S. aureus*-derived LTA (L2515) from Sigma-Aldrich Inc. (St. Louis, MO), *S. aureus*-derived PGN from Sigma-Aldrich Inc. ((Fluka) Buchs, CH) and *M. crenulata*-derived KLH from MP Biomedicals (Solon, Ohio), were determined. The natural antibody titres were determined essentially as described before (Van Knegsel *et al.*, 2007) and the cytokine detection was performed with capture ELISAs that were developed in-house. Repeatability in time was tested by calculating correlation coefficients in Statistical Analysis Software (SAS) 9.1. Variation between cows was tested using the mixed model in SAS with repeated measurements.

Results

Natural antibody levels against LPS, LTA, PGN and KLH were determined in milk and plasma samples of 20 cows to determine variability between cows, repeatability within a cow, and relation between milk and blood plasma. As an example Figure 1 shows the antibody titres against LPS per cow in plasma and in milk over time. The dots connected by a line represent the average of all cows over time, the others show individual cows. Figure 2 shows the antibody titres against LPS in milk per cow. The titres are represented as the average titre of a cow

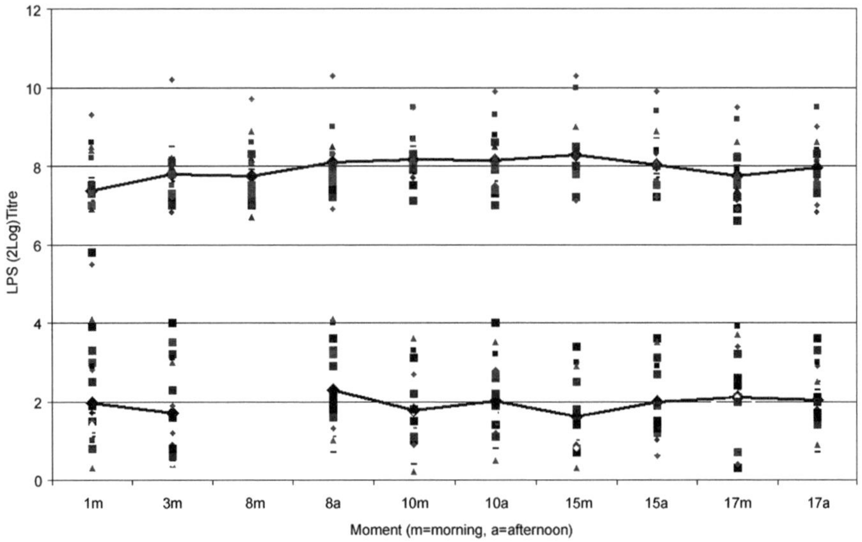

Figure 1. Antibody titres against LPS in plasma (upper lines) and milk (lower lines) of all cows per moment (day of experiment with m=morning and a=afternoon). Dots connected by a line show the averages of all cows, others are separate cows to show variation between cows.

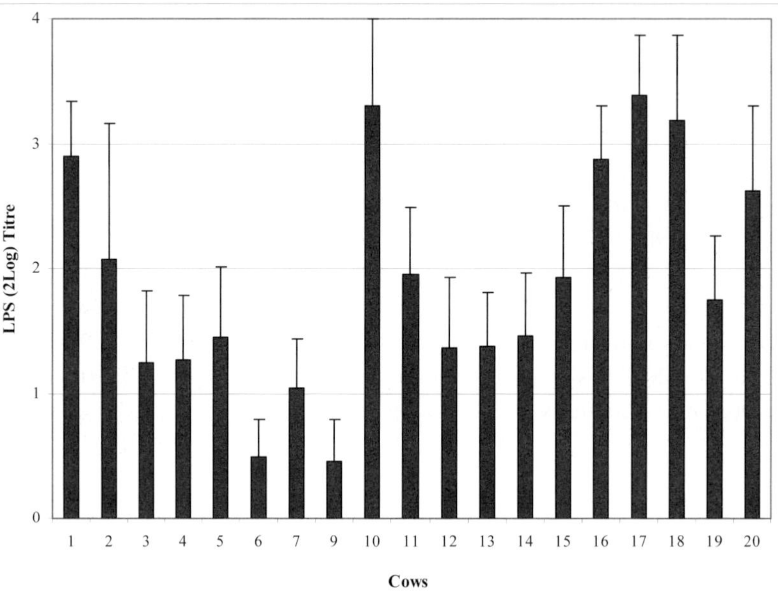

Figure 2. Antibody titres against LPS of all 20 cows in milk, averages over time. Error bars show standard deviations.

during the 3-weeks test period. Error bars represent the standard deviation for the different time points. Antibody titres showed significant differences between individual cows ($P<0.01$). Titres are quite stable over time (Figure 1). The repeatability coefficients for the antibody titres against LPS, LTA, KLH and PGN in time ranges from 0.72 to 0.87 (Table 1). Similar results were found for parameters measured in milk and in plasma. Repeatability coefficients for TNFα and IFNγ were even higher than the ones of antibody titres (Table 1). However, this is probably due to one cow which showed extreme values. When the observations of that cow were eliminated from the analysis, the correlation decreased to 0.66 (IFNγ in plasma), 0.61 (IFNγ in milk), 0.57 (TNFα in plasma), and 0.05 (TNFα in milk), of which TNFα in milk was very low. Table 2 shows the relation of antibody titres between milk and blood plasma by the correlation coefficients between them. Correlations varied between 0.49 and 0.76 with the lowest level for the antibody titres against the naïve antigen KLH.

Discussion

The overall aim of this project is to identify (immune) parameters in milk that correlate with resistance to mastitis in dairy cows. Based on literature, potentially useful parameters were selected. Before testing milk samples of nearly 2000 heifers with known mastitis history, six of these parameters (antibody titres to LTA and PGN from *S. aureus,* LPS from *E. coli* and KLH from *M. crenulata,* and TNFα and IFNγ levels) were tested in milk samples of 20

Table 1. Estimates of repeatability of antibody titres and TNFα and IFNγ levels in milk and plasma. Estimates as correlation between observations at different times during a 3 weeks period.

Parameter	Plasma	Milk
LPS	0.79	0.72
KLH	0.70	0.87
LTA	0.81	0.83
PGN	0.93	0.86
TNFα	0.99	0.84
IFNγ	0.99	0.99

Table 2. Estimates for correlation of antibody titres between milk and blood plasma.

Parameter	Correlation
LPS	0.60
KLH	0.49
LTA	0.76
PGN	0.69

cows to determine variability between cows, repeatability within a cow, and the relation between milk and blood plasma. The differences between cows in antibody and cytokine levels demonstrate the existence of variation between cows. This is important, because if there is no variation between cows the parameter can not be used as indicator for resistance to mastitis. A number of factors contribute to this variation including the variation in age and stage of lactation between cows. Repeatability estimates for the (natural) antibodies, measured as correlation between observations on the same cows over time, were in general high (Table 1). These results reveal that these immune parameters show a good degree of repeatability, but they are not equal to one, which would reflect a situation of complete repeatability. Our repeatability estimates for immune parameters are similar to estimates for repeatability of milk production (Mayeres *et al.*, 2004; Olori *et al.*, 1999). Especially Mayeres *et al.* (2004) show that test day milk records are predictive for future milk production. This implies that in our situation, with similar repeatability's, a single measurement of immune parameters gives a good indication of immune status of the cow. Repeatability for TNFα and IFNγ in the entire dataset was very high. This high repeatability found in the entire data set reduced considerably when observations on a single cow were eliminated from the analysis. They were still reasonable, except for repeatability of TNFα in milk, which was very low. The reason for this is yet unknown.

Although values in blood were higher than in milk, the values of the antibody titres in milk were considerably representative for the ones in blood, except for KLH titres which had a lower correlation coefficient between milk and blood. This implies that to a certain extent antibody titres in milk reflect antibody titres in blood plasma. The repeatability coefficients for the antibody titres and cytokine levels, and the significant variation of these parameters between cows, warrant further evaluation on a large number of milk samples, to determine their relationship with mastitis incidence.

Future work

The cytokine and natural antibody levels are being tested on milk samples of nearly 2000 heifers collected for the 'Milk Genomics' (MG) project. The aim of the MG project was to identify genetic variation and heritability for milk fat and protein composition (Dutch Milk Genomics Initiative, 2008). From these cows genetic (e.g. known pedigree) and phenotypic information (e.g. SCC, mastitis incidence) is available. Although the MG project was not set up for research concerning natural resistance to mastitis, it can be used for it because of the available information and the observational origin. Parameters indicative for natural resistance will be analysed for their heritability. This will reveal if they can be used as parameters for selective breeding.

Conclusion

Antibodies against LPS, LTA, KLH and PGN were found to be variable between cows and consistent within cows when measured repeatedly within a short period of time. This makes them suitable for further evaluation on milk samples of the nearly 2000 heifers with known mastitis incidence, to determine if they are useful parameters for natural resistance or susceptibility to mastitis. Furthermore, to a certain extent antibody titres in milk reflect the ones in blood plasma. Initial repeatability's of TNFα and IFNγ were very high. After deletion of one extreme cow from the dataset the repeatability's decreased, but were still reasonable, except for TNFα in milk. Despite of this, they will all be measured in the MG milk samples, because of their key functions in regulation of immune responses. The data will be used to determine the degree of heritability of the parameters and to study the predictive value for mastitis. This will make clear if they can be used as indicators for natural resistance and as parameters in the selective breeding of cows with increased resistance to mastitis.

Acknowledgements

This study is part of the five-year udder health program of the Dutch Udder Health Centre and was financially supported by the Dutch Dairy Board, CRV and the Dutch Agriculture and Horticulture Organisation (LTO Noord).

References

Bannerman, D.D., Paape, M.J., Lee, J-W., Zhao, X, Hope, J.C. and Rainard, P., 2004. *Escherichia coli* and *Staphylococcus aureus* elicit differential innate immune responses following intramammary infection. Clin. Diagn. Lab. Imm. 11: 463-472.

Dutch Milk Genomics Initiative, 2008. Available at: www.milkgenomics.com. Accessed 12 June 2008.

Lee, J-W., Bannerman, D.D., Paape, M.J., Huang, M.K. and Zhao, X., 2006. Characterization of cytokine expression in milk somatic cells during intramammary infections with *Escherichia coli* or *Staphylococcus aureus* by real-time PCR. Vet. Res. 37: 219-229.

Mayeres, P., Stoll, J., Bormann, J., Reents, R. and Gengler, N., 2004. Prediction of daily milk, fat, and protein production by a random regression test-day model. J. Dairy Sci. 87: 1925-1933.

Olori, V.E., Hill, W.G., McGuirk, B.J. and Brotherstone, S., 1999. Estimating variance components for test day milk records by restricted maximum likelihood with a random regression animal model. Livest. Prod. Sci. 61: 53-63.

Rainard, P. and Riollet, C., 2006. Innate immunity of the bovine mammary gland. Vet. Res. 37: 369-400.

Shuster, D.E., Kehrli, M.E. Jr., Rainard, P. and Paape, M., 1997. Complement fragment C5a and inflammatory cytokines in neutrophil recruitment during intramammary infection with *Escherichia coli*. Inf. Imm. 65: 3286-3292.

Van Knegsel, A.T., De Vries Reilingh, G., Meulenberg, S., Van den Brand, H., Dijkstra, J., Kemp, B. and Parmentier, H.K., 2007. Natural antibodies related to energy balance in early lactation dairy cows. J. Dairy Sci. 90: 5490-5498.

2006), with a significant detriment to the dairy industry. Antibiotic treatment often results in relapsing infection and efficacious vaccines are currently not available (Barkema *et al.*, 2006). Persistent or difficult-to-treat infections may relate to the ability of this pathogen to form a slow growing population termed small colony variants (SCVs) that can survive within professional and non-professional phagocytic cells and subsequently modulate immune responses (Sinha and Herrmann, 2005). While *S. aureus* SCVs have been described in human medicine, they have been overlooked in veterinary medicine.

Traditionally, *S. aureus* has been regarded as extracellular pathogen. However, the ability of this pathogen to survive within phagocytes (Voyich *et al.*, 2005, Hébert *et al.*, 2000) and nonprofessional phagocytic cells including cultured bovine aortic endothelial cells (BAEC) (Vann and Proctor, 1987) and a bovine mammary epithelial cell line (MAC-T) (Bayles *et al.*, 1998) has been documented. Internalisation within host cells appears to shield persistent strains of *S. aureus* from host defence and antibiotic treatment (Van Belkum, 2006). In addition, the intracellular milieu appeared to favour the selection and/or survival of small colony variants (SCVs) (Atalla *et al.*, 2008), which seem to survive within the host for long periods of time without triggering a cell-mediated immune response (CMIR). However, the association between specific strains of *S. aureus* especially those of the SCV phenotype and persistent infection of the bovine mammary gland is unknown. Therefore, the current objectives are to: (1) test the hypothesis that *S. aureus* strains associated with chronic mastitis are of the SCV phenotype, (2) test the hypothesis that bovine *S. aureus* SCV establish a mild intramammary infection and different *in vivo* local and systemic clinical signs compared to its parent strain 3231 and other genetically characterised strains, including a Newbould *hemB* SCV mutant and Newbould 305, (3) evaluate delayed-type hypersensitivity (DTH) as an indication of cell mediated immune response *in vivo* and (4) characterise innate and adaptive host response gene expression to bovine *S. aureus* SCV Heba3231 and its isogenic wild type parental strain. Unraveling the complex interaction between a microbial pathogen and the host is the fundamental basis of understanding microbial pathogenesis. While regulation of virulence genes of *S. aureus* strains has been extensively studied *in vitro*, there is a need to understand how specific microbial virulence factors influence the host response and the outcome of infection.

Materials and methods

Isolation of **S. aureus** *small colony variant (SCV) from milk*

Foremilk samples were collected from Canadian Holstein cows identified with persistent and recurrent *S. aureus* mastitis. Quarter milk samples were cultured on Columbia agar supplemented with 5% sheep blood (CBA, Difco) and MacConkey agar plates (Difco). Identification of positive *S. aureus* colonies was based on morphological (large highly hemolytic colonies on CBA), biochemical (catalase and positive, rapid coagulase production with 18 hr incubation) and genetic characterisation (*nuc* gene, Brakstad *et al.*, 1992). Enrichment of SCVs from the population of *S. aureus* isolates was done as described previously (Sadowska *et al.*, 2002). Briefly, overnight fresh cultures of the typical *S. aureus* strains in brain heart infusion (BHI, Difco) broth were adjusted to 5×10^6 or 5×10^7 cfu/ml and each dilution was incubated overnight (ON) with 0.25, 0.5 or 1.0 μg/ml gentamicin sulfate (Sigma).

Phenotypic and genetic characterisation of S. aureus *SCV*

The SCV isolate that was identified as *S. aureus* was analysed for growth curve characteristics compared to its wild type parent strain and the prototype Newbould 305 as described previously (Atalla *et al.*, 2008). Auxotrophy for hemin, menadione and thymidine was done by plating on chemically defined medium (CDM) (Van de Rijn and Kessler, 1980) and Mueller Hinton agar (MH, BBL), supplemented with 1, 2, and 5 μg/ml of hemin (Sigma), 1, 2, 5, and 10 μg/ml of menadione (Sigma) and 100 μg/ml of thymidine (Sigma) (Kahl *et al.*, 1998). Antimicrobial susceptibility for *S. aureus* SCV isolates, their parent strains and the prototypic strain Newbould 305 was determined by identifying the minimal inhibitory concentrations (MICs) of gentamicin, erythromycin, oxacillin, rifampicin, vancomycin and trimethoprim /sulfamethoxazole (TMP/SMX) (Atalla *et al.*, 2008). An intracellular persistence assay was performed using a primary culture of bovine aortic endothelial cells (BAEC) and bovine mammary epithelia cell line (MAC-T cells) (Bayles *et al.*, 1998, Vann and Proctor, 1987).

Comparative genomic hybridisation using microarray was used to determine the genome relatedness of the parental 3231 isolate and its derivative SCV Heba3231 (Atalla *et al.*, 2008). Gene expression analysis of the SCV Heba3231 and the parent strain 3231 was performed as described previously (Moisan *et al.*, 2006).

Experimental intramammary infection (IMI)

Twenty lactating Holstein dairy cows with no previous history of mastitis (5 cows/treatment group) at the University of Guelph herd were selected for the study. Selection of each group of cows was based on low somatic cell count (SCC) and negative bacterial culture. Following afternoon milking the teat end was swabbed with 70% ethanol. Cows were challenged with $\sim5\times10^3$ cfu/ml bacteria (3 quarters/cow) and infused with 5 ml pyrogen-free PBS, pH 7.4 (left hind quarter) followed by teat dipping in 1% iodine. Each group of infected cows was monitored and given a clinical score for the first 5 days post-infection based on rectal temperature, appetite, udder uniformity, milk appearance, bacterial culture, and somatic cell counts (SCC). A clinical scoring system was used following a modified format of Wenz *et al.* (2001). Cows with a total score of 0-2, 3-5, or 6-10 were classified as having mild, moderate or severe IMI, respectively. All cows were examined for chronic infection up to day 36 post-infection.

Delayed type hypersensitivity (DTH)

On day 24 post-infection each group of cows was injected intradermally with 0.1 ml of 5×10^8 cfu/ml UV killed homologous *S. aureus* strain, 0.1 ml of 2.5 mg/ml of PHA, and 0.1 ml sterile pyrogen-free PBS in the neck region. Double skin-fold thickness measurements were made at 0, 6 and 24 h as described previously (Hernández *et al.*, 2005).

Genetic characterisation of host response

Total RNA was extracted from blood mononuclear cells using Trizol reagent (Invitrogen) according to the manufacture's instruction. Reverse transcription of total RNA was done using oligo primer and Superscript III Reverse Transcriptase (Invitrogen) according to the manufacture's instructions. Each cDNA was analysed for innate recognition, proinflammatory cytokines and chemokines, type I and II immune response and regulatory genes. Real time quantification was performed in the lightCycler 000 instrument (Roche Diagnostics) using the SYBR green dye.

Results

Isolation of **S. aureus** *small colony variant (SCV) from milk*

Stable SCV phenotype (SCV Heba3231) was recovered after single passage of 5×10^6 cfu/ml in BHI broth containing 1 μg/ml gentamicin. The SCV Heba3231 had atypical phenotypic characteristics including slow growth, pin point and non-hemolytic colonies on CBA, delayed coagulase reaction. Antimicrobial susceptibility testing showed that the SCV Heba3231 was resistant to gentamicin (≥16 times) relative to its parent strain 3231 but was almost as sensitive as its parent strain and the prototype Newbould 305 to erythromycin, oxacillin, rifampicin, vancomycin and TMP/SMX. Supplementation of MH plates with 1 μg/ml hemin enhanced the growth of SCV after 18 hr of incubation. Although the two wild types hemolytic strains 3231 and Newbould 305 were internalised by cultured BAEC as was SCV Heba3231, the number of internalised SCV was as much as 40-fold higher than the number of the parent strain. Infection of BAEC or MAC-T cells with $\sim2\times10^7$ cfu SCV Heba3231 showed slight detachment from the monolayers after 3.5 hr. In contrast, co-incubation with strains Newbould 305 and the parent strain 3231 resulted in massive damage to the BAEC, demonstrated by rounding, detachment of monolayer cells and densely mottled cell membranes. Genetic characterisation showed strong similarities between strain 3231 and SCV Heba3231 supporting that both strains are derivates of the same clone (Atalla *et al.*, 2008). Transcription profiling showed reduced gene expression of *hla* (α-toxin) and *coa* (coagulase). This reduced expression correlated well with the non-hemolytic nature of SCV Heba3231 and the slow development of the coagulase test (Atalla *et al.*, 2008).

Experimental intramammary infection (IMI)

Intramammary challenge with the SCV Heba3231 induced mild clinical mastitis indicated by mild localised signs and virtual absence of systemic response. Similar observation was seen among those cows infected with the Newbould *hemB* mutant. On the other hand, IMI of cows with both 3231 and Newbould 305 wild type strains induced systemic and localised clinical signs and were classified as severe and moderate clinical mastitis, respectively, as determined by the disease severity scoring system.

Bacterial shedding of SCV Heba3231 was generally low throughout the study compared to other *S. aureus* strains. Milk samples from cows infected with both SCV Heba3231 and Newbould *hemB* had low SCS compared to their wild type parental strains. However, SCS of all treatment groups were significantly ($P<0.05$) higher during the first week post-infection and the chronic phase of infection compared to day 0 before challenge.

Delayed-type hypersensitivity (DTH)

Cows tested with SCV Heba3231 and its parent strain 3231 developed significant DTH compared with the prototypic strain Newbould 305. Cows tested with *hemB* induced immediate cutaneous hypersensitivity that stayed the same for 24 hr. Cows tested with the Newbould 305 failed to induce DTH.

Genetic characterisation of host response using QRT-PCR

Genetic characterisation of innate and adaptive immune response gene expression is ongoing. Expression levels for each gene of interest is normalised to B2-microglobulin gene at each time point (day 0 before IMI, day 2 and day 36 post-infection) which is used as the internal control house keeping gene.

Discussion

Persistent intramammary infection may be related to the ability of SCVs to survive within host cells and to cause minimal perturbation in cell physiology and minimal stimulation of host defences. Internalisation of *S. aureus* SCV within host cells provides protection against both host defence and antibiotic treatment. Slow growing bacteria may release small amounts of antigens that are insufficient to induce appropriate immune responses, thereby aiding SCV of *S. aureus* to establish persistent infection within its host. Slow growth rate, reduced or no hemolytic activity, slow coagulase production, presence of mixed culture with the wild phenotype and the high tendency to exhibit unstable phenotype explains why SCV are often misidentified and overlooked in diagnostic settings. This necessitates more attention to milk samples from herds with recurrent mastitis. The persistence of SCV within BAEC may explain why an antibody-mediated immune response alone is not always effective and emphasises the necessity of combined cell-mediated immune response and antibody against persistent strains of this pathogen (Tao and Mallard, 2007). Challenging cows with the naturally occurring *S. aureus* SCV Heba3231 and the disrupted mutant Newbould *hemB* elicited mild clinical mastitis and mild increase of milk SCC compared to their isogenic wild type parental strains. Mild clinical mastitis in response to both SCVs is mainly related to their phenotypic and genetic properties (Atalla *et al.*, 2008). Phenotypic DTH responses were greatly varied among cows infected with the persistent strain 3231 and SCVHeba3231 compared to the prototype Newbould 305 and *hemB*. The capacity of specific strains of S. *aureus* for intracellular survival seem to have a role in the observed cell-mediated immune response at day 24 post-infection in those cows infected with 3231 and SCV Heba3231. Transcriptional analysis of innate and adaptive host response genes is expected to be different in response to SCV Heba3231 compared to 3231. In conclusion, understanding innate and adaptive host response at the molecular and phenotypic level should provide better understanding of the pathophysiology of bovine mastitis following infection with persistent strains of *S. aureus*.

Acknowledgments

This research was financed by NSERC, Alberta Milk, Dairy Farmers of New Brunswick, Nova Scotia, Ontario and Prince Edward Island, Novalait Inc., Dairy Farmers of Canada, Canadian Dairy Network, AAFC, PHAC, Technology PEI Inc., Université de Montréal and University of Prince Edward Island through the Canadian Bovine Mastitis Research Network.

References

Atalla, H.N., Gyles,C., Jacob,C.L., Moisan, H., Malouin, F., and Mallard, B., 2008. Characterization of a *Staphylococcus aureus* Small Colony Variant (SCV) Associated with Persistent Bovine Mastitis. Foodborne Pathogen and Disease (In press).

Barkema, H.W., Schukken, Y.H. and Zadoks, R.N., 2006. Invited Review: The role of cow, pathogen, and treatment regimen in the therapeutic success of bovine *Staphylococcus aureus* mastitis. J. Dairy Sci. 89: 1877-1895.

Bayles, K.W., Wesson, C.A., Liou, L.E., Fox, L.K., Bohach, G.A. and Trumble, W.R., 1998. Intracellular *Staphylococcus aureus* escapes the endosome and induces apoptosis in epithelial cells. Infect. Immun. 66: 336-342.

Brakstad, O.G., Aasbakk, K. and Maeland, J.A., 1992. Detection of *Staphylococcus aureus* by polymerase chain reaction amplification of the nuc gene. J. Clin. Microbiol. 30: 1654-1660.

Hebert, A., Sayasith, K., Senechal, S., Dubreuil, P. and Lagace, J., 2000. Demonstration of intracellular *Staphylococcus aureus* in bovine mastitis alveolar cells and macrophages isolated from naturally infected cow milk. FEMS Microbiol. Lett. 193: 57-62.

Hernandez, A., Yager, J.A., Wilkie, B.N., Leslie, K.E. and Mallard, B.A., 2005. Evaluation of bovine cutaneous delayed-type hypersensitivity (DTH) to various test antigens and a mitogen using several adjuvants. Vet. Immunol. Immunopathol. 104: 45-58.

Kahl, B., Herrmann, M., Everding, A.S., Koch, H.G., Becker, K., Harms, E., Proctor, R.A. and Peters, G., 1998. Persistent infection with small colony variant strains of Staphylococcus aureus in patients with cystic fibrosis. J. Infect. Dis. 177: 1023-1029.

Moisan, H., Brouillette, E., Jacob, C.L., Langlois-Begin, P., Michaud, S. and Malouin, F., 2006. Transcription of virulence factors in *Staphylococcus aureus* small-colony variants isolated from cystic fibrosis patients is influenced by SigB. J. Bacteriol. 188: 64-76.

Olde Riekerink, R.G., Barkema, H.W., Veenstra, S., Poole, D.E., Dingwell, R.T. and Keefe, G.P., 2006. Prevalence of contagious mastitis pathogens in bulk tank milk in Prince Edward Island. Can. Vet. J. 47: 567-572.

Sadowska, B., Bonar, A., Von, E.C., Proctor, R.A., Chmiela, M., Rudnicka, W. and Rozalska, B., 2002. Characteristics of *Staphylococcus aureus*, isolated from airways of cystic fibrosis patients, and their small colony variants. FEMS Immunol. Med. Microbiol. 32: 191-197.

Sinha, B. and Herrmann, M., 2005. Mechanism and consequences of invasion of endothelial cells by *Staphylococcus aureus*. Thromb. Haemost. 94: 266-277.

Tao, W. and Mallard B., 2007. Differentially expressed genes associated with *Staphylococcus aureus* mastitis of Canadian Holstein cows. Vet. Immunol. Immunopathol. 120: 201-211.

Van Belkum, A., 2006. Staphylococcal colonization and infection: homeostasis versus disbalance of human (innate) immunity and bacterial virulence. Curr. Opin. Infect. Dis. 19: 339-344.

Van de Rijn, I. and Kessler, R.E., 1980. Growth characteristics of group A streptococci in a new chemically defined medium. Infect. Immun. 27: 444-448.

Vann, J.M. and Proctor, R.A., 1987. Ingestion of *Staphylococcus aureus* by bovine endothelial cells results in time- and inoculum-dependent damage to endothelial cell monolayers. Infect. Immun. 55: 2155-2163.

Voyich, J.M., Braughton, K.R., Sturdevant, D.E., Whitney, A.R., Said-Salim, B., Porcella, S.F., Long, R.D., Dorward, D.W., Gardner, D.J., Kreiswirth, B.N., Musser J.M. and DeLeo, F.R., 2005. Insights into mechanisms used by *Staphylococcus aureus* to avoid destruction by human neutrophils. J. Immunol. 175: 3907-3919.

Wenz, J.R., Barrington, G.M., Garry, F.B., Dinsmore, R.P. and Callan, R.J., 2001. Use of systemic disease signs to assess disease severity in dairy cows with acute coliform mastitis. J. Am. Vet. Med. Assoc. 218: 567-572.

Immunisation of dairy heifers with a *Staphylococcus aureus* bacterin reduces infection level and somatic cell counts at time of calving

S.C. Nickerson[1], E.P. Hovingh[2] and P.W. Widel[3]
[1]Animal and Dairy Science Dept., University of Georgia, Athens, GA, USA
[2]Veterinary and Biomedical Science Dept., Pennsylvania State University, University Park, PA, USA
[3]Boehringer Ingelheim Vetmedica, Inc., St. Joseph, MO, USA
Corresponding author: scn@uga.edu

Abstract

Use of a *Staphylococcus aureus* bacterin to prevent intramammary infections (IMI) in dairy heifers was evaluated. At 6 to 18 months of age, Holstein heifers were processed for vaccination and collection of mammary secretions. Fifty-three heifers were immunised with a commercial bacterin and 53 heifers served as unimmunised controls. The vaccine was a lysed culture of polyvalent *S. aureus* somatic antigens of 5 phage types in an aluminum hydroxide base. Two weeks after processing and at 6-month intervals until calving, vaccinates were processed for boosting. At 2-month intervals after trial initiation and through calving, mammary secretion samples were collected for bacteriological culture and somatic cell counts (SCC). Efficacy data showed that the percentage of heifers with *S. aureus* IMI at calving was lower in vaccinates (13.3%) compared with controls (34.0%); a reduction of 60.9%. The SCC in samples collected at calving from uninfected heifers for vaccinates and controls were 66,095 and 132,754/ml, and for infected heifers, SCC were 441,764 and 892,176/ml; reductions of approximately 50%. Likewise, average first lactation SCC were lower in vaccinates than controls (49,000 vs. 60,000/ml). The 305-day lactation milk yield for the first lactation demonstrated an 8.6% increase in vaccinates vs. controls (11,217 vs. 10,332 kg). In addition, the 305-day lactation kilograms of fat and protein were higher in vaccinates than controls (fat: 408.04 vs. 338.96 kg; protein: 329.77 vs. 315.23 kg). Evaluation of the number of days in milk for the first lactation demonstrated that vaccinates persisted 13 days longer than unvaccinated controls (349 vs. 336 days), and culling was reduced by one-third in vaccinates (16.9%: vaccinates, 24.5%: controls). Results demonstrated that administration of a commercial bacterin to breeding age and pregnant heifers reduced prevalence of *S. aureus* mastitis and SCC at calving, and increased first lactation performance.

Keywords: milk production, somatic cell count, vaccination

Introduction

Staphylococcus aureus mastitis continues to be a major challenge for the dairy industry because this disease is difficult to treat with antimicrobial drugs, especially during lactation. In some herds, *S. aureus* mastitis is prevalent in unbred and bred heifers, which serve as sources for infecting the milking herd. Such intramammary infections (IMI) in young dairy animals are associated with local inflammation, induration, and extremely high somatic cell counts (SCC), and have been found in heifers as early as 6 months of age (Boddie *et al.*, 1987). Likewise, histological analyses have shown that *S. aureus* infections adversely affect the development of milk-producing tissues of heifers (Trinidad *et al.*, 1990a).

Although intramammary therapy during gestation (Owens *et al.*, 1994; Trinidad *et al.*, 1990b) and during the immediate prepartum period (Oliver *et al.*, 1992, 2004) has been successful, the most efficient means of controlling mastitis is to prevent this disease in young dairy animals. Vaccination has been attempted to increase adult cows' immunity to *S. aureus* and to prevent establishment of these bacteria in the bovine mammary gland. Early vaccine formulations were shown to increase the spontaneous cure rates of *S. aureus* IMI in cows as well as to lessen the severity of infection but did not prevent new cases of mastitis (Adlam *et al.*, 1981; Brock *et al.*, 1975). More recently, various toxoids and adjuvants have been incorporated into experimental pseudocapsular vaccine formulations, and have been shown to be effective in preventing new *S. aureus* IMI when administered to dairy heifers (Giraudo *et al.*, 1997; Nickerson *et al.*, 1999; Nordhaug *et al.*, 1994; Sears *et al.*, 1990). In view of these successes, the present study was designed to evaluate a commercial *S. aureus* bacterin when administered to Holstein heifers as a primary immunisation at 6 to 18 months of age.

Materials and methods

One hundred six Holstein heifers from the James River Correctional Center dairy herd Goochland, VA, USA were used. This herd had a 9,979-kg rolling herd average milk production with an average SCC of ~200,000/ml. Previous microbiological culture of heifer mammary secretions indicated that approximately 35% of animals were infected with *S. aureus*.

At approximately 6 to 18 months of age, heifers were processed through a restraining chute to collect aseptic quarter mammary secretion samples for microbiological analyses following procedures outlined by the National Mastitis Council (Hogan *et al.*, 1999). Fifty-three heifers were vaccinated with Lysigin® (Boehringer Ingelheim Vetmedica, Inc., St. Joseph, MO, USA) using a dose of 5 ml intramuscularly that was administered in the semimembranosus muscle of the rear leg, and the other 53 heifers served as unvaccinated controls. The vaccine was a lysed culture of polyvalent *S. aureus* somatic antigens representing 5 phage types in an aluminum hydroxide adjuvant base, including serotypes 5, 8, and 336, the most common *S. aureus* serotypes associated with clinical mastitis. Fourteen days after the initial processing, the vaccinated group was again processed through the chute and boosted with Lysigin®. All animals were maintained on pasture and rotated by age group through calving. At 6-month intervals after the initiation of the trial and through time of calving, the vaccinated group was again processed through the chute for boosting.

At 2-month intervals after the trial initiation and through calving, mammary secretion samples were collected for bacteriological culture and for the determination of electronic SCC (A/SN Foss, Hillerod, Denmark). Microbiological examination of quarter samples collected from bred heifers over gestation demonstrated that 19.8% of heifers (9.4% of quarters) were infected with *S. aureus*, 68.9% of heifers (34.3% of quarters) were infected with coagulase-negative staphylococci (CNS), 6.6% of heifers (2.3% of quarters) were infected with environmental streptococci, and 1% of heifers (0.3% of quarters) were infected with coliforms.

At time of calving, heifers were enrolled in the Dairy Herd Improvement Program (DHIA) and data were recorded for milk yield, percentages and actual pounds fat and protein, days in milk, and SCC. Data on vaccine efficacy were examined in terms of mean percentage reduction in rate of new *S. aureus* or CNS IMI achieved among immunised heifers compared with the rate among unimmunised controls at the time of calving; differences between the percentage of heifers becoming infected among treatments was tested with the standard normal approximation (Steel and Torrie, 1980).

Results and discussion

Immunisation with Lysigin® did not cause any adverse reactions at the injection site or systemically. Minimal swelling (<2.5 cm) was occasionally observed, which disappeared within 48 hours of administration. Vaccine efficacy data showed that the percentage of heifers with *S. aureus* IMI at freshening was lower in vaccinates (13.3%) compared with controls (34.0%); a reduction of 60.9% ($P<0.01$). Likewise, an examination of health records showed that the percentage of heifers that were culled or died during the trial was reduced by approximately one-third by vaccination: 16.9% in vaccinates and 24.5% in controls ($P>0.05$). The vaccinated group also experienced a slight, insignificant reduction in mastitis caused by CNS. At freshening, IMI with CNS were lower in vaccinates (64.2%) compared with controls (69.8%); a reduction of 8.1%.

Somatic cell counts in samples collected during first week of lactation irrespective of infection status were 45% lower in vaccinates compared with controls (287,317 vs. 522,345/ml). Somatic cell counts in samples collected during first week of lactation from uninfected heifers for vaccinates and controls were 66,095 and 132,754/ml, respectively; a 50.2% reduction; and for infected heifers, SCC were 441,764 and 892,176/ml, respectively; a 50.5% reduction. Somatic cell counts in samples collected during the prepartum period were highest for *S. aureus* (6.730×10^3), followed by the environmental streptococci (3.850×10^3), and CNS (3.510×10^3).

An examination of the 305-day lactation milk yield for the 1st lactation of both vaccinated and unvaccinated control heifers demonstrated an approximate 8.6% increase in vaccinates vs. control (11,217 vs. 10,332 kg, respectively) or a difference of 886 kg. On a complete lactation basis, vaccinated animals produced 839 kg more milk than controls (12,537 vs. 11,698 kg, respectively); an increase of 7.3%.

The percentage of 305-day lactation fat was higher in vaccinates than controls (3.64 vs. 3.27%, respectively); however, the percentage of 305-day lactation protein was slightly higher in controls than vaccinates (3.06 vs. 2.95, respectively). Actual 305-day kilograms of both fat and protein were higher in vaccinates than controls (fat: 408 vs. 339 kg, respectively; protein: 330 vs. 315 kg, respectively). Likewise, on a complete lactation basis, actual kilograms of both fat and protein were higher in vaccinates than controls (fat: 460 vs. 393, respectively; protein: 370 vs. 353, respectively).

An examination of the number of days in milk for the first lactation demonstrated that vaccinates persisted 13 days longer than the unvaccinated controls (349 vs. 336 days). In addition, average first lactation SCC were 11,000 cells/ml lower in vaccinates compared with controls (49,000 vs. 60,000/ml.

Conclusions

Results of this investigation demonstrated that vaccinating dairy heifers according to the prescribed protocol with a commercial USDA licensed *S. aureus* bacterin, Lysigin®, reduced the number of new *S. aureus* IMI at time of calving by 60.9%, lowered the SCC by 50%, and decreased the culling rate by approximately one-third. In addition, overall milk yield, production of fat and protein, and number of days in milk were greater in vaccinated heifers compared with controls.

The decrease in frequency of new *S. aureus* IMI at calving (60.9%) in vaccinates using Holstein heifers is higher than the 44.7% reduction observed in a Louisiana trial using the same vaccine in Jersey heifers (Nickerson *et al.*, 1999). In both trials, SCC at calving were reduced by approximately 50%. The 60.9% efficacy found in the present trial is also higher than the 40.2% efficacy observed by Giraudo *et al.* (1989), the 46% efficacy observed by Nordhaug *et al.* (1994), and the 52% efficacy observed by Sears *et al.* (1990). However, it is difficult to compare among the latter three trials as the vaccine formulations were all quite different.

The question becomes: Is it economically feasible to use this vaccination protocol on young dairy heifers? Based on an average of 1,864 more lb milk per vaccinated heifer, which translates to 18.64 hundredweights (cwt) of milk (1,864/100), at the current price of US$ 25.00/cwt, an increased income of US$ 466.00/heifer would be realised (18.64 cwt x US$ 25.00/cwt = US$ 466.00). If each heifer was vaccinated beginning at 6 months of age until calving, this would entail vaccinations at (1) 6 months, (2) a booster 2-weeks later, and subsequently at (3) 12 months, (4)18 months, and (5) 24 months, or a total of 5 immunisations through calving. At $1.50/dose, this cost would total $7.50, which when subtracted from the increased income from milk production, would yield a net income of US$ 458.50 per heifer (US$ 466.00 - US$ 7.50). This figure does not include the costs of labour involved in the immunisation process; however, it is evident that vaccination is well worth the cost of the vaccine. Not only does it reduce new infections in first calf heifers at parturition, it may also reduce the introduction of *S. aureus* to the milking herd.

References

Adlam, C., Kerry, K.B., Edkins, S. and Ward, P.D., 1981. Local and systemic antibody responses in cows following immunization with staphylococcal antigens in the dry period. J. Comp. Path. 91: 105-113.

Boddie, R.L., Nickerson, S.C., Owens, W.E. and Watts, J.L., 1987. Udder microflora in nonlactating heifers. Agri-Practice 8: 22-25.

Brock, J.H., Steel, E.D. and Reiter, B., 1975. The effect of intramuscular and intramammary vaccination of cows on antibody levels and resistance to intramammary infection by *Staphylococcus aureus.* Res. Vet. Sci. 19: 152-158.

Giraudo, J.A., Calzolari, A., Rampone, H., Rampone, A., Giraudo, T., Bogni, C., Larriestra, A. and Nagel, R., 1997. Field trials of a vaccine against bovine mastitis. 1. Evaluation in heifers. J. Dairy Sci. 80: 845-853.

Hogan, J.S., González, R.N., Harmon, R.J., Nickerson, S.C., Oliver, S.P., Pankey, J.W. and Smith, K.L., 1999. Testing procedures. In: Laboratory handbook on bovine mastitis. National Mastitis Council, Inc., Madison, WI, USA, pp. 205-217.

Nickerson, S.C., Owens, W.E., Tomita, G.M. and Widel, P.W., 1999. Vaccinating dairy heifers with a *Staphylococcus aureus* bacterin reduces mastitis at calving. Large Animal Practice 20: 16-20.

Nordhaug, M.L., Neese, L.L., Norcross, N.L and Gudding, R., 1994. A field trial with an experimental vaccine against *Staphylococcus aureus* mastitis in cattle. 1. Clinical parameters. J. Dairy Sci. 77: 1267-1275.

Oliver, S.P., Lewis, M.J., Gillespie, B.E. and Dowlen, H.H., 1992. Influence of prepartum antibiotic therapy on intramammary infections in primigravid heifers during early lactation. J. Dairy Sci. 75: 406-414.

Oliver, S.P., Ivey, S.J., Gillespie, B.E., Lewis, M.J., Johnson, D.L., Lamar, K.C., Moorehead, H., Dowlen, H.H., Chester, S.T. and Hallberg, J.W., 2004. Influence of prepartum intramammary infusion of pirlimycin hydrochloride or penicillin-novobiocin on mastitis in heifers during early lactation. J. Dairy Sci. 87: 1727-1731.

Owens, W.E., Nickerson, S.C., Washburn, P.J. and Ray, C.H., 1994. Prepartum antibiotic therapy with a cephapirin dry cow product against naturally occurring intramammary infections in heifers. Vet. Med. B 41: 90-100.

Sears, P.M., Norcross, N.L., Kenny, K., Smith, B., Gonzalez, R.N. and Romano, M.N., 1990. Resistance to *Staphylococcus aureus* infections in staphylococcal vaccinated heifers. In: Proceedings of the international symposium on bovine mastitis. March 23-27, 1990. Indianapolis, IN, USA, pp. 69-74.

Steel, R.G.D. and Torrie, J.H., 1960. Principles and procedures of statistics. McGraw-Hill Inc., New York, NY.

Trinidad, P., Nickerson, S.C. and Adkinson, R.W., 1990a. Histopathology of staphylococcal mastitis in unbred dairy heifers. J. Dairy Sci. 73: 639-647.

Trinidad, P., Nickerson, S.C., Alley, T.K. and Adkinson, R.W., 1990b. Efficacy of intramammary treatment in unbred and primigravid dairy heifers. J. Am. Vet. Med. Ass. 197: 465-470.

Meta-analysis of the effect of oral selenium supplementation on milk selenium concentration in cattle

A. Ceballos[1], J. Sánchez[2], H.W. Barkema[3], H. Stryhn[1], J.B. Montgomery[1] and J.J. Wichtel[1]
[1]Dept. of Health Management, Atlantic Veterinary College, University of Prince Edward Island. Charlottetown, PE C1A 4P3, Canada
[2]Canadian Food and Inspection Agency. Charlottetown, PE C1E 1E3, Canada
[3]Dept. of Production Animal Health, Faculty of Veterinary Medicine, University of Calgary. Calgary, AB, T2N 4N1, Canada
Corresponding author: aceballos@upei.ca

Abstract

Soils in many regions of the world have low selenium (Se) content. Consequently, forages and crops grown on these soils may provide inadequate dietary Se for grazing animals and humans. Results of recent surveys in different countries reported a significant proportion of cattle appear to receive inadequate dietary Se, and that deficiency has been associated with several economically important diseases, such as mastitis. Selenium supplementation has been used to enhance Se status but results are still controversial. Milk Se concentration is an indicator of animal/herd Se status, and reflects the responsiveness to supplementation. A systematic review and meta-analysis were performed on 42 studies published between 1977 and 2007 to summarise all available scientific evidence of the effect of oral Se supplementation on milk Se concentration in cattle. The literature search was based on electronic and non-electronic databases. Fixed- and random-effects models of meta-analysis were performed, and a meta-regression was carried out to evaluate the heterogeneity among studies. The overall effect of oral Se supplementation was an increase of milk Se concentration in 0.16 (95% CI: 0.117, 0.207) μmol/l (P<0.05). Separate analyses for two sources of Se indicated that Se yeast had a larger effect as compared to sodium selenite/selenate. On average, cows supplemented with Se-yeast had a milk Se concentration of 0.33 (95% CI: 0.190, 0.476) μmol/l higher than in cows supplemented with sodium selenite/selenate. Dose of Se had a quadratic association to milk Se concentration, and dose explained 74% of the between study variance. Begg's (P<0.01) test and visual analysis suggested a weak evidence of publication bias. This information provides a basis for tailoring daily requirements of Se for lactating cattle.

Keywords: nutrition, minerals, selenium, systematic reviews

Introduction

Soils in many regions of the world have low Se content; consequently, feedstuffs grown on these soils may provide inadequate dietary Se for grazing animals and humans. Selenium nutritional requirements for beef and dairy cattle have been set at 0.1 ppm and 0.3 ppm, respectively (NRC

2000, 2001). Thus, feeding systems to increase milk Se content have been developed (Guyot *et al.*, 2007) but variable results are still found. After using different sources of Se, doses of Se and routes of administration, studies have described either non significant effects (Stowe *et al.*, 1988) or increased milk Se concentrations by as much as sevenfold (Guyot *et al.*, 2007).

Studies in the 1970s indicated that a relatively small proportion of Se was transferred into milk after feeding inorganic forms of Se such as sodium selenite. Supplementation with inorganic forms increased milk Se content when cows were fed rations low in naturally occurring Se forms, but there was less impact when cows were fed rations higher in naturally occurring Se (Conrad and Moxon, 1979). Even though many experiments have shown that Se supplementation results in an increase in Se content of milk, not all attempts have been successful (Stowe *et al.*, 1988; Gierus *et al.*, 2003).

A low milk Se concentration has been linked to decreased expression of selenoproteins that have a pivotal role in the antioxidant and immune defence of the mammary tissue (Bruzelius *et al.*, 2007; Sordillo *et al.*, 2007), and the consumption of animal products derived from animals grazing on low-Se areas can influence the Se status of entire human communities, putting humans at risk of overt deficiency (WHO/FAO, 2004). Accordingly, there is a need to summarise the response to different sources of supplementary Se, and its transfer into milk to assist in the design of effective supplementation programs. Clear guidelines as to how Se supplements should be administered to cattle, in particular to enhance milk Se concentration, have not been available.

Narrative reviews have indicated a beneficial effect of Se supplementation on milk Se concentration (Conrad and Moxon, 1980; Weiss, 2005). However, traditional narrative reviews, which have been widely used in veterinary literature, do not use either a systematic or statistical method to identify, assess, and synthesise the information they are gathering, and are prone to bias (Sargeant *et al.*, 2006). Systematic reviews appraise critically, summarise and attempt to reconcile all published evidence concerning to a particular intervention, minimise systematic and random errors, and may or may not include a quantitative statistical analysis (meta-analysis) of the results of two or more studies (Jadad *et al.*, 1997). The objective of this study was to summarise, through a systematic review and a meta-analysis, all available scientific evidence related to the effect of oral Se supplementation on milk Se concentration in cattle.

Material and methods

An electronic and non-electronic literature search was conducted to identify primary studies carried out between January of 1970 and March of 2008. The databases AGRICOLA, CAB abstracts, MEDLINE, PubMed, Science Direct, Web of Science, and WorldCat Basic Search were covered. Primary studies published in English, French, Italian, Portuguese, Spanish and German, were included. There was no restriction to peer-reviewed journals, and the eligible publications included abstracts, conference proceedings, book chapters and theses. Proceedings of the most relevant meetings concerning animal science were also scanned for references. In addition, different groups of investigators were emailed asking for unpublished studies related to the intervention of interest, and finally, the potential studies were combined with a set of studies recovered from the trial database of Alltech Inc (Nicholasville, KY, USA).

Manuscripts were excluded if the title or abstract had an indication of pertaining to species different than cattle, or pertaining to supplementation trials enrolling animals other than first-calving heifers or multiparous cows, or if the milk Se concentration was not evaluated. Additionally, studies were excluded if cows were supplemented with sources other than sodium selenite, sodium selenate or Se yeast, since these forms are the most widely used for oral supplementation in cattle (Weiss, 2005).

The mean difference in milk Se concentration between Se-supplemented and unsupplemented cows was the outcome of interest. The precision of the estimate was based on its standard error (SE) or standard deviations (SD) of treated and control groups. Milk Se concentration data between 28 and 170 days were considered for the meta-analysis. All results were transformed to μmol/l. For unit standardisation, 78.96 g/mol was considered for Se molecular weight, and 1,030 g/l for milk density. Clinical trials were included regardless of whether they were conducted in a randomised fashion.

When an exact calculation of the SD was not possible, missing SD was imputed as pooled SD (SD_p) from all the other available studies included in the meta-analysis (Furukawa *et al.*, 2006). Two independent investigators extracted the information using a structured data-collection form, and the first author solved the discrepancies after re-reviewing the manuscript.

Meta-analyses and meta-regression

The effect of Se supplementation on milk Se concentration in cattle was evaluated carrying out fixed and random-effects meta-analyses. Random-effects meta-analysis was reported given the observed heterogeneity amongst studies. Meta-analysis was presented graphically using a forest plot (Egger *et al.*, 2001). Statistical (Begg's and Egger's tests) and graphical methods (funnel plot) were used to evaluate possible publication bias. The 'Trim and Fill' method was used to estimate and correct for an eventual publication bias (Egger *et al.*, 2001).

A meta-regression analysis was conducted to estimate the extent to which one or more covariates explained heterogeneity in the treatment effects. Meta-regression of factors related to study quality and study design on the factor of interest was performed using the method-of-moments estimation (Egger *et al.*, 2001). Unconditional analyses of trial precision, continent where the study was performed, study population, parity, type of production, source and dose of Se, stage of lactation, and frequency of administration, were evaluated. Analyses were carried out in Stata Statistical Software, release 10 (StataCorp, College Station, TX, USA).

Results

The search identified 139 potential references containing the keyword combination either in their titles or abstracts. Twenty-three manuscripts could not be recovered. From the remaining 116 references, 77 were excluded from the analysis because of the following reasons: 12 were not clinical trials; 24 did not report the outcome of interest; 9 had reported duplicate data of other studies; 11 described results of parenteral Se supplementation; 19 manuscripts compared two sources or different doses of Se, therefore, the control group was no unsupplemented; one report described the results of administering two sources of Se to the same animal; and one report described the results of oral and parenteral administration of Se to the same animal.

Three manuscripts reported the outcome of interest but no data were recorded because supranutritional doses of Se were used. Three manuscripts did not report milk Se concentration for the period between 28 and 170 days from treatment, and were excluded from the analyses. Consequently, 33 manuscripts containing the results of 42 studies provided data that fulfilled all criteria and were used to perform the meta-analyses. Twenty-eight manuscripts were published in peer-reviewed journals, three published as abstracts, one appeared in conference proceedings, and one was published as book chapter. Studies were categorised according to the continent where they were performed: 15 in America, 13 in Europe, and 5 in Australia/ New Zealand.

Out of the 33 references, 25 reported a positive effect of Se supplementation (Hidiroglou *et al.*, 1985, 1987b; Salih *et al.*, 1987; Hidiroglou and Proulx, 1988; Aspila, 1991; Charmley *et al.*, 1993; Cuesta *et al.*, 1993; Grace *et al.*, 1997; Hemken *et al.*, 1998; Knowles *et al.*, 1999; Ortman and Pehrson, 1999; Batchelor, 2002; Gierus *et al.*, 2002; McDowell *et al.*, 2002; McIntosh and Royle; 2002; Bis Wencel, 2003; Wiewiora *et al.*, 2003; Brzoska and Brzoska, 2004; Waldron *et al.*, 2004; Muniz-Naveiro *et al.*, 2005; Juniper *et al.*, 2006; Guyot, *et al.*, 2007; Heard *et al.*, 2007; Paschoal *et al.*, 2007; Phipps *et al.*, 2007), four did not show a significant effect (Ammerman *et al.*, 1980; Hidiroglou *et al.*, 1987a; Stowe *et al.*, 1988; Gierus, *et al.*, 2003), and four did not report the significance of the effect (Perry *et al.*, 1977; Conrad and Moxon, 1979; Syrjala Qvist and Aspila, 1993; Malbe *et al.*, 1995). All these four manuscripts reported, however, a numerically positive effect of Se supplementation on milk Se concentration.

Meta-analysis and meta-regression

The average treatment effect obtained was 0.16 μmol/l (95% CI: 0.117, 0.207). The results from each trial, the average effect of treatment, its 95% CI, and the prediction interval are shown in Figure 1. Begg's test for publication bias was significant ($P<0.001$), while the Egger's test did not suggest a significant bias ($P=0.28$). However, the 'Trim and Fill' method did not impute any study, and the overall estimate of the effect remained the same.

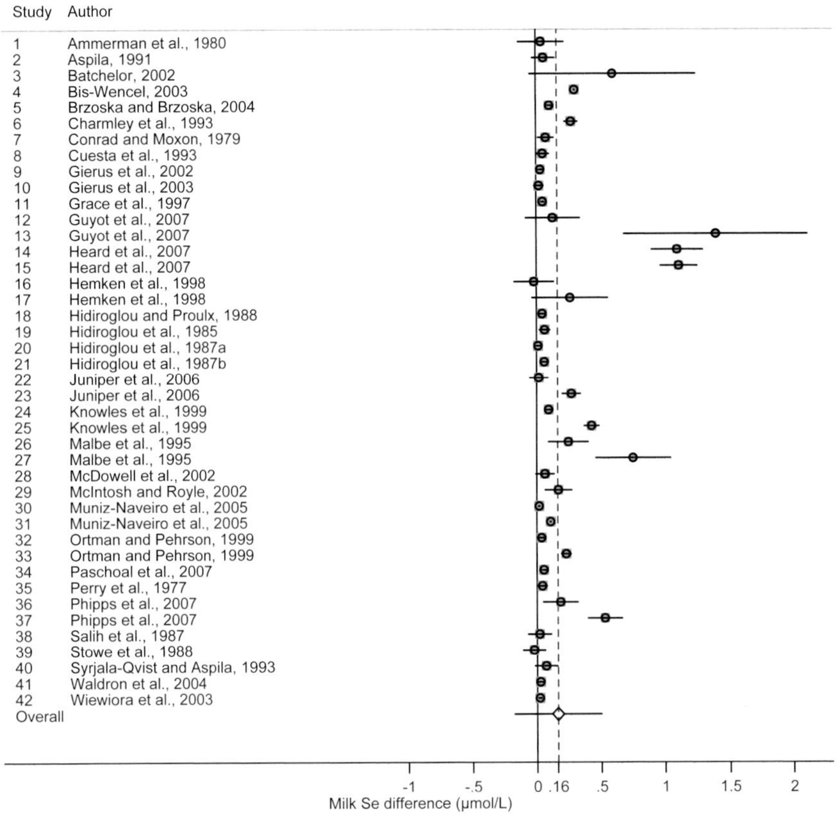

Figure 1. Forest plot of the effect of oral selenium supplementation on milk selenium concentration (μmol/l) difference in cattle. The average estimate of the effect was derived from the random-effects meta-analysis. The length of the horizontal line represents the 95% confidence interval (CI) for the effect size from each study, the center of the square (□) represents the point estimate from that study, and the area of the square is proportional to the weight assigned to the study. The dashed line is the average effect of treatment (0.16 μmol/l) obtained from the analysis, while the solid vertical line marks the value where Se supplementation would have no effect. The diamond (◊) at the bottom of the dashed line shows the 95% CI for the overall effect (0.117, 0.207), and the horizontal line beside the diamond represents the prediction interval (95%: -0.17, 0.50 μmol/l) for the milk Se difference in future studies.

None of the variables related to study quality and study design showed a significant association with the outcome of interest. However, the effect of Se supplementation on milk Se concentration was less when cows were part of a randomised clinical trial (P=0.15). A significant (P<0.01) association with the outcome of interest was found for the continent where the study was performed, source of Se and dose of Se (Table 1). Studies that administered Se yeast (6 mg/

Table 1. Meta-regression based on 42 studies of Se supplementation in cattle. Coefficients (β), 95% confidence interval (95% CI), P-values, and the method-of-moments estimator of the between-study variance (τ^2) are presented.

Factor	***β***	**95% CI**	***P***	τ^2
Null model	0.162	0.083, 0.241	<0.01	0.019
Random allocation	-0.115	-0.276, 0.045	0.15	0.019
Continent			<0.01	0.019
America	Baseline			
Europe	0.100	-0.051, 0.253	0.19	
Australia/New Zealand[a]	0.379	0.167, 0.591	<0.01	
Stage of lactation				0.011
Dry period[b]	Baseline		0.13	
Early lactation (<100 DIM)	0.133	-0.047, 0.314	0.14	
Late lactation (>100 DIM)	0.168	-0.004, 0.339	0.06	
Milk yield (n=9[c])	-0.035	-0.094, 0.025	0.21	0.038
Source				0.027
Sodium selenite/selenate	Baseline			
Selenium yeast	0.333	0.190, 0.476	<0.01	
Dose	-0.087	-0.160, -0.015	0.02	0.005
Quadratic term	0.012	0.006, 0.017	<0.01	

[a] Only studies performed in Australia/New Zealand were reported.
[b] Dry period corresponds to starting Se supplementation before calving.
[c] Milk production was reported only in 9 studies.

head/day) had, on average, a milk Se concentration of 0.11 μmol/l higher than unsupplemented cows. Dose of Se accounted for a large proportion of the between-study variance (74%).

Discussion

A meta-analysis based on the results of the 42 studies meeting all selected criteria estimated an average increase in milk Se concentration of 0.16 μmol/l in response to oral Se supplementation (Figure 1). Results varied considerably among studies: continent, source of Se and dose of Se were significant contributors to this variation.

The critical examination for the presence of publication bias, or other bias types, is an integral part of the meta-analysis process. In this case, Begg's test indicated weak evidence of publication bias, but Egger's test was not significant, and the 'Trim and Fill' test did not impute any study.

Supplementation with Se yeast resulted in a higher milk Se concentration compared to using inorganic forms. The effect of Se yeast decreased about 41% but remained positive after controlling for dose of Se. Studies where Se yeast was used tended to supplement at higher doses than did studies where inorganic sources were given, and studies performed in Australia/New Zealand used even higher doses of both sources than did in American or European studies. Particular characteristics of soils, forages, and cattle production in America and Europe compared to Australia/New Zealand, and Se yeast characteristics, may account for the different strategies used in the design of trials on Se supplementation. Recently, a narrative review suggested that Se concentration was increased by 90% when cattle were fed Se yeast compared to an inorganic source (Weiss, 2005). The biological properties of Se yeast may also account for the observed response in milk Se concentration. Moreover, Se yeast is better transferred to milk than inorganic Se sources, probably because of the amino acid composition of milk proteins. Milk has approximately two times higher methionine concentration when compared to blood protein; therefore, it is two times more likely that Se-met will be incorporated into milk protein than blood protein (Weiss, 2005).

Conclusion

An increase of 0.16 μmol/l in milk Se concentration might be expected, on average, after oral Se supplementation in cattle. The mean difference might be expected to lie between -0.17 and 0.50 μmol/l (95% certainty) if future clinical trials are conducted to evaluate the effect of oral Se supplementation on milk Se concentration.

High variation between studies was observed due in part to geographic factors, and characteristics of the study design such as Se source, and dose of Se. A weak evidence of publication bias was observed. Higher doses of Se are required to achieve an adequate milk Se concentration to enhance antioxidant and immune defence of the mammary gland. Seleno-amino acids from Se yeast are metabolised by mechanisms distinct from those of inorganic forms and may be the form of choice for enhancing milk Se concentration.

References

Ammerman, C.B., Chapman, H.L., Bouwman, G.W., Fontenot, J.P., Bagley, C.P. and Moxon, A.L., 1980. Effect of supplemental selenium for beef cows on the performance and tissue selenium concentrations of cows and suckling calves. J. Anim. Sci. 51: 1381-1386.

Aspila, P., 1991. Metabolism of selenite, selenomethionine and feed-incorporated selenium in lactating goats and dairy cows. J. Agric. Sci. Fin. 63: 1-74.

Batchelor, J., 2002. Supplementing selenium to pasture-based dairy cows. Sel-Plex 136. Alltech Inc, Nicholasville, KY, USA.

Bis Wencel, H., 2003. Mineral elements level in milk of the cows with mineral dietary supplementation. Ann. Univ. M.C. Sklod. Sect. EE 21: 259-264.

Bruzelius, K., Hoac, T., Sundler, R., Onning, G. and Akesson, B., 2007. Occurrence of selenoprotein enzyme activities and mRNA in bovine mammary tissue. J. Dairy Sci. 90: 918-927.

Brzoska, F. and Brzoska, B., 2004. Effect of dietary selenium on milk yield of cows and chemical composition of milk and blood. Ann. Anim. Sci. 4: 57-67.

Charmley, E., Nicholson, J.W.G. and Zee, J.A., 1993. Effect of supplemental vitamin E and selenium in the diet on vitamin E and selenium levels and control of oxidized flavor in milk from Holstein cows. Can. J. Anim. Sci. 73: 453-457.

Conrad, H.R. and Moxon, A.L., 1979. Transfer of dietary selenium to milk. J. Dairy Sci. 62: 404-411.

Conrad, H.R. and Moxon, A.L., 1980. Selenium requirements for dairy cows. Ohio Report Res. Dev. 65: 8-9.

Cuesta, P.A., McDowell, L.R., Kunkle, W.E., Bullock, F., Drew, A., Wilkinson, N.S. and Martin, F.G., 1993. Serum selenium and vitamin E, and selenium concentration in liver, milk and hair as affected by supplementation to beef cattle. Int. J. Anim. Sci. 8: 257-262.

Egger, M., Smith, G.D. and Altman, D.G., 2001. Systematic reviews in health care: Meta-analysis in context. BMJ Books, London, UK.

Furukawa, T.A., Barbui, C., Cipriani, A., Brambilla, P. and Watanabe, N., 2006. Imputing missing standard deviations in meta-analyses can provide accurate results. J. Clin. Epidem. 59: 7-10.

Gierus, M., Schwarz, F.J. and Kirchgessner, M., 2002. Selenium supplementation and selenium status of dairy cows fed diets based on grass, grass silage or maize silage. J. Anim. Phys. Anim. Nutr. 86: 74-82.

Gierus, M., Schwarz, F.J. and Kirchgessner, M., 2003. Investigation on selenium supplementation for dairy cows in late pregnancy. Zuchtungskunde 75: 88-100.

Grace, N.D., Lee, J., Mills, R.A. and Death, A.F., 1997. Influence of Se status on milk Se concentrations in dairy cows. N.Z. J. Agric. Res. 40: 75-78.

Guyot, H., Spring, P., Andrieu, S. and Rollin, F., 2007. Comparative responses to sodium selenite and organic selenium supplements in Belgian Blue cows and calves. Livest. Sci. 111: 259-263.

Heard, J.W., Stockdale, C.R., Walker, G.P., Leddin, C.M., Dunshea, F.R., McIntosh, G.H., Shields, G.H., McKenna, A., Young, G.P. and Doyle, P.T., 2007. Increasing selenium concentration in milk: Effects of amount of selenium from yeast and cereal grain supplements. J. Dairy Sci. 90: 4117-4127.

Hemken, R.W., Harmon, R.J. and Trammell, S., 1998. Selenium for dairy cattle: A role for organic selenium. Feed Compounder 18: 22-24.

Hidiroglou, M., and Proulx, J., 1988. Evaluation of a long-acting selenium and copper preparation for intraruminal administration to cattle. Ann. Rech. Vet. 19: 187-191.

Hidiroglou, M., Proulx, J. and Jolette, J., 1985. Intraruminal selenium pellet for control of nutritional muscular dystrophy in cattle. J. Dairy Sci. 68: 57-66.

Hidiroglou, M., McAllister, A.J. and Williams, C.J., 1987a. Prepartum supplementation of selenium and vitamin E to dairy cows: Assessment of selenium status and reproductive performance. J. Dairy Sci. 70: 1281-1288.

Hidiroglou, M., Proulx, J. and Jolette, J., 1987b. Effect of intraruminally administered, selenium soluble-glass boluses on selenium status in cows and their calves. J. Anim. Sci. 65: 815-820.

Jadad, A.R., Cook, D.J. and Browman, G.P., 1997. A guide to interpreting discordant systematic reviews. Can. Med. Ass. J. 156: 1411-1416,

Juniper, D.T., Phipps, R.H., Jones, A.K. and Bertin, G., 2006. Selenium supplementation of lactating dairy cows: effect on selenium concentration in blood, milk, urine, and feces. J. Dairy Sci. 89: 3544-3551.

Knowles, S.O., Grace, N.D., Wurms, K. and Lee, J., 1999. Significance of amount and form of dietary selenium on blood, milk, and casein selenium concentrations in grazing cows. J. Dairy Sci. 82: 429-437.

Malbe, M., Klaassen, M., Fang, W., Myllys, V., Vikerpuur, M., Nyholm, K., Sankari, S., Suoranta, K. and Sandholm, M., 1995. Comparisons of selenite and selenium yeast feed supplements on Se-incorporation, mastitis and leucocyte function in Se-deficient dairy cows. J. Vet. Med. A 42: 111-121.

McDowell, L.R., Valle, G., Cristaldi, L., Davis, P.A., Rosendo, O. and Wilkinson, N.S., 2002. Selenium availability and methods of selenium supplementation for grazing ruminants. In: Proceedings of 13th Annual Florida Ruminant Nutrition Symposium, Gainesville, FL, p. 86.

McIntosh, G.H. and Royle, P.J., 2002. Supplementation of cows with organic selenium and the identification of selenium-rich protein fractions in milk. In: Biotechnology in the feed industry: Proceedings of Alltech's 18th annual symposium. T.P. Lyons, and K.A. Jacques, (eds.) Nottingham University Press, Nottingham, UK, pp. 233-238.

Muniz-Naveiro, O., Dominguez-Gonzalez, R., Bermejo-Barrera, A., Cocho de Juan, J.A., Fraga-Bermudez, J.M., Goris-Pereiras, A., Lopez-Santamarina, A., Martinez-Lede, I., Valledor-Puente, J., Fernandez-Couto-Gomez, L. and Bermejo-Barrera, P., 2005. Selenium content and distribution in cow's milk supplemented with two dietary selenium sources. J. Agric. Food Chem. 53: 9817-9822.

National Research Council, 2000. Nutrient requirements of beef cattle. 7th rev. ed. Natl. Acad. Press, Washington, DC, USA.

National Research Council, 2001. Nutrient requirements of dairy cattle. 7th rev. ed. Natl. Acad. Press, Washington, DC, USA.

Ortman, K. and Pehrson, B., 1999. Effect of selenate as a feed supplement to dairy cows in comparison to selenite and selenium yeast. J. Anim. Sci. 77: 3365-3370.

Paschoal, J.J., Zanetti, M.A., Del Claro, G.R., de Melo, M.P., Pugine, S.P. and Cunha, J.A., 2007. Fatty acid profile and oxidative stability of milk from Holstein cows fed with extruded soybean and organic selenium. Pesquisa Agropecuaria Brasileira 42: 1793-1799.

Perry, T.W., Peterson, R.C. and Beeson, W.M., 1977. Selenium in milk from feeding small supplements. J. Dairy Sci. 60: 1698-1700.

Phipps, R.H., Grandison, A.S., Jones, A.K., Juniper, D.T. and Bertin, G., 2007. Selenium supplementation of lactating dairy cows: Effects on total selenium content and speciation in blood, milk, and cheese. J. Dairy Sci. 90 (Suppl. 1): 599.

Salih, Y., McDowell, L.R., Hentges, J.F., Mason Jr., R.M. and Wilcox, C.J., 1987. Mineral content of milk, colostrum and serum as affected by physiological state and mineral supplementation. J. Dairy Sci. 70: 608-612.

Sargeant, J.M., Rajic, A., Read, S. and Ohlsson, A., 2006. The process of systematic review and its application in agri-food public-health. Prev. Vet. Med. 75: 141-151.

Sordillo, L.M., O'Boyle, N., Gandy, J. C., Corl, C.M. and Hamilton, E., 2007. Shifts in thioredoxin reductase activity and oxidant status in mononuclear cells obtained from transition dairy cattle. J. Dairy Sci. 90: 1186-1192.

Stowe, H.D., Thomas, J.W., Johnson, T., Marteniuk, J.V., Morrow, D.A. and Ullrey, D.E., 1988. Responses of dairy cattle to long-term and short-term supplementation with oral selenium and vitamin E. J. Dairy Sci. 71: 1830-1839.

change. For example, the plasma concentration of α-tocopherol decreases during the last month prepartum (Goff and Stabel, 1990) and oxidative stress increases around parturition (Bernabucci *et al.*, 2002). Given its importance as an antioxidant, one could expect that the concentration of vitamin E in tissues undergoing great change would influence the local degree of oxidative stress. However, to our knowledge, there are no reports on oxidative damage products in liver and mammary gland, nor studies of correlations between the concentrations in these organs and blood. The aim of this study was to investigate the relationship between vitamin E and oxidative damage measured in blood, mammary gland and liver tissue in periparturient Holstein Friesian Heifers.

Materials and methods

Animals

The experiment, carried out from March until June 2006, used sixteen pregnant Holstein heifers. The control group and the vitamin E group both comprising 8 cows. Vitamin E (3,000 IU/day) was supplied on a corn-based carrier (100 grams/day) mixed through the corn silage every afternoon. The vitamin E supplementation was provided at a high 3,000 IU per animal per day to try to prevent the expected decrease in vitamin E blood concentration just before calving. The control group received an equal portion of this carrier (100 grams/day) without vitamin E, also mixed through the corn silage every afternoon. Supplementation started 8 weeks before predicted calving date and lasted until 2 weeks after calving.

Sampling procedures

During the experiment, heifers were sampled weekly except for the two weeks before expected calving date, when they were sampled twice weekly. Samples were collected with BD vacutainer systems and SST™ II Advance tubes (Plymouth, UK) at 8 am and kept at 6-10 °C before they arrived at the laboratory. Blood samples were centrifuged for 15 minutes at 4465 RPM (3500 g), at 4 °C. Sera were frozen at -80 °C until analysis. Serum was analysed for vitamin E, cholesterol and MDA. Liver biopsies were taken at weeks -5 and -1 relative to expected calving day and week 2 of lactation. Blood samples and milk samples (after calving) were obtained simultaneously for correlation analysis. The biopsy areas (80 cm^2) between the 11th and 12th costae and at the level of the greater trochanter were clipped, scrubbed with an antiseptic solution and disinfected. A local anesthetic was given subcutaneously (7 ml Lidocaïne-HCL 2% with adrenaline, Alfasan Nederland b.v., Woerden) before a stab incision was made. Approximately 400 mg liver tissue (wet weight) was collected with a 17Gx200mm biopsy needle. This was immediately frozen in liquid nitrogen (-196 °C). After thawing, PBS was added to biopsy material (5:1) and this was homogenised. Homogenised samples were then centrifuged at 15,800 G and refrozen at -80 °C until analysis. Samples were analysed for vitamin E, cholesterol, MDA and total protein content. Liver concentrations were corrected for differences due to the homogenisation process by calculating all concentrations per mg protein. Milk was obtained from all heifers immediately after calving, the first two milkings after calving and at day 3, 7 and 14 at 6 am. A blood sample was collected simultaneously directly after calving and on days 7 and 14 for correlation with milk analysis. Milk samples were stored at -80 °C until analysed for vitamin E, MDA and somatic cell count.

Laboratory analysis

Vitamin E (α-tocopherol) was measured with HPLC with both UV and fluorescence detection using a kit from Chromsystems, Munich, Germany. Cholesterol and total protein concentration were determined routinely on a clinical autoanalyzer (Hitachi 912, Roche Diagnostics, Almere, Netherlands) using kits from Roche Diagnostics, Almere, Netherlands. MDA was measured with an isocratic HPLC system of Varian Ass. using a kit from Chromsystems, Munich, Germany. A 10 cm C18 cartridge was used (Varian Ass.) with a flow rate of 1.0 ml/min at ambient temperature (25 °C). Fluorescence detection (Jasco) occurred with excitation at 515 nm and emission at 553 nm. All analyses were done at The National Institute for Public Health and the Environment (RIVM), Bilthoven, The Netherlands. The somatic cell count was determined with flow cytometry according to the standard method ISO 13366-2 148-2 of International Organisation for Standardisation/International Dairy Federation version 2006. These analyses were done at Milk Control Station (Zutphen, The Netherlands).

Statistical analysis

To find trends in time and differences between treatments, vitamin E and oxidative damage in blood, liver tissue and milk were studied in mixed models, with group and group × time interaction as fixed effects and cow as random effect. Blood samples were divided into 6 time intervals related to calving date. Time interval 1 is the start of supplementation, time interval 2 is two weeks later, time interval 4 was defined as the mean concentration of week -2, -1.5, -1 and -0.5, time interval 5 was at calving and time interval 6 was defined as the mean concentration of week 1 and 2 after parturition. Group × time interaction in blood was tested against the base line (time interval 3), defined as the mean concentration of week -5, -4 and -3. Group × time interaction in liver and milk was tested against the final measurement at day 14 after parturition. To investigate the relationship between MDA and vitamin E in blood, liver and milk, partial correlation coefficients were calculated between MDA and vitamin E at compartment level, corrected for group and repeated measures. Data were log10 transformed to create normally distributed concentrations. For all analyses significance was set at $P \leq 0.05$, and all analyses were carried out in SPSS 12.0.1 for Windows.

Results

Group and group x time interaction

The results of differences between treatments and time trends are summarised in Table 1 and Figure 1, 2 and 3. The vitamin E concentration and the vitamin E: cholesterol ratio in blood were higher in the supplemented group (*P*<0.01). In the control group vitamin E concentrations start to decrease in the two weeks before parturition (*P*=0.029). In both groups, vitamin E concentrations decreased at calving (control group *P*=0.044, vitamin E group *P* = 0.036) and increased after calving (control group *P*=0.007, vitamin E group *P*=0.016). The vitamin E: cholesterol ratio increased two weeks before calving in the supplemented group (*P*=0.024) and remained steady after parturition, while in the same period this ratio decreased in the non-supplemented group and increased (*P*<0.01) after parturition. In both groups, MDA concentrations increased (control group *P*=0.039, vitamin E group *P*<0.01) at calving, but only in the supplemented group did they decrease after parturition (*P*<0.01).Vitamin E concentration and the ratio of vitamin E to cholesterol in liver tissue were higher in the supplemented group (*P*<0.01 resp. *P*=0.02). MDA concentrations decreased in the supplemented group (*P*=0.003) and tended to increase in the control group. Vitamin E concentrations in milk tended to be higher in the supplemented group. MDA concentrations in both groups were high in the first

Table 1. Results (P values) of linear mixed models.

Blood	**time x group**	**group**
Vitamin E(μmol/l)	0.001	0.002
Cholesterol (mmol/l)	0.001	0.202
Ratio vitamin E: cholesterol (mmol/l)	0.001	0.001
Malondialdehyde (μg/l)	0.001	0.542
Liver tissue	**time x group**	**group**
Vitamin E (nmol/gP)	0.780	0.001
Cholesterol (mmol/gP)	0.111	0.418
Ratio vitamin E: cholesterol (mmol/gP)	0.319	0.020
Malondialdehyde (μg/gP)	0.026	0.869
Milk	**time x group**	**group**
Vitamin E (μmol/l)	0.146	0.117
Malondialdehyde (μg/l)	0.000	0.570
Somatic cell count	0.029	0.228

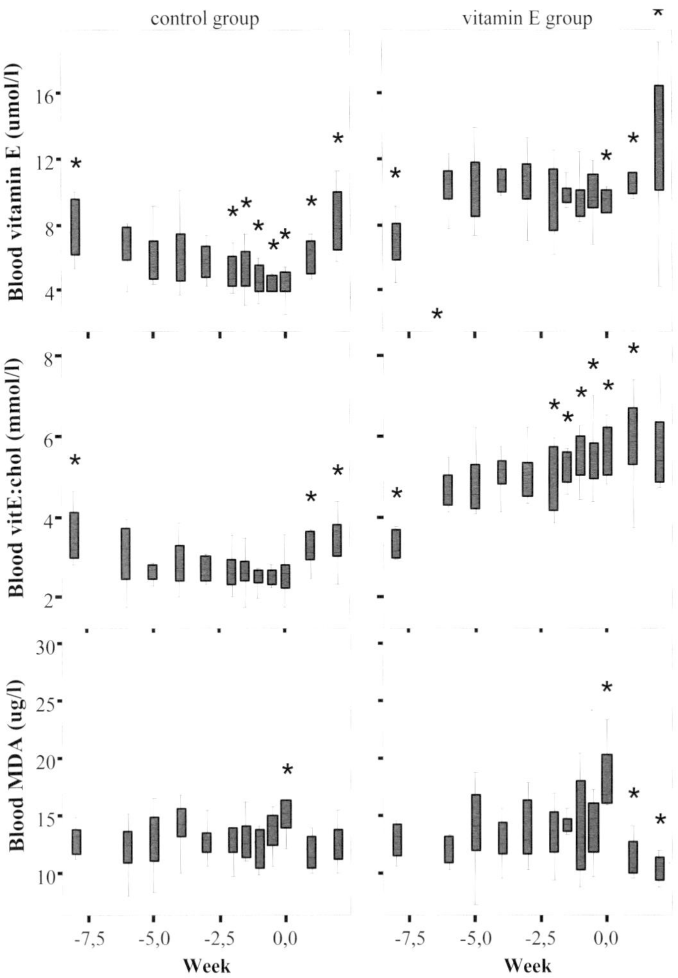

Figure 1. Blood vitamin E, the ratio vitamin E: cholesterol (vitE:chol) and malondialdehyde (MDA) in control and vitamin E group during experimental period. Displayed are medians and quartiles.
**Significant group x time interaction compared to the base line (P<0.05).*

three milkings (P<0.01) and decreased in the following period. SCC in the control group was high in the first three milkings and decreased afterwards. In the supplemented group, fewer SCC fluctuations were observed and SCC tended to be lower.

Table 2. Results of partial correlation corrected for group and repeated measures. Displayed are the correlation coefficients (r) between different parameters within blood, liver and milk.

Blood	**Vitamin E**	**Cholesterol**	**MDA**	
Vitamin E (µmol/l)	x			
Cholesterol (mmol/l)	0.725[a]	x		
MDA[1](µg/l)	-0.033	-0.048	x	
Ratio vitE: chol[2](mmol/l)	x	x	-0.004	
Liver tissue	**Vitamin E**	**Cholesterol**	**MDA**	
Vitamin E (nmol/gP)	x			
Cholesterol(mmol/gP)	-0.214	x		
MDA(µg/gP)	-0.286[d]	0.327[c]	x	
Ratio vitE: chol (mmol/gP)	x	x	-0.392[b]	
Milk	**Vitamin E**	**Fat%**	**MDA**	**Ratio vitE: fat%**
Vitamin E (µmol/l)	x			
Fat percentage (%)	-0.197	x		
MDA(µg/l)	0.176	-0.085	x	
Ratio vitE: fat%[3] (µmol/%)	x	x	0.223[c]	x
SCC[4]	0.003	0.313[b]	-0.036	-0.102

[a] (P<0.001); [b] (P<0.01); [c] (P<0.05); [d] (P<0.10).
[1] Malondialdehyde.
[2] Ratio vitamin E: cholesterol.
[3] Ratio vitamin E: fat percentage.
[4] Somatic cell count.

blood vitamin E concentration prepartum; other research, with 1,000 IU/day, found lower concentrations in prepartum supplemented cows (Smith *et al.*, 1997).Vitamin E supplementation in our study also resulted in higher vitamin E concentrations in liver tissue, which has also been reported in cattle, mice and rats (Ferre *et al.*, 2001). The ratio vitamin E:cholesterol is a commonly used as blood value. In liver tissue, the ratio was also higher in the supplemented group, and the results show less individual variation in comparison with absolute vitamin E concentrations in liver tissue. No reports are available on the usefulness of this ratio in liver tissue. Absolute vitamin E concentration in milk tended to be higher in supplemented cows.

MDA is one of the lipid-peroxidation products and is thus often used as indicator of oxidative damage. In previous studies, increased blood concentrations of MDA or precursors of MDA (TBARS) have also been found in periparturient cows (Bernabucci *et al.*, 2005). The data of this study confirmed that, based on MDA blood concentrations, periparturient heifers experience oxidative stress, and that the effect of vitamin E on MDA differs between the blood, liver and the mammary gland. Vitamin E supplementation could not prevent the rise in blood MDA at calving, but the lower MDA blood concentrations of supplemented cows in the two weeks after calving suggest a role of vitamin E in recovering from parturition related oxidative stress. Given the important role of the liver in dealing with metabolic changes, oxidative damage and the influence of vitamin E at liver level could be more important than concentrations measured in blood. Our data confirm this; vitamin E supplementation reduced oxidative damage in liver, while no obvious effects of supplementation were found in milk and blood MDA concentrations. MDA concentration in the liver was not correlated to absolute vitamin E concentrations, but was correlated to the ratio vitamin E: cholesterol. A rise in ratio vitamin E: cholesterol also implies a decrease in lipid peroxidation in liver tissue. This ratio may then be a better value for evaluating the anti-oxidant capacity of vitamin E in liver tissue. The importance of MDA in milk is even more difficult to evaluate. The question is whether it is formed or excreted in the mammary gland. The high concentrations at the beginning of lactation could support either theory. The MDA from blood might be excreted in the mammary gland and the high blood concentrations at calving may cause high concentrations of MDA in milk. But the change from non-lactating to lactating could also cause high levels of oxidative damage products in the mammary gland. We did not find that vitamin E had a positive effect on MDA concentrations in milk. This is explainable if milk MDA is a reflection of values in blood, because no effect of vitamin E on MDA was found in blood, either. In milk, the somatic cell count (SCC) group × time interaction was different, due to two cows with SCC>1,000,000 in the control group. SCC is an indicator of mastitis, and a low SCC generally represents good mammary health (Smith *et al.*, 1997). Higher SCC in cows with low dietary vitamin E concentration compared to cows with high dietary vitamin E has also been reported by various other authors.

Conclusion

We concluded that periparturient dairy heifers experience oxidative stress. Overall, we found that the influence of vitamin E supplementation on oxidative damage differ in the blood, liver and mammary gland. Vitamin E supplementation reduces oxidative damage in the liver, but has no obvious effect on milk and blood MDA concentrations. And vitamin E supplementation seems to influence mammary gland health in a positive way.

Acknowledgements

This study is part of the five-year udder health program of the Dutch Udder Health Centre and was financially supported by the Dutch Dairy Board.

References

Bernabucci, U., Ronchi, B., Lacetera, N. and Nardone, A., 2005. Influence of body condition score on relationships between metabolic status and oxidative stress in periparturient dairy cows. J. Dairy Sci. 88: 2017-2026.

Ferre, N., Camps, J., Paul, A., Cabre, M., Calleja, L., Osada, J. and Joven, J., 2001. Effects of high-fat, low-cholesterol diets on hepatic lipid peroxidation and antioxidants in apolipoprotein E-deficient mice. Mol. Cell. Biochem. 218: 165-169.

Goff, J.P. and Stabel, J.R., 1990. Decreased plasma retinol, alpha-tocopherol, and zinc concentration during the periparturient period: effect of milk fever. J. Dairy Sci. 73: 3195-3199.

Miller, J.K., Brzezinska-Slebodzinska, E. and Madsen, F.C., 1993. Oxidative stress, antioxidants, and animal function. J. Dairy Sci. 76: 2812-2823.

Smith, K.L., Hogan, J.S. and Weiss, W.P., 1997. Dietary vitamin E and selenium affect mastitis and milk quality. J. Anim. Sci. 75: 1659-1665.

The usefulness of a new udder health index to decrease mastitis incidence

Y. de Haas[1,2], G. de Jong[2], W. Ouweltjes[1], J. ten Napel[1] and J.J. Windig[1]
[1]Animal Sciences Group, P.O. Box 65, 8200 AB Lelystad, the Netherlands
[2]CRV, P.O. Box 454, 6800 AL Arnhem, the Netherlands
Corresponding author: Yvette.deHaas@wur.nl

Abstract

Genetic selection for udder health in the Netherlands is currently based on indirect traits combined in an udder health index. This index has an accuracy of 0.74 for young unproven bulls. Genetic trends of udder health over the years are horizontal despite a strong selection on milk yield and the negative genetic correlation with udder health. Although this indicates that the unfavourable effect of selection on milk yield on udder health is counteracted, there is room for improvement by constructing a better udder health index. A new index is proposed to reduce both clinical and subclinical mastitis in equal proportions that consists of (1) average SCC in early lactation (5-150 days), (2) average SCC in late lactation (151-400 days), (3) absence or presence of a test-day SCC above 150,000 cells/ml, (4) proportion of test-day SCC above 150,000 cells/ml and (5) number of patterns of peaks in SCC. This index results in an accuracy of 91% for young unproven bulls, which implies more distinction between the best and worst sires with respect to their udder health breeding values. With the new index udder health breeding values are estimated for bulls and cows using the national database for a test run. Average breeding vales of bulls and cows vary from -9 to +6% for bulls and from -4 to +6% for cows. Both the higher accuracy and the presence of genetic variation improves possibilities to select sires and dams that improve udder health genetics, and to realise a favourable genetic trend in the future.

Keywords: breeding, clinical mastitis, selection index, somatic cell count

Introduction

Mastitis is one of the most frequent and costly diseases in the dairy industry. Beside management, breeding is an important tool to reduce the incidence of clinical mastitis (CM). The advantage of reducing CM by breeding is that it results in a permanent change in the genetic composition of the dairy herd (Shook, 1989). Several studies have shown that selection for production alone causes negative effects on udder health (Heringstad *et al.*, 2003). This caused a growing interest in broadening national selection indices to include functional traits such as health and reproduction (Miglior *et al.*, 2005). In most national indices summarised by Miglior *et al.* (2005) log-transformed somatic cell count (SCS) was the main trait contributing to udder health. The current Dutch udder health index consists of this SCS, completed with milking speed and conformation traits (De Jong and Lansbergen, 1996). This index has an accuracy of 0.74 for young unproven bulls, indicating that there is still room for improvement. The aim of this study was firstly to define alternative traits for somatic cell count (SCC) and to link them genetically to cases of clinical and subclinical mastitis (SCM). This research has been described in detail by De Haas *et al.* (2008). Secondly, it is examined which combination of SCC-traits can be used best for a new udder health index. Thirdly, breeding values (BV) for CM and SCM are estimated based on this proposed index to determine genetic variation and genetic trends.

Alternative SCC-traits

Several studies have shown that the frequency of cases of CM is much higher in the first part of the lactation than in the second part (Emanuelson *et al.*, 1988; Barkema *et al.*, 1998). Therefore, the hypothesis was that SCC in the first half of the lactation is more informative as a mastitis-indicator, than SCC including the second half of the lactation. It is beneficial for genetic selection as well to reduce the period of collecting sufficient data, because information becomes available sooner and reliable genetic selection can occur at an earlier age. The first group of SCC-traits consisted of test-day SCC averaged over different lengths of lactations. Cell counts were averaged per lactation over the test-day records up to 400, 350, 300, 250, 200, 150, and 100 days (De Haas *et al.*, 2008; Ouweltjes, unpublished data).

However, an average does not do fully describe the dynamic variation in SCC. The most desirable cow would respond very quickly to an intramammary infection (IMI) and then return to normal levels of SCC. Such a picture is not reflected in an average. Therefore, SCC was summarised in a more biologically intuitive way by taking patterns of peaks in SCC into account in the second group of SCC-traits (De Haas *et al.*, 2008; Ouweltjes, unpublished data). Patterns of peaks in SCC distinguish between lactations with short or long periods of increased SCC on the basis of recovery within two test-day records. The first pattern was a quick rise in SCC followed by an immediate decrease in SCC. This pattern is often associated with cases of CM caused by environmental pathogens (Smith and Hogan, 1993), and was therefore referred to as 'environmental pattern' (P_ENV). The second pattern captured longer periods of increased SCC, and can often be associated with cases of CM caused by contagious pathogens (Fox and Gay, 1993). Therefore it was referred to as 'contagious pattern' (P_CONT). The patterns were analysed both individually and combined into all patterns of peaks (P_ALL), without specification of the exact peak.

The third group of SCC-traits were defined based on excessive cell counts. Excessive test-day SCC was assumed as it was originated from an IMI. Each test-day SCC was classified individually as a binary trait. A test-day SCC above 150,000 cells/ml was registered as 1; otherwise it was registered as 0. Four SCC-traits were defined based on excessive test-days to describe the dynamics of SCC during lactation (De Haas *et al.*, 2008; Ouweltjes, unpublished data). The hypothesis was that the dynamics differ between healthy and mastitic cows.

'Suspicion of IMI' distinguished between presence (1) or absence (0) of a test-day SCC above 150,000 cells/ml in a lactation. 'Extent of IMI' was calculated as the proportion of all recorded test-days in a lactation that excess 150,000 cells/ml. 'Severity of IMI' was only calculated for the 'suspected' group. It expressed whether the cell count was moderately (0) or severely (1) increased, with a threshold at 250,000 cells/ml. 'Length of IMI' and was also calculated only within the 'suspected' group, and was defined as the number of test-day recordings during the longest streak of consecutive cell counts above 150,000 cells/ml.

Data

Three different datasets (A, B and C) were available with different ways of recording CM (De Haas *et al.*, 2008; Ouweltjes, unpublished data). After editing, dataset A contained 28,688 lactations from 21,673 cows in 394 herds. Dataset B contained 56,726 lactations of 30,145 cows in 272 herds and dataset C contained 70,216 lactations from 39,769 cows in 404 farms. For dataset A, information on CM was collected by NRS (Arnhem, the Netherlands) during the monthly milk recording. The milk-recording officers asked the farmers if a cow was mastitic on the day of milk recording, or if she experienced a case of CM in the period between the previous and current milk recording. For dataset B, data of cases of CM were recorded in on-farm PC management information systems. The farmers themselves collected information on (treatments of) CM and allowed us to upload and use these data. For dataset C, data from bacteriological culturing programs of GD Animal Health Service were used. All datasets contained farmer-diagnosed CM.

Statistical analyses

(Co)variance components were estimated with a generalised linear mixed model using ASREML (Gilmour *et al.*, 2006). Univariate analyses were carried out for CM, SCM and SCC-traits using a linear model. The model included random effects for sire and MGS and for cow (to account for the permanent animal effects across repeated lactations). Fixed effects included were an interaction between herd and year of calving, parity (with three classes) and month of calving (with twelve classes). Linear polynomials were included for age at calving and days at risk. Bivariate analyses were carried out to estimate correlations between CM, SCM and SCC-traits, using a linear model for all traits.

Results

Estimated heritabilities for all mastitis-traits were around 0.03. Heritabilities for SCC-traits ranged from 0.01, for patterns of peaks in SCC, to 0.13 for lactation-average SCC. Genetic correlations between SCC-traits and CM or SCM ranged from 0.55 to 0.99 for CM and from 0.55 to 0.98 for SCM (Table 1). Genetic correlations of CM were high with lactation-average SCC, and also with the patterns of peaks in SCC. Genetic correlations with lactation-average SCC over longer periods (i.e. >300 days) were higher for SCM (>0.85) than for CM (>0.66).

Table 1. Genetic correlations between udder health traits (clinical mastitis (CM) and subclinical mastitis (SCM)) and several alternative somatic cell count traits in three different datasets (dataset A, B and C).

	CM			SCM		
	A	B	C	A	B	C
SCS100	0.77	0.71	0.89	0.70	0.67	0.66
SCS150	0.82	0.73	0.92	0.77	0.75	0.70
SCS200	0.84	0.72	0.92	0.84	0.81	0.74
SCS250	0.87	0.69	0.89	0.88	0.87	0.79
SCS300	0.86	0.67	0.87	0.91	0.89	0.85
SCS350	0.86	0.66	0.87	0.93	0.90	0.88
SCS400	0.85	0.66	0.86	0.94	0.91	0.89
SCS151-400	0.79	0.55	0.75	0.98	0.95	0.96
Suspicion	0.75	0.66	0.80	0.98	0.94	0.97
Extent	0.61	0.64	0.86	0.79	0.85	0.92
Severity	0.62	0.88	0.92	0.73	0.70	0.76
Length	0.69	0.62	0.82	0.89	0.88	0.83
P_ALL	0.80	0.89	0.96	0.72	0.73	0.74
P_ENV	0.66	0.93	0.86	0.55	0.68	0.64
P_CONT	0.83	0.88	0.99	0.77	0.76	0.79

Correlations with traits describing the dynamics of SCC were also higher for SCM than for CM except for 'severity of IMI'. For P_ENV, genetic correlations were lower with SCM than with CM. Generally, if a genetic correlation with CM was relatively high, it was relatively low with SCM and vice versa.

Selection indices

To determine the optimal combination of SCC-traits selection index theory was used. In selection index theory, the selection goal (H) is defined as consisting of multiple traits weighted by their (economic) importance, e.g. $H = v_1x_1 + v_2x_2 + ... + v_nx_n$ with x is a trait and v is its weight. Here H was defined as 50% CM and 50% SCM, e.g. H = 0.5 CM + 0.5 SCM.

In selection index theory, the objective is to find an index (I) consisting of several observed indirect traits, e.g. $I = b_1x_1 + b_2x_2 + ... + b_nx_n$ with x is a trait and b is its weight, so that the correlation between the selection goal and index ($r_{H,I}$) is maximised. The optimum weight to maximise $r_{H,I}$ is given by $b = P^{-1}Gv$ where P is the genetic variance/covariance matrix of the observed traits and G is the genetic variance/covariance matrix of the traits forming the selection goal. The efficiency of two indices consisting of a different set of traits can be compared by calculating their $r_{H,I}$'s.

Statistical analyses

Two selection indices were used as benchmarks for comparisons with different combinations of SCC-traits. The first benchmark was a selection index with only direct observations on SCM, e.g. the minimal number of observed SCC-traits. The second benchmark was an index with the maximum number of SCC-traits possible. This consisted of a combination SCC5-400 and all other SCC-traits in the second and third group of SCC-traits, except P_ALL. Only one trait out of the first group of SCC-traits was used to avoid using non-independent traits containing partly the same information. For the same reason P_ALL was not used in the benchmark because this trait is a combination of P_ENV and P_CONT.

To select the best combination of traits, r_{HI} of different combinations were calculated. Because the number of possible combinations of the 15 traits is too large to analyse a stepwise approach was used. First, each trait was compared separately to the minimum and maximum benchmark. Second, combinations within the three groups of SCC-traits were analysed. Finally, promising combinations from the within set analyses were combined to find the optimum index.

Selection indices were calculated using the average of the genetic variance/covariance matrices of the three datasets. This reflects probably best the actual (co-)variances between the traits. For each trait, except CM, observations on 120 offspring were assumed. The most promising combinations selected on the basis of the average G were also evaluated using the G's of the separate datasets, to avoid selecting an inappropriate index for one of the datasets.

Results

The accuracy indicates how well the selection index predicts the breeding value of a young bull for the breeding goal. If only information on SCM was used to compose the index, its accuracy was 64% (Table 2). Combining SCM with SCC early and SCC late in lactation (i.e. between 5 and 150 days and between 151 and 400 days, respectively) considerably improved the accuracy to 85%. Further improvement came from the addition of 'suspicion of IMI' and 'extent of IMI'. The addition of the presence of peaks added another 1% to the accuracy of the index. All other traits had hardly any influence on the accuracy. If all traits except CM were used to compose the index the accuracy was 91%.

Addition of CM information further improved the index. However, improvement was relatively small for indices with four or more SCC-traits (Table 2). The accuracy of an index composed of SCM, early SCC, late SCC, suspicion of IMI, extent of IMI and any pattern of peaks in SCC improved by only 1.5% if all offspring had information on CM. Thus setting up an information

Table 2. Accuracy of breeding values predicted by udder health indices composed of different sets of SCC-traits. The accuracy is for a bull with 120 offspring with data on all traits, except for CM which varied in number of offspring with information.

No	Data used	No. of offspring with data on CM				Gain relative to no CM		
		0	30	60	120	30	60	120
1	Only SCM	0.64	0.68	0.72	0.76	6.7%	11.9%	18.8%
2	1 + Early and Late SCC	0.85	0.89	0.89	0.91	4.2%	4.9%	5.9%
3	2 + Suspicion and Extent	0.90	0.91	0.91	0.92	0.6%	1.1%	1.9%
4	3 + Peaks	0.91	0.91	0.92	0.92	0.5%	0.9%	1.5%
	Full set	0.91	0.92	0.92	0.93	0.4%	0.8%	1.4%

system for CM of all cows in the Netherlands will improve breeding for mastitis resistance only slightly.

Breeding values

Breeding values of udder health (i.e. both CM and SCM) in parity 1, 2 and 3 separately for bulls and cows were estimated using the national database. In total, 4,212,745 animals were included in the analyses.

Genetic variation in BVs of bulls and cows is present. For parity 1, the BVs for CM of bulls range from -5% to +5% around the population mean. For parities 2 and 3, the BVs range from -9% to +6% around the population mean. This indicates that an efficient selection against mastitis is possible. Slightly less genetic variation is shown for the BVs for CM of cows. Their estimated BVs are closer to the population mean, due to the lower reliability of their BVs caused by less offspring per cow.

For parity 1, the BVs for SCM of bulls range from -13% to +13% around the population mean. For parity 2, the BVs range from -14% to +12% around the population mean, and for parity 3 from -20 to +19%. Slightly less genetic variation is shown for the BVs for SCM of cows, but still in the range between -15 and +15%, especially in parity 3.

No clear trend in average BVs for CM of cows is shown, with only small differences between parities (Figure 1A). Genetic trends of udder health over the years are horizontal despite a strong selection on milk yield and the negative genetic correlation with udder health. This indicates that the unfavourable effect of selection on milk is counteracted, probably even most

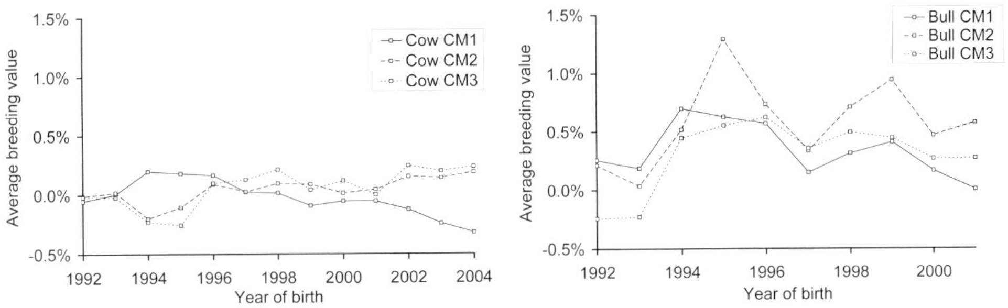

Figure 1. Trend in average breeding value (BV) for clinical mastitis (CM) in parity 1 to 3 of (A) Holstein-Friesian cows and (B) bulls. The average estimated BV for sires born in a certain year, with at least 100 offspring in milk, is shown. The average estimated BV for cows with records in the national milk recording, born in a certain year, is shown.

in parity 1. The estimated BVs for CM of bulls show many fluctuations between the years (Figure 1B), and no clear trend was present in any of the parities.

Average BVs for SCM of bulls and cows are slightly higher than the average BVs for CM. However, similar curves are shown for all parities, and no clear trend seems to be present. This absence of a real clear trend indicates that the current breeding strategy did counteract the negative effect of selection for higher milk production on the udder health status. However, a decreasing trend was not seen either, indicating that there is room for improvement for the future. For example by a more efficient mastitis index, as proposed in this study.

Conclusions

A new udder health index is proposed including (1) average SCC in early lactation (5-150 days), (2) average SCC in late lactation (151-400 days), (3) absence or presence of a test-day SCC above 150,000 cells/ml, (4) proportion of test-day SCC above 150,000 cells/ml and (5) number of patterns of peaks in SCC. This index results in an accuracy of 91% for young unproven bulls, implying that a better distinction can be made between the best and worst sires with respect to their genetics of udder health. Improved genetic selection for a better udder health is possible with the proposed new index.

Acknowledgements

The farmers are greatly acknowledged for providing information on occurrence of cases of clinical mastitis. This study is part of the five-year udder health program of the Dutch Udder Health Centre and was financially supported by the Dutch Dairy Board.

References

Barkema, H.W., Schukken, Y.H., Lam, T.J.G.M., Beiboer, M.L., Wilmink, H., Benedictus, G. and Brand, A. 1998. Incidence of clinical mastitis in dairy herds grouped in three categories by bulk milk somatic cell counts. J. Dairy Sci. 81: 411-419.

De Haas, Y., Ouweltjes, W., Ten Napel, J., Windig, J.J. and De Jong, G. 2008. Alternative somatic cell count traits as mastitis indicators for genetic selection. J. Dairy Sci. 91:2501-2511.

De Jong, G. and Lansbergen, L. 1996. Udder health index: selection for mastitis resistance. Interbull Bull. 12: 42-47.

Emanuelson, U., Danell, B. and Philipsson, J. 1988. Genetic parameters for clinical mastitis, somatic cell counts, and milk production estimated by multiple-trait restricted maximum likelihood. J. Dairy Sci. 71: 467-476.

Fox, L.K. and Gay, J.M. 1993. Contagious Mastitis. Vet. Clin. N. Am. – Food Anim. Pract. 9: 475-487.

Heringstad, B., Chang, Y.M., Gianola, D. and Klemetsdal, G. 2003. Genetic analysis of longitudinal trajectory of clinical mastitis in first-lactation Norwegian cattle. J. Dairy Sci. 86: 2676-2683.

Gilmour, A.R., Gogel, B.J., Cullis, B.R. and Thompson, R. 2006. ASREML User Guide Release 2.0 VSN International Ltd., Hemel Hempstead, HP1 1ES, United Kingdom

Miglior, F., Muir, B.L. and Van Doormaal, B.J. 2005. Selection indices in Holstein cattle of various countries. J. Dairy Sci. 88: 1255-1263.

Shook, G.E. 1989. Selection for disease resistance. J. Dairy Sci. 72: 1349-1362.

Smith, K.L. and Hogan, J.S. 1993. Environmental Mastitis. Vet. Clin. N. Am. – Food Anim. Pract. 9: 489-498.

Efficient breeding against mastitis by creative use of somatic cell counts

J.J. Windig[1], G. de Jong[2], W. Ouweltjes[1], J. ten Napel[1] and Y. de Haas[2]
[1]Animal Sciences Group, Wageningen UR, Animal Breeding and Genomics Centre, P.O. Box 65, 8200 AB Lelystad, the Netherlands
[2]CRV, P.O. Box 454, 6800 AL Arnhem, theNetherlands
Corresponding author: jack.windig@wur.nl

Breeding is an important tool to decrease mastitis incidence. Efficient breeding will result in a permanent change in the cows ability to resist and recover from mastitis infections, despite a high milk production. Information for breeding against mastitis can come directly from registration of mastitis, and indirectly from related traits such as SCC. Here we evaluate the efficiency of breeding against both clinical mastitis (CM) and subclinical mastitis (SCM) based on new traits derived from somatic cell counts (SCC). We also evaluate the gain in efficiency if direct information on CM is used. We looked at 10 SCC traits in three sets: SCC over a restricted lactation period (early vs. late), SCC-traits evaluating excessive SCC (e.g. number of SCC test days above threshold) and patterns of peaks in SCC. For different combinations of SCC-traits the accuracy (indicating how well the breeding goal is predicted) was determined. The breeding goal in our case was defined as reducing both SCM and CM in equal amounts. A combination of 5 SCC traits plus SCM resulted in an accuracy of 0.94. Adding information on CM improved the accuracy only slightly. Efficient breeding is thus possible by creative use of SCC only.

A dual purpose breed guarantees not a higher resistance against mastitis

K. Barth and K. Aulrich
Federal Research Institute for Rural Areas, Forestry and Fisheries, Institute of Organic Farming, Trenthorst 32, 23847 Westerau, Germany
Corresponding author: kerstin.barth@vti.bund.de

The standards of organic farming recommend using adopted breeds in animal production. Local breeds are supposed to be more resistant against production diseases due to their lower milk yield. Since December 2004 two breeds are kept in the same cowshed under equal management conditions on our experimental farm. In a long-term experiment the dual purpose breed Red-and-White-Holsteins (RW) and the milk oriented breed of Holstein-Friesian (HF) shall be compared with regard to their suitability for organic dairy farming. Animals are sampled at regular intervals and each case of disease is recorded. The results of cyto-bacteriological analyses and the monthly carried out California Mastitis Test (CMT) as well as the measurement of electrical conductivity (EC) are used for the decision about the antibiotic dry cow therapy (DCT). A first analysis evaluated the data of 28 HF and 21 RW cows. This evaluation revealed that the animals of the dual purpose breed were treated more often with antibiotics at drying off than the HF cows. On quarter level 73.3% and 58.4% of the RW and HF quarters, respectively, were treated. As expected, the quarters receiving DCT had higher EC readings and higher CMT scores. But we also observed differences between the breeds. The healthy and the treated quarters of RW showed significant higher readings of EC of foremilk and higher CMT scores than the HF: 6.0 and 6.3 mS/cm and 0.2 and 0.6, respectively. One explanation of our findings might be that the animals of the dual purpose breed lacked the udder form of a breed oriented to milk yield and higher milk flows. However, our findings do not support the popular (and maybe to simple) assumption that it is better to use older breeds in organic farming.

Effect of selenium supplementation on somatic cell count around calving and in lactating dairy cows

A. Ceballos[1], J. Neumann[2], A. Mella[2], J. Kruze[2], H.W. Barkema[3], J. Wichtel[1] and F. Wittwer[2]
[1]University of Prince Edward Island. 550 Univ Ave, Charlottetown, PE C1A4P3, Canada
[2]UACH, Isla Teja S/N, Valdivia, Chile
[3]University of Calgary, 3330 Hosp Dr NW, Calgary, AB T2N4N1, Canada
Corresponding author: aceballos@upei.ca

Mastitis remains the most costly disease in dairy cattle. It induces economic losses, mainly consisting of discarded milk, increased health costs and reduced milk quality. Several risk factors, including sub-optimal nutrition, contribute to mastitis. Thus, supplementing dairy cattle with specific micronutrients (e.g. selenium) and its effect on udder health has already described. However, it is unknown how organic oral supplements compare to long-acting inorganic supplements regarding to somatic cell counts (SCC) in milk around calving and in lactating cows. Two studies were conducted to investigate the effects of two commercial Se supplements on the SCC around calving, and across lactation in dairy cows. One hundred and forty heifers and 48 cows were fed a suboptimal Se diet. Two groups of heifers were supplemented using either oral or long-acting Se forms before calving, and a group of cows received a single injection of a long-acting Se form 45 days before calving. In the first group, milk samples from individual quarters were collected on a weekly basis until 28 DIM, and milk composite samples were monthly collected for the entire lactation from the second group of cows to evaluate SCC. Data were analysed using a multilevel mixed-effects model adding random-slopes for time. SCC around calving were lower in Se-supplemented groups ($P<0.05$), but SCC patterns were depending on milk production across lactation ($P=0.06$), suggesting a reduction of SCC in those cows with high milk production. The effects on intramammary infections and milk production are currently underway, and will be presented at the conference.

RRR-a-tocopheryl acetate provides protection against mastitis in transition cows

M.R. Peisker and Y. Dersjant-Li
ADM Specialty Ingredients (Europe) B.V., Stationsstraat 76, 1541 LJ Koog aan de Zaan, the Netherlands
Corresponding author: Ydersjantli@admworld.com

Nutritional management is one of the strategies for mastitis prevention. Supplementation of vitamin E can provide adequate amounts of antioxidants for neutrophils that assist in killing pathogens and provide protection against mastitis. Vitamin E supplementation around calving is associated with enhanced functionality of blood macrophages and neutrophils, and decreased incidence of placental retention and other reproductive disorders. In transition cows, plasma concentration of α-tocopherol should exceed 3 to 3.5 mg/l at calving. Lower plasma α-tocopherol concentrations are considered a significant risk factor for mastitis. Vitamin E can be supplemented as either natural source vitamin E (100% RRR-a-tocopherol) or as synthetic vitamin E (all-rac-a-tocopherol - 12.5% of RRR-stereoisomer). When all-rac-a-tocopheryl acetate is supplemented to cow's feed, RRR-a-tocopherol stereoisomer is the absolutely dominating form retained in cows` plasma (96%) and milk (86%). Plasma and neutrophil a-tocopherol concentration is significantly improved with RRR-a-tocopheryl acetate compared to all-rac-a-tocopheryl acetate supplementation during calving, indicating improvement of the immune system for protection against mastitis. Practical experiences have substantiated the positive effect of RRR-a-tocopherol in transition cows revealing improved cow health at and after calving and reduced occurrences of placenta retention, milk cell count and mastitis. The current recommendation for dietary supplementation of RRR-a-tocopheryl acetate is 2000 mg/cow/d - 30 days before calving and 1000 mg/cow/d - 30 days after calving.

Lymphocyte apoptosis during experimentally induced mastitis

P. Slama[1,2], Z. Sladek[1,2], D. Rysanek[2], T. Langrova[1,2] and M. Zouharova[2]
[1]Mendel University of Agriculture and Forestry in Brno, Department of Animal Morphology, Physiology and Genetics, Zemedelska 1, 613 00 Brno, Czech Republic
[2]Veterinary Research Institute, Immunology, Hudcova 70, 621 00 Brno, Czech Republic
Corresponding author: xslama@node.mendelu.cz

The aim of our study was to determine if apoptosis of lymphocytes is modulated by infections of *Staphylococcus aureus* and *Streptococcus uberis*. For this purpose, apoptosis of lymphocytes was studied in model of acute response of the bovine mammary gland caused by experimentally induced *S. aureus* and *S. uberis* mastitis of virgin mammary gland. The experiments were carried out in twenty mammary glands of five virgin Holstein × Bohemian Red Pied crossbred heifers. Before the experimental infection with *S. aureus* and *S. uberis*, the mammary glands were treated with phosphate buffered saline (PBS) as a control. The samples of leukocytes were obtained by lavages of the mammary glands in four intervals (24, 48, 72 and 168 hours) after the PBS application and after the experimental infections. Flow cytometry was used to determine apoptotic lymphocytes. After PBS instillation, the percentage of apoptotic lymphocytes increased within 24 hours. There was the highest proportion of apoptosis in that time point. Proportion of apoptotic lyphocytes subsequently return to the initial condition. The percentage of apoptotic lymphocytes was increasing gradually after stimulation of mammary glands with *S. aureus* and *S. uberis* and it was persisting at approximately equal level after 48 hours after the experimental infections. The results of this study demonstrate that the apoptosis of lymphocytes is modulated during experimental infections of the mammary gland with *S. aureus* and *S. uberis*. This study was supported by the Ministry of Agriculture of the Czech Republic (MZE 0002716201).

The resident leukocytes from bovine mammary gland: proportion of functional and dead cells

Z. Sladek and D. Rysanek
Veterinary research institute, Immunology, Hudcova 70, 621 00 Brno, Czech Republic
Corresponding author: sladekz@seznam.cz

The resident cells play an important role in immunological defense of the mammary gland. The presence of a high number of death cells may significantly compromise the functional capacity of these cells to mount an adequate immune response upon infection. We used a model of virgin mammary gland as a source of the resident leukocytes. The cell death was detected using Annexin V (An) and propidium iodide (PI) positivity in flow cytometry. The resident leukocytes were presented by neutrophils (12.9%), macrophages (50.1%) and lymphocytes (37.0%). The highest proportion of apoptotic cells (An+/PI-) was observed in macrophages (15.8%), followed by neutrophils (13.9%) and lymphocytes (1%). Moreover, the highest proportion of necrotic cells (An+/PI+) was observed in neutrophils (22.5%), followed by macrophages (11.4%) and lymphocytes (0.8%). These results indicated that all types of resident leukocytes displayed the higher proportion of living cells. It assumed that the resident cells have the great functional potential in reaction to invading pathogens. This study was supported by the Ministry of Agriculture (MZE 0002716201).

The bacterial cellular wall components are able to affect the apoptosis and the expression of surface receptors on heifer mammary gland neutrophils

T. Langrova[1,2]*, Z. Sladek*[1,2]*, D. Rysanek*[2] *and P. Slama*[1,2]
[1]*Mendel University of Agriculture and Forestry in Brno, Zemedelska 1, 613 00 Brno, Czech Republic*
[2]*Veterinary Research Institute, Hudcova 70, 621 00 Brno, Czech Republic*
Corresponding author: xlangrov@node.mendelu.cz

The present thesis studied apoptosis and expression of CD14 and CD44, surface receptors on neutrophils, which are important during inflammatory response. The aim of the experiment was to prove the effect of muramyldipeptide (MDP) and lipopolysaccharide (LPS) on the apoptosis and the expression of CD14 and CD44. During the incubation, a progressive increase in number of apoptotic neutrophils was observed. Incubation with MDP and LPS was accompanied with more gradual increase. A statistically significant higher proportion of CD14+ neutrophils were observed after 30 and 120 minutes of incubation with MDP. There were not detected statistically significant differences during incubation with LPS. After 30 and 120 minutes of incubation with MDP and 30 and 60 minutes of incubation with LPS were detected a statistically significant higher proportion of CD44+ neutrophils. The proportion of apoptotic neutrophils was the greatest after incubation without components of cellular wall, whereas after incubation with MDP and LPS it was manifested with more gradual increase. The results of this study indicate that the MDP and LPS may prolong the duration of an acute inflammation. Higher proportion of CD14+ and CD44+ neutrophils after 30 minutes of incubation with MDP indicates that reaction of neutrophils to LPS is slower than reaction to MDP. This progress of apoptosis and expression of CD14 and CD44 during incubation indicates that components of bacterial cellular wall have an ability to affect an expression of surface receptors on neutrophils under study. This study was supported by Ministry of Agriculture of the Czech Republic (MZE 0002716201).

Effect of intramammary injection of liposomal RbGM-CSF on milk and peripheral blood mononuclear cells of subpopulation in Holstein cows with naturally infected subclinical mastitis

Y. Kiku[1], T. Ozawa[1], S. Inumaru[1], S. Kushibiki[2], T. Hayashi[1,3] and H. Takahashi[1]
[1]National Institute of Animal Health, Tsukuba, Ibaraki, 305-0856, Japan
[2]National Institute of Livestock and Grassland Science, Tsukuba, Ibaraki, 305-0901, Japan
[3]Tokyo University of Science, Noda, Chiba, 278-8510, Japan
Corresponding author: yokiku@affrc.go.jp

Although the liposomal recombinant bovine granulocyte-macrophage colony-stimulating factor (rbGM-CSF) has a potential as the therapeutic agent for *Staphylococcus aureus* infection causing subclinical mastitis of dairy cows, the contribution of mononuclear cells in milk and blood to this treatment remains unclear. The present study was designed to investigate the effect of the intramammary injection of rbGM-CSF on milk and blood levels of mononuclear cells subpopulation and shedding pattern of total bacterial count in an udder infected with subclinical mastitis. Six Holstein cows were used. Seven days after the injections of the control solution, 0.4 mg/5ml saline of rbGM-CSF was injected into the cistern. Blood samples, and milk samples from injected quarters were collected before injection and for 2 weeks after injection. Using flow cytometry, we determined the expression of specific antigens on the surface of mononuclear leukocytes in milk and blood. The CMT score and total bacterial count in milk were decreased on day 7 and 14 after rbGM-CSF injection. The percentage of CD14+ cells in milk were increased on day 1 after the cytokine injection. Following an increase of the percentage of CD14+ cells, CD4+ and CD8+ cells were increased. In contrast, the percentages of CD3+, CD8+ and CD14+ cells in blood were increased on day 3 or 7. Our study demonstrates that the intramammary injection of rbGM-CSF accelerates the trafficking of CD14+ cells in an udder infected with subclinical mastitis, and these cells induce the enhancement of cellular immunity in the mammary gland.

Effect of intramammary injection of RbGM-CSF on neutrophils function of blood and milk in Holstein cows with subclinical mastitis

T. Ozawa[1], Y. Kiku[1], S. Inumaru[1], S. Hasegawa[2], S. Kushibiki[2], T. Hayashi[3] and H. Takahashi[1]
[1]National Institute of Animal Health, Tsukuba, Ibaraki, 305-0856, Japan
[2]National Institute of Livestock and Grassland Science, Tsukuba, Ibaraki, 305-0901, Japan
[3]Tokyo University of Science, Noda, Chiba, 278-8510, Japan
Corresponding author: ozatomo@affrc.go.jp

The aim of this study was to examine the effect of intramammary injected recombinant bovine granulocyte-macrophage colony-stimulating factor (rbGM-CSF, 400 μg/5 ml) on the expression of L-selectin (CD62L) and Mac-1 (CD11b) at the surface of blood and milk neutrophils using five Holstein cows of subclinical mastitis naturally infected with *Staphylococcus aureus*. The adhesion molecules were stained at the cell surface and analysed flow cytometrically. In addition, somatic cell count (SCC), blood leukocyte count, blood neutrophil count and milk *S. aureus* count were measured. The injection of rbGM-CSF caused the changes in CD62L and CD11b expression were opposed to each other, with a decrease of CD62L expression and an increase CD11b expression on milk neutrophils at 6 h, days 1 and 2 after injection. The expression of CD62L and CD11b of blood neutrophils changed with no significance. The milk *S. aureus* count decreased significantly at 6 h afterinjection, but increased back to preinjection levels on day 14 after injection. On the other hand, SCC markedly increased at 6 h, but decreased back to preinjection levels on day 1 and was lower on day 14 than preinjection levels. These results suggest that the intramammary injection of rbGM-CSF to the cows of subclinical mastitis induces the enhancement of function of milk neutrophils.

Phenotypic and genotypic variation of bovine immune responses in cohort dairy herds across Canada

K.A. Thompson and B.A. Mallard
University of Guelph, Pathobiology, Ontario Veterinary College, 50 Stone Road East, N1G 2W1, Guelph, Canada
Corresponding author: kthomp02@uoguelph.ca

Mastitis contributes economic loss to the dairy industry with human and animal health implications. Selection solely for production negatively impacts disease incidence. The immune system is tightly genetically regulated and controls response to infectious disease. Including estimated breeding values (EBVs) of immune response traits in a selection index has the potential to improve inherent animal health. Recently, cows ranked as high responders in a large US commercial dairy were shown to have lower disease scores. The objective here is to evaluate antibody-mediated (AMIR) and cell-mediated immune responses (CMIR) in 80 commercial cohort herds across Canada in order to determine effects on health and performance. In collaboration with the Canadian Bovine Mastitis Network (CBMRN) ~500 Holsteins were immunised with test antigens designed to stimulate AMIR and CMIR, respectively. To classify cows as high (H) or low (L) responders, serum antibody is measured by ELISA and skin-fold thickness measurements are taken to evaluate delayed-type hypersensitivity, a measure of CMIR. Genome scan is performed to provide insight into the genes associated with these phenotypes. Health and production records are available for correlation with IR classification on a country-wide scale. Preliminary results show measurable differences in response between cows, herds, and provinces, making it possible to identify H and L responders. Identifying H and L responders (both phenotypically and based on EBVs) and understanding the genetic diversity of these phenotypes may make it feasible to include immune response in breeding indices to improve health.

Cis-urocanic acid protects against mammary tissue injury during intramammary *Escherichia coli* infection

D.D. Bannerman[1], M. Rinaldi[1], B.T. Vinyard[1], J. Laihia[2] and L. Leino[2]
[1]U.S. Department of Agriculture, Agricultural Research Service, BARC-East, Bldg. 1040, Rm. 2, Beltsville, Maryland 20705, USA
[2]BioCis Pharma, Ltd., Itäinen pitkäkatu 4 B, Turku, 20520, Finland
Corresponding author: douglas.bannerman@ars.usda.gov

Cis-urocanic acid (cis-UCA), which is formed in response to ultraviolet radiation-induced photoisomerisation of the trans isomer that is naturally found in skin, is a potent anti-inflammatory molecule. In a previous in vitro study, cis-UCA has been demonstrated to downregulate bovine neutrophil generation of reactive oxygen species, which are known to induce tissue injury. The objective of the current study was to evaluate the in vivo effect of intramammary infusion of cis-UCA on inflammation and tissue injury during acute clinical mastitis, a disease characterised by the influx of large numbers of neutrophils. Immediately prior to and at various time points after experimental infection with Escherichia coli and subsequent treatment, milk samples were aseptically collected and analysed for various markers of inflammation and injury. A major finding of the current study was that two markers of mammary tissue injury, N-acetyl-beta-D-glucosaminidase (NAGase) activity and lactate dehydrogenase (LDH) concentration, were lower in cis-UCA treated quarters than in those treated with saline. Further, cis-UCA had no adverse effect on bacterial clearance, as demonstrated by the equivalent milk colony forming units of E. coli across treatment groups. These findings suggest that cis-UCA is able to reduce mastitis-associated tissue damage without compromising host immune defenses against bacterial infection.

Detection, diagnosis and treatment

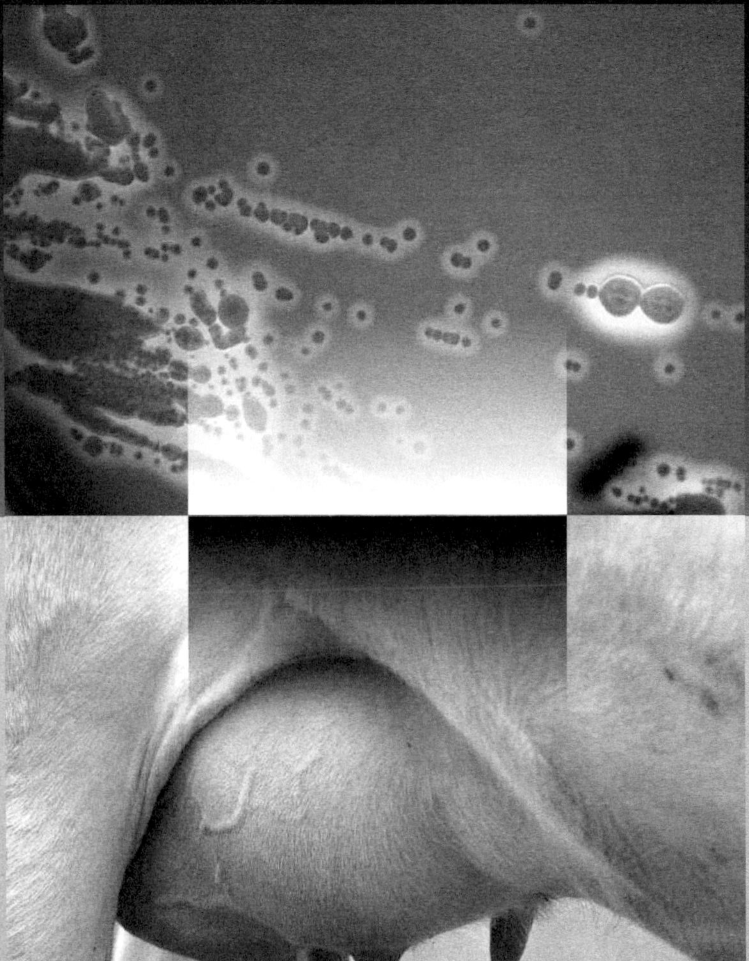

Epidemiologic association of *Staphylococcus aureus* virulence markers with intramammary infection chronicity

B.V. LeThanh[1,3], C.J. Lebeau[2,3], S. Messier[1,3], F. Malouin[2,3] and D. Scholl[1,3]
[1]University of Montreal, Faculty of Veterinary Medicine, 3200 rue Sicotte, Saint-Hyacinthe (QC) J2S 2M2, Canada
[2]University of Sherbrooke, Department of Biology, 2500 boul. Université, Sherbrooke (QC) J1K 2R1, Canada
[3]Canadian Bovine Mastitis Research Network
Corresponding author: daniel.scholl@umontreal.ca

Abstract

Despite effective techniques for controlling *Staphylococcus aureus* intramammary infection (IMI), it is still one of the most predominant causes of IMI in many dairy populations. The pathogen has an advantage due to many strains' ability to infect chronically and persistently without severe clinical signs. We hypothesised that the genetic profile of IMI-causing strains of *S. aureus* is associated with the likelihood of causing a chronic IMI versus an acute clinical IMI. To test this hypothesis, a prospective case-control study of 91 Canadian commercial dairy farms was initiated. The profiles of specific target genes are determined by multiplex PCR reactions on *S. aureus* isolated from chronic IMI (detected at the end of lactation [cases]) and from clinical IMI (controls) in the cohort. The preliminary analyses presented in this paper are of association of cases and controls with phenotypic expressions of haemolysis and biofilm formation, which are hypothesised to be related to expression of genes that are important in promoting subclinical chronic IMI. Isolates from 164 subclinical cases at the end of lactation and 82 clinical controls during lactation were studied. Expression of beta-haemolysis or weak beta-haemolysis was associated with subclinical infection (Odds ratio 2.1, 95% confidence interval 1.1 to 4.0). Isolates from subclinical IMI formed more biofilm than isolates from clinical IMI (P<0.01). Further examination of the *S. aureus* virulence genes and genotypes that are involved in controlling biofilm formation and beta-haemolysis is warranted in order to gain a more thorough understanding of how *S. aureus* establishes subclinical, and presumably chronic, infections. Knowing genetic markers for strains more likely to cause chronic IMI could enable targeted diagnostics, treatments or vaccination.

Keywords: beta-haemolysis, biofilm, genotyping, persistent infection, *Staphylococcus aureus*

Introduction

Staphylococcus aureus is one of the major pathogens causing bovine mastitis. Intramammary infection (IMI) by *S. aureus* is contagious and causes substantial financial losses. The pathogen has an advantage due to many strains' ability to infect chronically and persistently without severe clinical signs. It is known that some chronic *S. aureus* infections in humans are attributable to certain genetic virulence markers (Moisan *et al.*, 2006). A number of studies on *S. aureus* IMI have concentrated on the presence and role of different virulence factors (Aerestrup, 1995; Fitzgerald *et al.*, 1997; Middleton *et al.*, 2002) and the virulence factor relationship with the host (Zecconi *et al.*, 2005, 2006). We hypothesise that the likelihood of an *S. aureus* isolate causing a subclinical chronic IMI versus an acute clinical IMI is associated with its genetic profile and phenotypic expression of haemolysis and biofilm production.

Materials and methods

A case-control study of 91 farms participating in the National Cohort of Dairy Farms (NCDF) of the Canadian Bovine Mastitis Research Network during 2007 was conducted. These farms were from Ontario, Quebec, Alberta and the Atlantic provinces. Cases were those quarters with *S. aureus* IMI (≥100 colony forming units (cfu) per ml of milk in pure or mixed growth) within 30 days of dry-off with normal appearing milk. Controls were those quarters with *S. aureus* IMI (≥100 cfu per ml of milk in pure or mixed growth [2 colony types or more]) accompanied by abnormal milk, swollen quarters or fevers. Case and control IMI were enrolled sequentially as isolates and data became available through the CBMRN database and mastitis pathogen culture collection.

Mammary quarter milk samples were taken by study technicians using sterile technique and following a uniform protocol. Samples were frozen at -20 °C, submitted frozen to one of three milk bacteriology laboratories and kept frozen until bacteriological analysis. Bacteriological analyses were conducted following a uniform protocol for culture, identification and conservation of isolates. Culture and identification protocols were based on NMC guidelines. Haemolysis pattern of *S. aureus* on primary culture was recorded as alpha, beta, weak beta, or double zones of haemolysis or as non-haemolytic. Isolates were conserved in duplicate in the CBMRN Mastitis Pathogen Culture Collection at -80 °C in 1.5 ml of trypticase soy broth and 15% glycerol until further manipulations. All sampling, analysis, data capture and archiving, and isolate conservation procedures are documented in the CBMRN National Cohort Reference Manual (v. 10.9.07, CBMRN, St-Hyacinthe, QC).

The isolates available to date from case and control IMI selected via the NCDF database were sub-cultured from the culture collection vials, were inoculated on individual Columbia agar with 5% sheep blood plates and incubated for 18 hours at 35 °C. Two or three cfu were removed from these plates for biofilm formation testing and the plates transported under refrigeration to a collaborating laboratory for genetic analyses. The profiles of case and control *S. aureus* IMI isolates with respect to specific target genes will be determined by multiplex PCR reactions. The target genes were selected by earlier comparative genomic hybridisation studies of prototype and field *S. aureus* IMI strains that had been obtained from documented severe clinical IMI and chronic IMI cases (Jacob, 2008).

The cfu selected for biofilm formation testing were inoculated into BHI broth with 0.25% glucose and incubated for 18 to 24 hours at 35 °C. The broth culture was diluted 1:40 in BHI with 0.25 % glucose and 200μL replicates inoculated in four wells of a 96 well flat bottom tissue culture treated polystyrene microplate (353072, BD Falcon™ Clear 96-well Microtest™ Plate). The microplates were incubated 24 hours at 35 °C, washed 3 times with PBS 1x, air-dried at room temperature for 30 min., stained with 200 μl of crystal violet (0.1% in water) for 30 min. at room temperature, washed 3 times with water and allowed to dry at room temperature for 30 min. 150 μl of 95 % ethanol was added to each well, and the microplates were allowed to sit at room temperature for one hour and agitated occasionally to discolour the well contents. After discarding the ethanol, the optical density (OD) was determined at 570 nm wavelength by a 96 well automatic plate reader (EL800, Universal Microplate Reader – Bio-tek Instrument, Inc.) Each 96 well plate contained four replicates of 14 *S. aureus* case and control field isolates and four replicates of three reference bacterial strains: *S. epidermidis* ATCC35984, as a positive control for biofilm formation (Fox et al, 2005), *S. epidermidis* ATCC12228, as a negative control for biolilm formation (Fox et al, 2005), and *S. aureus* Newbold 305 as a known chronic IMI strain. Furthermore, each field isolate was assayed on two microplates. Any micro-well producing an OD beyond the microplate reader's maximum readable value of 3.0 was eliminated from calculations and statistical analyses. The average OD of replicates within microplate were calculated and the ratio of the field isolates' plate-average OD to the reference strains' plate-average OD were calculated. The ratios of the field isolates' plate-average OD to the respective reference strains' plate-average OD were averaged across the two microplate replications to obtain total average ratios of the field isolates to positive control, negative control, and Newbold 305.

Analyses of the associations between case or control status and the isolates' haemolysis expression and biofilm formation were carried out. Random effects of herd or quarter were not taken into consideration in these preliminary analyses. Plots of plate-average positive control and negative control pairs were examined to verify that positive control plate-average OD exceeded the corresponding negative control values. The differences between case and control field isolates' ratios to the three respective reference strains were tested by two sample t-tests for groups with unequal variances (Systat 10.0, SPSS Science Marketing Department, Chicago, IL.). Equality of the distribution of case and control isolates over all haemolysis patterns were tested by a χ^2 test of homogeneity with exact errors (StatXact 3.0. Cytel Software Corporation, Cambridge, MA). Case and control isolates' association with the presence of specific haemolysis patterns were analysed by estimated odds ratios and evaluating 95% mid-p exact confidence intervals.

Results

Phenotypic haemolysis differed between cases and controls (χ^2 = 11.29, exact P=0.02 with 4 degrees of freedom [df]). Alpha haemolysis occurred only among control isolates (2.4%) beta or weak-beta haemolysis was observed more frequently among case isolates (24% and 9.2%, respectively) than among control isolates (18% and 1.2%, respectively). Non-haemolysis was identically distributed between cases and controls (3.7%). Beta and weak beta haemolysis together were associated with case status, being two times more likely to occur in subclinical IMI at the end of lactation than in clinical IMI at any time during lactation (Table 1).

Biofilm formation by the positive control strain was greater than by the negative control strain bacteria or Newbold 305. Because a subjectively large number of negative control total average biofilm OD values were greater than their corresponding positive control values, our negative control was judged to be inappropriate negative control in this study. The ratio of biofilm formed by the case and control IMI *S. aureus* isolates to their corresponding positive controls (range = 0.90 to 1.63) and Newbold 305 references were moderately skewed (mean = 0.51, median = 0.40, and mean = 1.16 and median = 0.96, respectively), suggesting non-normal distribution of the biofilm ratios. Nevertheless, because non-parametric statistical analyses were quantitatively equivalent to the two-sample t-tests; only the latter t-test results are presented. The case group isolates' positive control biofilm ratios were distributed over a wider range and had a higher mean than the control group isolates' positive control biofilm ratios (Figure 1). Similarly, the case group isolates' biofilm formation relative to Newbold305 was also wider ranging and on average higher than that of the control group (Figure 1). Both of these differences were statistically significant (Table 2).

Table 1. Estimated odds ratios and confidence intervals of association of phenotypic haemolysis expression of S. aureus *isolated from intramammary infections with presentation as subclinical infection at end-of-lactation versus acute clinical infection at any time during lactation.*

Haemolysis		**Frequency**		**Odds ratio**	**95% confidence interval**[3]
Phenotype	**Present**	**Cases**[1]	**Controls**[2]		
Alpha	Yes	0	2	0.0	0.0, 1.7
	No	164	80		
Beta	Yes	40	15	1.4	0.8, 2.9
	No	124	67		
Beta and weak beta	Yes	55	16	2.1	1.1, 4.0
	No	109	66		
Double zone	Yes	103	61	0.6	0.3, 1.0
	No	61	21		

[1] Cases: Apparently subclinical S. aureus intramammary infection within 30 days of dry-off.
[2] Controls: Clinical S. aureus intramammary infection at any time during lactation with visible abnormality to the infected quarter or systemic abnormality.
[3] Mid-p exact confidence limits.

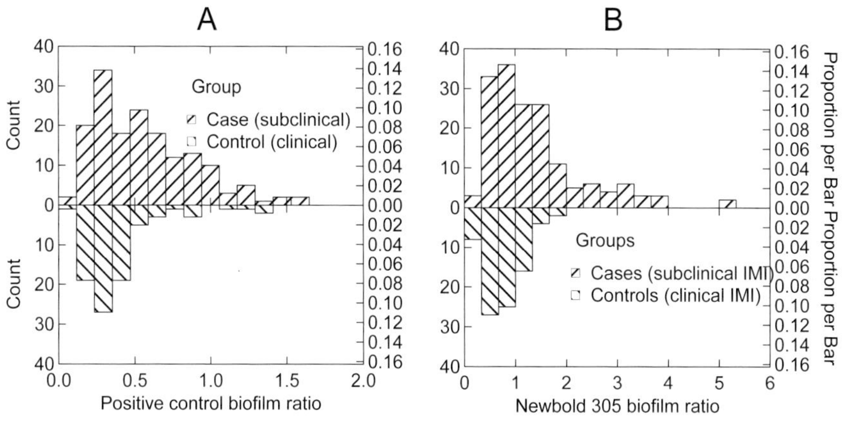

Figure1. Biofilm formation as a ratio to positive control (A) and to Newbold 305 (B) of Staphylococcus aureus *isolates from subclinical (cases) and clinical (controls) intramammary infections.*

Table 2. Differences in biofilm formation of S. aureus *isolated from subclinical intramammary infections (IMI) before dry-off (cases) or from clinical IMI during lactation (controls)as a ratio to a positive control biofilm-forming bacteria1 and to Staphylococcus aureus Neubold 305.*

Biofilm ratio denominator	**Mean (SD)**		**95% C.I. of mean differences**	**T–statistic[2] (df)**	***P***
	Cases (n=164)	**Controls (n=82)**			
Positive control[1]	0.56 (0.33)	0.39 (0.26)	0.10, 0.25	4.46 (203.5)	<0.01
Newbold 305	1.36 (0.94)	0.79 (0.36)	0.41, 0.74	6.85 (232.8)	<0.01

[1] *Staphylococcus epidermidis* (ATCC35984).
[2] Two-sample t-test with separate group variances.

Discussion

The objective of the analyses presented here were to explore the hypothesis that strains of *S. aureus* that cause bovine IMI vary in their tendency to cause subclinical, and presumably persistent, IMI, and that there exists phenotypic and genotypic markers these tendencies. An understanding of the molecular mechanisms for such a tendency and the ability to identify bacteria these bacteria or to preferentially prevent IMI by these bacteria would aid in the targeted reduction of chronic *S. aureus* IMI and a diminution of chronic subclinical IMI as a reservoir of the agent within herds. The present results are preliminary analyses of two phenotypic characteristics of the bacteria isolated from subclinical and clinical IMI occurrences. Although clustering of IMI within cows and within herds have not been taken into consideration in the analyses, the number of herds relative to the number of IMI suggest that a group effect of herd is not likely to qualitatively alter statistical results. Moreover, the sampling design eliminated repeat infections and multiple quarter IMI per cow was not substantial (data not shown).

The low level of alpha haemolysis among our isolates is different than reported elsewhere. Matsunaga *et al.* (1993), for example, observed 74% of 58 clinical *S. aureus* isolates producing alpha haemolysis after 18 hours of incubation on blood agar. The low proportion expressing alpha haemolysis means that the gene coding for alpha-haemolysin, *hla,* was infrequently present or was not expressed at primary culture. Haveri *et al.* (2007) found that 96% of isolates in a population of clinical IMI in Finland possessed *hla.* It was at one time suggested that alpha-haemolysin is a risk factor of gangrenous *S. aureus* mastitis (Anderson, 1983), but it is certainly not a necessary cause for clinical mastitis (Akineden *et al.*, 2001).

The beta haemolysis we observed was also lower than others' observations. Larsen *et al.* (2005) observed that 52% to 98% *S. aureus* isolated from mastitis in ten countries expressed beta-haemolysis, although case definitions from which the isolates were obtained were not presented. Assuming comparability between those populations studied and our study population, there is either more geographic variation to phenotypic beta-haemolysis expression than previously believed, phenotypic beta-haemolysin expression is influenced by *in-vitro* methodology, or *hlb* expression is quite variable. Our observation that phenotypic beta-haemolysis differs among our subclinical and clinical IMI isolates suggests a role for beta-haemolysin in establishing subclinical IMI or that beta-haemolysin expression is an incidental result of the expression of other virulence genes that render a strain more likely to cause subclinical. One might assume that a larger proportion of our pre-dry-off subclinical IMI are chronic than of our clinical IMI. In contrast to our results, Matsunaga *et al.* (1993) found 61% beta-haemolysis in isolates from acute and chronic cases, with no difference between the two. The role of beta-haemolysin in *S. aureus* mastitis pathogenesis is still not well elucidated, but our data make it clear that it is neither a necessary or sufficient cause for chronic *S. aureus* IMI. Under the conditions of our milk sampling regimen and milk bacteriology methods, beta-haemolysin production either increases the chance that the infection will be chronic and perhaps persistent, or it is incidental to gene expression controls that do play a role in establishing subclinical IMI. This might suggest activation of the *agr* complex in a particular way. Our phenotypic data do not permit distinguishing between differences in presence of *hlb,* the beta-haemolysin gene, or in control of the *hlb* expression.

Biofilm formation has often been suspected to play a role in *S. aureus'* ability to cause chronic IMI. Genetic control of biofilm formation involves a complex of genes (Oliviera *et al.*, 2006).

Our data show that the amount of biofilm formation is associated with *S. aureus* IMI being subclinical versus having a moderate to severe clinical presentation. Because many isolates from subclinical infections produced an amount of biofilm equivalent to the clinical isolates, it is clear that elevated biofilm production is not strictly essential for an infection to become chronic. It is also not clear to what extent *in-vivo* biofilm formation after cryopreservation and subculturing represents *in-vitro* biofilm formation. Further examination of the *S. aureus* virulence genes and genotypes that are involved in controlling biofilm formation is warranted in order to gain a more thorough understanding of how *S. aureus* establishes subclinical, and presumably chronic, infections. This understanding would also provide targets for strain-specific diagnosis of IMI by problematic strains and will provide a basis for exploring the host's role in *S. aureus* IMI presenting subclinically and becoming chronic.

References

Aerestrup, F.M., Dangler, C.A. and Sordillo, L.M., 1995. Prevalence of coagulase gene polymorphism in *Staphylococcus aureus* isolates causing bovine mastitis. Can. J. Vet. Res. 59: 124-128.

Akineden, O., Annemuller, C., Hassan, A.A., Lammler, C., Wolter, W. and Zschöck, M., 2001. Toxin genes and other characteristics of *Staphylococcus aureus* isolates from milk of cows with mastitis. Clin. Diagn. Lab. Immunol. 8: 959-964.

Anderson, J.C., 1983. Veterinary aspects of staphylococci. In: Staphylococci and Staphylococcal infections, vol. 1. Easmon, C.S.F. and Adlam, C. (Eds.) London: Academic Press, pp. 193-241.

Fitzgerald, J.R., Meaney, W.J., Hartigan, P.J., Smyth, C.J. and Kapur, V., 1997. Fine-structure molecular epidemiological analysis of *Staphylococcus aureus* recovered from cows. Epidemiol. Infect. 119: 261-269.

Fox, L.K., Zadoks, R.N. and Gaskins, C.T., 2005. Biofilm production by *Staphylococcus aureus* associated with intramammary infection. Vet. Microbiol. 107: 295-299.

Haveri, M., Roslö, A., Rantala, L. and Pyörälä, S., 2007. Virulence genes of bovine *Staphylococcus aureus* from persistent and nonpersistent intramammary infections with different clinical characteristics. J. Appl. Microbiol. 103: 993-1000.

Jacob, C. L., Lefebvre, B., Poirier, E., Roy, J.-P., Scholl, D., Malouin, F. 2008. Comparative Genomics and Virulence Potential of Staphylococcus aureus Isolates from Chronic Mastitis. American Society of Microbiology. 108th General Meeting. June 1- 5, 2008. Boston, MA. USA. Z-020.

Larsen, H.D., Aarestrup, F.M. and Jensen, N.E., 2002. Geographical variation in the presence of genes encoding superantigenic exotoxins and β-hemolysin among *Staphylococcus aureus* isolated from bovine mastitis in Europe and USA. Vet. Microbiol. 85: 61-67.

Matsunaga, T., Kamata, S., Kakiichi, N, and Uchida, K., 1993. Characteristics of *Staphylococcus aureus* isolated from peracute, acute and chronic bovine mastitis. J. Vet. Med. Sci. 55: 297-300.

Middleton, J.R., Fox, L.K., Gay, J.M., Tyler, J.W. and Besser, T.E., 2002. Use of pulsed-field gel electrophoresis for detecting differences in *Staphylococcus aureus* strain populations between dairy herds with different cattle importation practices. Epidemiol Infect 129, 387-395.

Moisan, H., Brouillette, E., Jacob, C.L., Langlois-Bégin, P. Michaud, S. and Malouin, F., 2006. Transcription of virulence factors in *Staphylococcus aureus* small-colony variants isolated from cystic fibrosis patients is influenced by sigb. J. Bact. 188: 64-76.

Oliveira, M., Bexiga, R., Nunes, S.F., Carneiro, C., Cavaco, L.M., Bernardo, F. and Vilela, C.L., 2006. Biofilm-forming ability profiling of *Staphylococcus aureus* and *Staphylococcus epidermidis* mastitis isolates. Vet. Microbiol. 118: 133-140.

Zecconi, A., Binda, E., Borromeo, V. and Piccinini, R., 2005. Relationship between some *Staphylococcus aureus* pathogenic factors and growth rates and somatic cell counts. J. Dairy Res. 72: 203-208.

Zecconi, A., Cesaris, L., Liandris, E., Daprà, V. and Piccinini, R., 2006. Role of several *Staphylococcus aureus* virulence factors on the inflammatory response in bovine mammary gland. Microbial. Pathogen. 40: 177-183.

Identification of bacteria associated with mastitis and poor hygiene in bovine farm tank milk

J.L.W. Rademaker
NIZO food research, P.O. Box 20, 6710 BA Ede, the Netherlands
Corresponding author: Jan.Rademaker@nizo.nl

Abstract

The presence of bacteria associated with poor farm hygiene and bovine mastitis was determined in farm tank milk using DNA-based methods. Random samples of raw farm (bulk) tank milk with high somatic cell counts (HSCC >400,000 cells/ml; n=25), high total bacterial counts (HTBC >100,000 cells/ml; n=25) and low (L)TBC (<10,000 cells/ml; n=42) were analysed. Sixteen samples tested positive with one or more quantitative real-time PCR assays targeting six groups of bacteria. Three positive test results were obtained from samples with HTBC. Thirteen positive tests were obtained from samples with HSCC. SCC is a key indicator of milk quality and is often used as an indirect measure of the overall amount of mastitis that a herd is experiencing. The three samples with HTBC tested PCR-positive for *Pseudomonas, Escherichia coli,* and *Enterococcus.* All LTBC samples tested negative. The thirteen PCR positive samples with HSCC all tested positive for *Pseudomonas*. In addition, these samples tested positive for bacteria that can be associated with mastitis and/or poor hygiene; two samples for *Staphylococcus aureus,* six samples for *Streptococcus uberis,* three samples for *E. coli,* and finally three samples for *Enterococcus.* In one sample *S. uberis* and *E. coli* were found. No samples were tested positive for *Streptococcus agalactiae*. In conclusion, bacterial flora associated with poor hygiene or mastitis was identified in 16 samples of raw farm tank milk. This supports the suitability of the use of DNA markers in a real-time PCR assay for specific analysis of the microbiological quality of raw milk. The high incidence of *Pseudomonas* in samples with HSCC indicates that these bacteria may be involved in a (secondary) infection of mastitis.

Keywords: diagnosis, monitoring, pathogens, PCR, *Pseudomonas*

Introduction

The aim of this study was to evaluate DNA markers in real time PCR assays, which target micro-organisms in raw milk, for rapid identification of the cause of increased bacterial counts in raw farm tank milk. Cows with mastitis may shed large numbers of bacteria whereas herds suspected of incling cows with clinical mastitis are usually identified by a high somatic cell count (HSCC). Fast identification of causes of increased bacterial numbers would offer new opportunities for accurate control measures and optimisation of farm management. Bacteria known to be associated with poor cattle housing hygiene (the genus *Pseudomonas*, *Enterococcus* and *Escherichia coli*) as well as micro-organisms associated with mastitis (*Staphylococcus aureus*, *Streptococcus agalactiae* and *Streptococcus uberis*) were therefore selected to be used as targets in real-time PCR assays.

Material and methods

Milk samples and DNA extraction

Random anonymous samples of raw farm (bulk) tank milk with a high somatic cell count (HSCC >400,000 cells/ml; n=25 encoded HSCC001-HSCC25), high total bacterial counts (HTBC >100,000 cells/ml; n=25 encoded HTBC001-HTBC025) and LTBC (<10.000 cells/ml; n=42), obtained from QLIP (earlier known as Melk Controle Station; Zutphen, the Netherlands), were analysed. From these samples, DNA was extracted from 1 ml milk that was cleared with 200 µl sterile 18% sodium citrate solution. After centrifugation and removal of the supernatant and fat layer, 200 µl Instagene was added to the pellet and treated according to the manufacturer's recommendation.

Real-time PCR tests

Six quantitative real-time PCR-tests based on literature were set up in our laboratory using an Applied Biosystems 7500 Fast Real-time PCR System in '9600 emulation mode' using TaqMan Universal PCR Master Mix (Applied Biosystems part number 5304437), primers at 200 nM and probes at 100 nM.

- *Pseudomonas*: A 65-bp fragment of the *Pseudomonas* SSU rRNA gene was amplified using a forward primer Pf (5'-GGGTGGTGGAATTTCCTGTGT), a reverse primer Pr (5'-GAAGCGGTGACCACAAGGAA) and an MGB-probe Pp (5'-GTGAAATGCGTAGATATAG) described earlier (Lloyd-Jones *et al.*, 2005). The applied temperature profile was: 2 min at 50 °C, 10 min at 95 °C, followed by 40 cycles of 15 s at 95 °C and 1 min at 60 °C.
- *Enterococcus*: A circa 130-bp fragment of the LSU rDNA, described as generic for all described species of the genus *Enterococcus*, was amplified using the forward primer ECST748F (5'-AGAAATTCCAAACGAACTTG), reverse primer ENC854R (5'-CAGTGCTCTACCTCCATCATT) and probe GPL813TQ (5'-6FAM-TGGTTCTCTCCGAAATAGCTTTAGGGCTA-TAMRA) as reported earlier (Haugland *et al.*, 2005). The applied temperature profile was: 2 min at 50 °C, 10 min at 95 °C, followed by 40 cycles of 15 s at 95 °C and 1 min at 60 °C.
- *Escherichia coli*: An *E. coli* specific fragment of the SSU rRNA gene was amplified using the forward primer EcoliFW (5'-CATGCCGCGTGTATGAAGAA), and the reverse primer EcoliRV (5'-CGGGTAACGTCAATGAGCAAA) and detected with the probe EcoliFAM (5'-6FAM-TATTAACTTTACTCCCTTCCTCCCCGCTGAA-TAMRA) as described earlier (Huisdens *et al.*, 2002). The applied temperature profile was: 2 min at 50 °C, 10 min at 95 °C, followed by 40 cycles of 15 s at 95 °C and 1 min at 60 °C.

Described below are three quantitative real-time PCR tests, specific for mastitis-causing pathogens, carried out simultaneously in one multiplex PCR-reaction. The applied temperature profile was: 2 min at 50 °C, 10 min at 95 °C, followed by 40 cycles of 15 s at 95 °C and 1 min at 60 °C as described earlier (Gillespie and Oliver, 2005):

- *Staphylococcus aureus*: A *S. aureus* specific genetic marker was detected using StaphAu-fwd primer (5'-TCAACGATATTCTTCACGACTAA), StaphAu-rev primer (5'-CCAGCTTCGGTACTACTAAAG) and probe StaphAu-probe (5'-6FAM-TCAAGACGGCTTTTACATACAGAACACA-BHQ2) as described earlier (Gillespie and Oliver, 2005).
- *Streptococcus agalactiae*: A fragment of the *cfb* gene encoding the Christie-Atkins-Munch-Petersen factor specific for *S. agalactiae* was detected using forward primer StrepAgal-fwd (5'-AGCTCTATTAGAAGTACATGCT), reverse primer StrepAgal-rev (5'-CATTTGCTGGGCTTGATTATT) and probe StrepAgal-probe (5'-TexasRed-ATCAAGTGACAACTCCACAAGTGGTAA-BHQ1) as described earlier (Gillespie and Oliver, 2005).
- *Streptococcus uberis*: The plasminogen activator gene of *S. uberis* was detected using forward primer StrepUberis-fwd (5'-AGAGGAATTCATCATGTTTTAACA), reverse primer StrepUberis-rev (5'-AATTGTAGAAGAACCATTTGATGT), and probe StrepUberis-probe (5'-Cy5-AGCGTCTAACAACTCGGCCTTTG-BHQ2), as described earlier (Gillespie and Oliver, 2005).

Reference cultures

From the NIZO culture collection 30 strains were selected (see Table 1) as positive and negative controls for the real-time PCR methods. A volume of 100 μl from fully-grown cultures of these strains was used for the DNA extraction using 200 μl Instagene according to the manufacturer's instructions.

PCR test detection limit and conversion to colony forming units per ml

The detection limit was determined using a dilution series of freshly cultured *Pseudomonas fluorescens* NIZO1372 cells. The concentration in colony forming units (cfu) per ml was determined using a plate count method. Based on these results the detection limits of the other bacteria (groups) were estimated. The detection limit of the different PCR tests is circa 10^2-10^3 cfu/ml.

Results and discussion

Six quantitative real-time PCR-tests targeting *Pseudomonas, E. coli, Enterococcus, S. aureus, S. uberis* en *S. agalactiae* were evaluated for specificity using 30 reference strains. All PCR tests showed a high specificity and no cross-reaction (Table 1), with the exception of the *S. aureus* and *S. uberis* PCR tests that showed a low cross-reaction with *S. agalactiae* DNA. All

Table 2. Number of raw farm tank milk samples tested positive with one or more real-time PCR tests.

	All tests	*Enterococcus*	*Pseudomonas*	*S. aureus*	*S. uberis*	*S. agalactiae*	*E. coli*
LTBC (n=42)	-	-	-	-	-	-	-
HTBC (n=25)	3	3	3	-	-	-	1
HSCC (n=25)	13	3	13	2	6	-	3

LTBC: Low Total Bacterial Count (Bactoscan count), <10,000 cfu/ml; HTBC: High Total Bacterial Count (Bactoscan count), >100,000/ml; HSCC: High Somatic Cell Count, >400,000 cells/ml.

high concentrations, of 4×10^4 up to 2×10^7 cfu/ml. This may even suggest that these bacteria could result from a (secondary) infection of mastitis, as has been described earlier (Hillerton and Berry, 2005; Rendos *et al.*, 1975; Watts, 1988).

The use of DNA markers in a real-time PCR is applicable for specific analysis of the microbiological quality of raw milk and may have potential for mastitis diagnostics based on (individual) cow milk samples. In 16 samples of raw farm tank milk it was possible to identify two or three bacteria (groups) which can be associated with poor hygiene, insufficient refrigeration, or mastitis. Apparently, other dominant bacteria (groups) were present in the 22 out of 25 samples milk with a HTBC that were negative for all six PCR tests. To obtain a more complete picture of the dominant bacterial flora, additional tests for dominant bacterial (groups) are necessary to complement the set of six tests used in this study. More research into the association of bacteria with their specific origins of contamination is important for use of the current approach to optimise farm management.

Conclusion

Several dominant bacterial groups were found with real-time PCR tests applied to evaluate farm tank milk samples with high somatic and bacterial cell count. *Pseudomonas* was found most often and in high concentrations (10^4-10^7 cfu/ml). Remarkably this genus was found particularly in samples with HSCC, possibly as a result of infection. The shown ability to detect *S. aureus* and *S. uberis* and to differentiate these species in samples with a HSCC demonstrates the potential of these tests for mastitis diagnostics in milk. In 22 out of 25 samples with a HTBC and in 12 out of 25 samples with HSCC no positive responses in six PCR tests were observed; apparently many bacterial groups remained undetected.

In conclusion, the dominant bacterial flora associated with poor hygiene or mastitis was identified in 16 samples of raw milk. This supports the suitability of the use of DNA markers targeted in a real-time PCR assay for specific analysis of the microbiological quality of raw milk. Moreover the results may suggest that *Pseudomonas* is a genus that is underestimated in standard mastitis testing, or is in a different way associated with mastitis or other causes of HSCC.

Acknowledgements

I gratefully acknowledge Jan Hoolwerf and Arjen Wagendorp for excellent technical support and Meike te Giffel, Marjon Wells-Bennik and Frank Driehuis for critically reading this manuscript.

References

Gillespie, B.E. and Oliver, S.P., 2005. Simultaneous Detection of Mastitis Pathogens, *Staphylococcus aureus, Streptococcus uberis,* and *Streptococcus agalactiae* by Multiplex Real-Time Polymerase Chain Reaction. J. Dairy Sci. 88: 3510-3518.

Haugland, R.A., Siefring, S.C., Kristen, L.J., Brenner, P. and Dufour, A.P., 2005. Comparison of *Enterococcus* measurements in two recreational beaches by quantitative polymerase reaction and membrane filter culture analysis. Water Res. 39: 559-568.

Hillerton, J.E. and Berry, E.A., 2005. Treating mastitis in the cow – a tradition or an archaism. J. Appl. Microbiol. 98: 1250-1255.

Huisdens, X.W., Linskens, R.K., Meuwissen, S.G., Vandenbroucke-Grauls, C.M. and Savelkoul, P.H., 2002. Quantification of bacteria adherent to gastrointestinal mucosa by real-time PCR. J. Clin. Microbiol. 40: 4423-4427.

Lloyd-Jones, G., Laurie, A.D. and Tizzard, A.C. 2005. Quantification of the *Pseudomonas* population in New Zealand soils by fluorogenic PCR assay and culturing techniques. J. Microbiol. Meth. 60: 217-224.

Rendos, J.J., Eberhardt, R.J. and Kesler, E.M., 1975. Microbial populations of the teat ends of dairy cows and bedding materials. J. Dairy Sci. 58: 1492-1500

Watts, J.L., 1988. Etiological agents of bovine mastitis. Vet. Microbiol. 16: 41-66.

Analytical detection limit of the PathoProof™ Mastitis PCR Assay determined using two different experimental approaches

M.T. Koskinen, J. Holopainen, L. Salmikivi, H. Lehmusto, S. Niskala and J. Kurkela
Finnzymes Oy, Keilaranta 16A, 02150 Espoo, Finland
Corresponding author: mikko.koskinen@finnzymes.fi

Abstract

The PathoProof Mastitis PCR Assay is a real-time PCR based reagent kit for identification of all major mastitis-causing pathogens. Here, we report on the analytical bacterial detection limit of the assay using two different experimental approaches. We first used purified DNA to prepare a standard dilution series from 450 to less than one genome copy of the assay's bacterial targets and determined how many copies of each target could be detected by the test with >95% probability. In our second experiment, we measured sensitivity of the entire assay, including the DNA extraction procedure from raw milk samples. For this experiment, ten mastitis milk samples, shown to be negative for the tested targets, were randomly chosen, spiked with known quantities of the target bacterial colony forming units (cfu) and analysed using the assay. When sensitivity was measured based on the dilution series of purified DNA, the analytical detection limit of the test was as low as 5.6 bacterial genomes per PCR reaction. When using mastitis milk samples spiked with the bacterial targets, the detection limit was as low as <200 cfu's per one milliliter of milk. Both experiments showed much variation in the detection limit of the test between the different bacterial targets. In conclusion, the results of this study demonstrate that the PathoProof Mastitis PCR Assay can detect low quantities of bacterial DNA, which is important for the mastitis testing laboratories now complementing or replacing bacterial culture based testing schemes with the assay. Variation in the detection limit between the different bacterial targets is explained by a combination of the biological characteristics of the bacteria and details related to the molecular specifications of the assay. This presentation discusses these variables as well as some of the challenges involved in detection limit validation of a PCR test in a controlled manner when using raw bovine milk as a sample matrix.

Keywords: detection limit, diagnosis, DNA extraction, PCR

Introduction

Intramammary infection (IMI), also commonly known as mastitis, is the most frequently occurring and economically the most important infectious disease in dairy cattle. Bacterial culture has long served as the golden standard for mastitis testing. However, several studies have suggested that Polymerase Chain Reaction (PCR)-based assays could be useful to complement or to replace the conventional bacteriological IMI identification methods (e.g.

Riffon *et al.*, 2001). Among the primary arguments in favour of PCR assays are their short throughput times, potential for objective and user-independent identification of bacteria and antibiotic resistance genes, and ability for sensitive detection of growth-inhibited and dead bacteria. A modification of PCR, known as real-time PCR, may offer further benefits to quantify the microbial load in the milk samples, to facilitate automation of the laboratory workflow, and to reduce the risk of PCR cross-contaminations in the laboratory. Among the first commercially available PCR-based mastitis tests is the 'PathoProof Mastitis PCR Assay', which uses real-time PCR to identify a total of 11 mastitis-causing bacterial species or species groups and the blaZ gene coding for staphylococcal β-lactamase production, i.e. penicillin resistance (Finnzymes Oy, Espoo, Finland). Here, we report on experiments assessing the analytical bacterial detection limit of the assay based on two different approaches: (1) detection limit in bacterial genome copy equivalents in PCR reaction; and (2) detection limit in bacterial colony forming units in milk originating from cows with clinical mastitis.

Materials and methods

Real-Time PCR Assay

The PathoProof™ Mastitis PCR Assay included all necessary reagents for DNA extraction and real-time PCR. The assay targeted the following bacterial species and groups: (1) *Staph. aureus*; (2) *Staph.* spp. including *Staph. aureus, Staph. intermedius* and all major mastitis-causing CNS; (3) *Streptococcus agalactiae*; (4) *Str. dysgalactiae*; (5) *Str. uberis*; (6) *Escherichia coli*; (7) *Enterococcus* spp. including *E. faecalis* and *E. faecium*; (8) *Klebsiella* spp. including *K. oxytoca* and *K. pneumoniae*; (9) *Corynebacterium bovis*; (10) *Arcanobacterium pyogenes* and *Peptoniphilus indolicus*; (11) *Serratia marcescens*; and (12) β-lactamase penicillin resistance gene. The assay identified *Staph.* spp., *Enterococcus* spp., *Klebsiella* spp. and *A. pyogenes / P. indolicus* to their species group levels, i.e. for example *E. faecalis* and *E. faecium* were identified in the same real-time PCR reaction and instrument channel.

The assay's protocol involved four separate multiplex real-time PCR reactions, each of which targeted three bacterial species or species groups and an internal amplification control (IAC). The following real-time PCR instruments were used for: ABI 7500 Fast Real-Time PCR System (Applied Biosystems), Bio-Rad Chromo 4 (Bio-Rad Laboratories) and Stratagene Mx Pro 3000P (Agilent Technologies). A negative control (dH_2O) was included in every real-time PCR run and each multiplex PCR reaction, for confirmation that cross-contaminations had not occurred in the laboratory.

Detection limit in genome copy equivalents

DNA was extracted and purified from culture isolates representing the target species of the PathoProof Mastitis PCR Assay. DNA concentration of the extracts was measured using

standard spectrophotometric procedures. The DNA concentrations were converted to genome copy numbers as follows:
N (copies) = [Na * m (g)] / [M (g/mol) * L (bp)]
Na = $6.022*10^{23}$ (Avogadro´s constant)
M = 649 g/mol per base pair

A 10x dilution series of the extracted DNA was prepared in dH_2O. The dilutions were calculated to contain 450-0.6 genome copies / µl concentration of bacterial DNA. Each dilution (for each bacterial target) was analysed with the assay in 24 replicate reactions. The positive and negative results obtained for the dilutions were used to calculate the detection limit of the assay in bacterial genome copies per PCR.

Detection limit in cfu/ml of milk

The PathoProof Mastitis PCR Assay was used to analyse fresh milk samples from cows with clinical mastitis. Based on the results, ten mastitis milk samples providing negative results were selected for each bacterial species targeted by the assay. Culture isolates representing the target species of the assay were used to prepare a dilution series of bacteria in dH_2O. The dilutions were used to spike the ten milk samples that were shown to be negative for the respective target species. The dilutions were then cultured on blood agar plates to find out the number of cfu's spiked into the PCR reactions. It should be noted that the initial cfu amounts in the cultures used for preparing the dilution series were not known prior to plating. Hence, the exact amounts of cfu's present in the spiking experiments had some variation.

Results and discussion

The detection limit of the PathoProof Mastitis PCR Assay in genome copy equivalents was 5.5-50 bacterial genomes per PCR reaction, depending on the bacterial species targeted by the kit ($P \leq 0.05$; Table 1). In other words, these copy numbers of bacterial DNA pipetted into the real-time PCR reaction were detected with >95% probability (at least 23 of the 24 replicate reactions provided positive results). Figure 1 exemplifies, for *Staph. aureus,* the frequency of positive results across the 24 replicate reactions as a function of the number of genome copies present in PCR. Variation observed in the genome copy detection limits of the different bacteria can be due to at least two factors. First, the purity of the DNA used in the experiment (amount of PCR inhibitors) perhaps varied between the targets, leading to variation in PCR inhibitor concentration and/or inaccurate spectrophotometric readings in determination of the initial bacterial genome copy numbers. Second, the PCR efficiencies of the different target amplicons are different. It is not surprising that the effect of these two possibilities becomes apparent especially with low genome copy numbers (late Ct values) and in demanding multiplex PCR reactions (each multiplex PCR reaction of the assay has four target amplicons).

Table 1. Analytical detection limit of the PathoProof PCR Assay in bacterial genome copies per PCR reaction.

Bacterial target of the assay	Analytical sensitivity in bacterial genome copy number per PCR ($p<0.05$)
Staph. aureus	16.7
Enterococcus spp.	50
C. bovis	16.7
β-lactamase gene	50
E. coli	50
Str. dysgalactiae	16.7
Staphylococcus spp.	16.7
Str. agalactiae	5.6
Str. uberis	16.7
Klebsiella spp.	5.6
S. marcescens	50
A. pyogenes / P. indolicus	50

In our experiments, the lowest dilution of bacterial CFUs spiked into mastitis milk turned out to correspond to 200-810 cfu/ml of milk (variation between the target species was due to initial variation in bacterial concentrations used for preparing the dilution series). When analysing the samples with the PathoProof Mastitis PCR Assay, the results confirmed a clear association between the Ct values of the assay and the amount of bacteria spiked. In other words, the higher the amount of bacteria present in the milk samples, the lower the Ct value obtained with the assay (results are exemplified for *Staph. aureus* in Figure 1). This was the case for all bacterial targets, confirming the assay's accuracy in bacterial quantification.

The PathoProof Mastitis PCR Assay provided positive results for milk samples in the lowest cfu dilution for all bacterial targets, except for *Serratia marcescens*. While the real-time PCR efficiency for *S. marcescens* is excellent (~100%; data not shown) and 50 genome copies per PCR were detected in this study (Table 1), the spiking experiments for the species failed for an unknown reason. The experiment is currently being repeated for *S. marcescens* and will not be discussed further in this presentation. The lowest Ct values obtained for the lowest cfu dilution varied between 27.7 (*Staph.* spp.) and 36.5 (*K. oxytoca*). The average Ct values obtained for the different bacterial targets versus the CFU count in mastitis milk are shown in Figure 2.

Ct value variation across the ten milk samples for each CFU dilution was substantial within each bacterial target, as exemplified for *Staph. aureus* in Figure 3. This effect was most

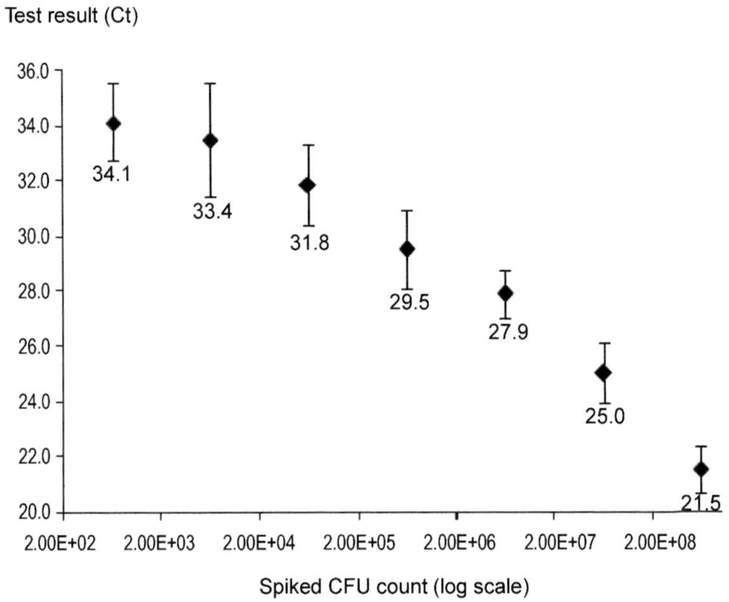

Figure 1. Association of Ct values provided by the PathoProof Mastitis PCR Assay with CFU count in mastitis milk for Staph. aureus. *Each point represents the average Ct value across the ten mastitis milk samples spiked using one bacterial dilution. For* Staph. aureus, *the dilution series corresponded to 630...6.3x108 cfu/ml of milk. The error bars are standard deviations of the Ct values across the ten mastitis milk samples.*

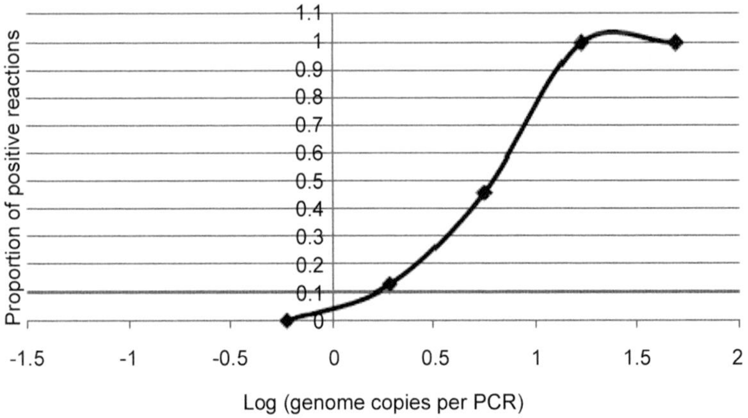

Figure 2. Average Ct values obtained from the PathoProof PCR Assay for the different cfu dilutions spiked into mastitis milk. For the sake of clarity, the dilutions within each category have been rounded to 500...5000000 cfu/ml, although the dilutions in each category had some variation (in the lowest dilution '500 cfu/ml' the values varied between 200 and 810 cfu/ml).

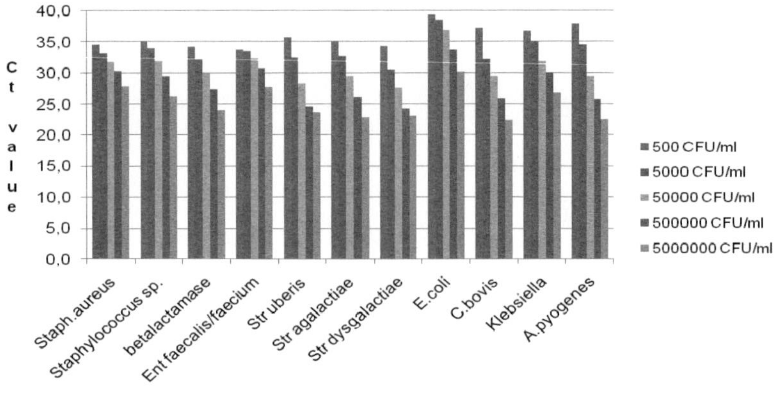

Figure 3. Analytical detection limit of the PathoProof Mastitis PCR Assay in bacterial genome copies per PCR reaction for Staph. aureus. *'Proportion of positive reactions' indicates the percentage of positive results from 24 replicate runs of the assay with the given genome copy numbers added into the PCR reactions. For* Staph. aureus *the analytical detection limit corresponds to 16.7 genomes per PCR.*

likely primarily due to variation in the composition of the different mastitis milk samples. Also variation in Ct between the different species was substantial within each CFU dilution (Figure 2). When interpreting this result, it must be remembered that all of the milk samples were different, i.e. the 10 milk samples used e.g. for *Staph. aureus* experiment were different than those used e.g. for *E. coli,* perhaps explaining some of the differences. Another possible explanation is that some species targeted by the assay (e.g. *Staph. aureus*) can include multiple (up-to hundreds) of genomes per one colony, while for some others (e.g. *E. coli*) this is not the case. As the PCR assay identifies bacterial DNA instead of colonies, this variable can alone result in 100-fold differences in cfu detection limits of the PCR test for the different pathogens. Furthermore, as explained above, the PCR efficiencies for the different target amplicons have some variation, which may influence the Ct values observed, especially in the late cycles. Finally, it is also possible that the different species are harvested with slightly different efficiency by the DNA extraction procedure applied by the assay.

Detection limits of commercially available real-time PCR-based pathogen identification kits are commonly measured in genome copy equivalents per PCR reaction. While this is a simple and straightforward measure suitable for estimating the efficiency of the PCR step, we argue that it has limited relevance in the case of mastitis and in the case of any application involving samples containing high amounts of PCR inhibitors. In IMI identification, the sample matrix is typically milk, which exhibits a range of PCR inhibitors and much variation in composition across all clinical and subclinical cases. Therefore, DNA extraction is an integral step determining the detection limit of an assay.

In this study, we have taken the approach of using bacterial cells spiked into multiple mastitis milk samples, and investigating how many cfu's are detected per ml of milk. This approach has the benefit that it makes use of cells that undergo the entire assay including DNA extraction (use of pure genomic DNA would not mimic the 'real-life' situation as well, as DNA may behave differently in extraction procedures than bacterial cells). However, this approach has a number of variables that make comparison of the results between the target species difficult, some of which are discussed above. Furthermore, correlating the results observed in this study with the detection limit of the conventional bacterial culture methods in real IMI testing schemes has an added complication that bacterial cells may have decreased viability to grow in culture when arriving to a laboratory. Perhaps due to this reason, up-to 50% of milk samples have been reported to exhibit no growth in culture (e.g. Makovec and Ruegg, 2003). In the current study, dilution series of bacterial cells prepared in water was used for calculating the number of cfu's, which likely decreased cfu detection limit estimates for the PCR assay in comparison to real clinical milk samples undergoing transportation to a laboratory.

In conclusion, while the results of this study demonstrate that the PathoProof PCR Assay has potential to identify as few as ~5 bacterial genomes per PCR or ~200 cfu of bacteria per ml of milk, variation exists between the pathogens targeted by the test. While the assay has been demonstrated to provide quantitative results (Figure 1), comparison of the Ct values against CFU numbers in milk is far from simple and may not even be possible. It must be emphasised that an analytical detection limit of a molecular assay should not be mixed with its clinical sensitivity. The assay's clinical sensitivity is best studies by field trials whereby the same mastitis milk samples are analysed using bacterial culturing and the PCR test. Such experiments are currently underway in many countries.

References

Riffon, R., Sayasith, K., Khalil, H., Dubreuil, P., Drolet, M. and Lagace, J., 2001. Development of a rapid and sensitive test for identification of major pathogens in bovine mastitis by PCR. J. Clin. Microbiol. 39: 2584-2589.

Makovec, J.A. and Ruegg, P.L., 2003. Results of milk samples submitted for microbiological examination in Wisconsin from 1994 to 2001. J. Dairy Sci. 86: 3466-3472.

Phenotypic and molecular identification of *Streptococcus* species isolated from milk of intramammary infected dairy cows in Austria

M. Gonano[1] and P. Winter[1,2]
[1]Institute of Milk Hygiene, Milk Technology and Food Science, Department for Farm Animals and Veterinary Public Health, University of Veterinary Medicine Vienna, Veterinärplatz 1, 1210 Vienna, Austria
[2]Institute for Veterinary Disease Control, Austrian Agency for Health and Food Safety, Robert Kochgasse 17, 2340 Moedling, Austria
Corresponding author: petra.winter@ages.at

Abstract

Streptococcal species, especially *Streptococcus uberis,* are one of the most significant pathogens causing intramammary infections in dairy cattle and responsible for considerable economic loss. The identification of streptococci concentrates on serological Lancefield grouping and analysis of biochemical activity. But it is well known that different species are able to express the same Lancefield group antigen or are not serological groupable. To study the distribution of *Streptococcus* species we collected 195 gram-positive and catalase negative cocci on blood-agar plates isolated from subclinical and clinical mastitis cases in dairy cows in Austria. After serogrouping and identification to the species level by API 20 Strep kit, the strains were investigated by a multiplex PCR to differentiate seven relevant streptococcal species. Not type-able isolates were transferred to another PCR to examine the enterococci and lactococci strains. Phenotypic and molecular identification was in accordance in 54.9% of the strains. Biochemical typing revealed to following distribution: 37.4% enterococci, 27.7% *S. uberis,* 10.3% lactococci, 8.2% *S. dysgalactiae,* 4.6% *Aerococcus* spp., 3.6% *S. agalactiae* and 2.6% other streptococci. PCR identification was more precise: 20.5% enterococci, 44.1% *S. uberis,* 13. % lactococci, 7.2% *S. dysgalactiae,* 3.1% *S. bovis,* 1.5% *S. agalactiae,* 1.0% *S. canis,* 0.5% *S. parauberis* and 8.7% non type-able strains. This shows that a reliable biochemical differentiation of *Streptococcus* species is difficult and fails to detect *S. uberis* infections. Conventional routine diagnostics have to be improved to give precise information on species level for establishing farm specific mastitis prevention programs.

Keywords: API Strep, diagnosis, pathogens, PCR, *Streptococcus uberis*

Introduction

Mastitis remains the most economically important disease of dairy cattle throughout the world, with the three streptococcal pathogens, *Streptococcus agalactiae, S. dysgalactiae, S. uberis* and *Staphylococcus aureus* being among the most significant pathogens involved. Although mastitis control programmes, based on improved milking practice and teat dipping have achieved dramatic reductions in the incidence of contagious mastitis caused by *S. agalactiae* and *Staphylococcus aureus,* these measures have had little impact on environmental pathogens, notably *S. uberis* and *Escherichia coli* (Tomita *et al.*, 2008).

A correct identification to species level of the bacterial pathogens causing bovine mastitis is of clinical and epidemiological interest. This knowledge helps in the development of preventive strategies and special treatment schemes. In routine bacteriological laboratories, mastitis causing bacteria are usually identified by conventional identification systems, which are more time-consuming and less precise. The inability to identify 1-10% of isolates because of atypical test results is reported by numerous authors (Zschöck *et al.*, 2005).

The present study was designed to gain more knowledge about the mastitis causing streptococci and to compare the conventional method and a multiplex PCR method for identification and differentiation of streptococci isolated from bovine intramammary infections in Austrian dairy herds.

Material and methods

In total, 195 gram-positive and catalase negative isolates were obtained from quarter milk samples of dairy cattle in Austria. The cows were suffering either from subclinical or clinical mastitis in at least one quarter. Clinical mastitis was defined as the presence of clots in milk or visible signs of inflammation in the mammary glands. Cows were considered to have subclinical mastitis if the quarter somatic cell count was >250,000 cells/ml (California Mastitis Test showed +++ reactions) but had no clinical signs of mastitis. Quarter milk samples were plated onto Columbia agar (containing 5% sheep blood). Agar plates were incubated for 48 h at 37 °C and examined after 24 h and 48 h of incubation. Bacterial examination was conducted according to NMC (1999) recommendations.

Conventional and biochemical examination

195 gram positive and catalase negative isolates were further differentiated by means of Lancefield serogrouping (streptococcal grouping kit, Oxoid, Basingstone, UK), esculin reactions and hemolysis. Biochemical tests were performed on all streptococcal isolates with the API 20 STREP system as recommended by the manufacturer (BioMérieux, Marcy l`Etoile, France). Fermentations were read after 4 h and 24 h. Data were analysed by using the apiweb™ system (Version V7.0). Strain identification to the species level was divided into four subgroups, by using the manufacturer defined variables (%id and *T*-value): (1) excellent species identification, %id of ≥99.9% and a *T*-value of ≥0.75, (2) very good species identification, %id of ≥99.0% and a *T*-value of ≥0.5, (3) good species identification, id% of ≥90% and a *T*-value of ≥0.25 and (4) acceptable species identification, %id of ≥80% *T*-value of ≥0. Isolates with a %id ≤80% were classified as not acceptable or as isolates with low selectivity.

Additionally following reference strains were comparatively investigated: *Streptococcus agalactiae* (DSM 2134), *Streptococcus bovis* (DSM 20480), *Streptococcus canis* (DSM 20715), *Streptococcus dysgalactiae* ssp. *dysgalactiae* (DSM 20662), *Streptococcus dsygalactiae* ssp. *equisimilis* (DSM 6176), *Streptococcus parauberis* (DSM 6631), *Streptococcus porcinus* (DSM 20725) and *Streptococcus uberis* (DSM 20569) obtained from the German collection of Microorganisms and Cell Cultures (DSM).

Molecular biological examination

Genomic DNA was isolated from 1-ml volumes of an overnight culture at 37°C in BHI using the Nucleospin® Tissue kit (Macherly-Nagel, Düren, Germany) in accordance with the manufacturers instructions. The concentration was determined in a Hoefer DyNA Quant 200 apparatus (Pharmacia, Biotech, San Francisco, CA, USA) and adjusted with ddH_2O to a final concentration of 0,1 ng/µl. Species identification of Streptococci was done in two different sets of multiplex PCR with species specific primers for *S. agalactiae, S. bovis, S. canis, S. dsygalactiae, S. equi, S. porcinus, S. uberis* and *S. suis* (type I + type II) as published previously (Kawata *et al.*, 2004). Primers were obtained from MWG Biotech (Ebersberg, Germany). Strains without a species specific amplification product in multiplex PCR were transferred to a PCR for detection of *Enterococcus spp.* and to a PCR for *Lactococcus spp.* using genus-specific primer pairs, according to Deasy *et al.* (2000). All PCR amplifications were carried out in a GeneAmp®System 9700 (Applied Biosystems, Foster City, CA, USA).

Results

The examined isolates were obtained from 79 clinical mastitis cases (40.5%) and from 116 subclinical mastitis cases (59.5%).

Isolate identification by routine diagnostic

The identification by means of Lancefield serogrouping revealed following distribution: 3 (1.5%) isolates of serogroup B, 27 (13.9%) of serogroup C, 40 (20.5%) of serogroup D and 2 (1.0%) of serogroup G. A total of 123 (63.1%) isolates showed no agglutination with the used serogroups (A, B, C, D, F, G). Out of this isolates 19 (15.5%) showed negative β- hemolysis combined with positive esculin reaction and were assigned to the species *S. uberis.*

Isolate identification by API 20 STREP system

All reference strains, except *S. parauberis* (DSM 6631) were correctly identified to species level. API 20 STREP testing revealed that out of 195 isolates tested, 90 (46.2%) belonged to the Genus *Streptococcus*, 73 (37.4%) isolates were identified as *Enterococcus* spp., 20 (10.3%) as *Lactococcus* spp., 9 (4.6%) as *Aerococcus* spp., 2 (1.0%) as *Granulicatella spp.* and the remaining one (0.5%) as *Leuconostoc* spp. The API 20 STREP system yielded excellent, very good, good and acceptable species identification for 46 (23.6%), 45 (23.1%), 69 (35.4%) and 16 (8.2%) isolates. Nineteen isolates (9.7%) were classified as low selective, respectively as not acceptable.

Isolate identification by PCR

All reference strains revealed a unique amplified DNA fragment. An amplificat of 1100 bp was obtained for *S. parauberis* DSM 6631, with the primers used in Multiplex PCR. By PCR based methods 112 (57.4%) *Streptococcus* spp., 40 (20.5%) *Enterococcus* spp., and 26 (13.3%) *Lactococcus* spp. were identified. Seventeen (8.7%) isolates remained not identified, they belonged to non target species in PCR.

Multiplex PCR of 112 *Streptococcus* spp. showed following distribution: 86 (76.8%) *S. uberis*, 14 (12.5%) *S. dysgalactiae*, 3 (2.7%) *S. agalactiae*, 6 (5.4%) *S. bovis*, 2 (1.8%) *S. canis*, 1 (0.9%) *S. parauberis*. One isolate (0.9%) was determined as *S. parauberis*, because it displayed the same amplicon size (1100 bp) as the reference strain of *S. parauberis* (DSM 6631). Comparison of the *S. parauberis* gene for 23S rRNA (accession no. X68036 in the GenBank database) to the used oligonucleotide primers published by Kawata *et al.* (2004), showed a sequence homology of 100% and 95% to the forward primer of *S. uberis* and the reverse primer of *S. canis*. As expected, none of the mastitis isolates developed a species-specific amplicon for *S. suis* or *S. equi*. One-hundred-twenty isolates (61.5 %) shared the same genus in PCR and API 20 STREP results. Out of the 112 detected *Streptococcus* spp. only 63 (56.2%) isolates performed an equal result.

Based on the PCR identification out of the 79 clinical mastitis cases, 36 were caused by *S. uberis*, 15 by enterococci and 10 by lactococci, respectively.

Discrepancy between the different methods

The distribution of *Streptococcus* and *Enterococcus* species identified by API Strep and multiplex PCR is described in Table 1 and 2. The identification of enterococci by routine diagnostics was not in accordance in 22 strains (55.0 %, Table 1). Comparing the results achieved by routine diagnostics, biochemical and molecular biological identification a discrepancy of 43.0 and 84.9% can be seen for *S. uberis*, respectively (Table 2). Reliable results can be obtained in routine diagnostics for *S. agalactiae* (0%) and *S. dysgalactiae* (28.5%).

Discussion

Our results showed, Lancefield serogrouping is an accurate method for typing group B streptococci or *S. agalactiae* and also group G streptococci or *S. canis*, because of their relative consistent serological properties (Facklam, 2002). Nevertheless serogrouping is not a helpful tool in mastitis diagnostics, because the major group of isolated streptococci belongs to *S.*

Table 1. Identification of genus Enterococcus spp. by serogrouping, API 20 Strep and PCR and the identified discrepancy (n, %).

Species	Number (%) of identified isolates				
	Routine diagnostic	API 20 Strep	PCR	Discrepancy	
				API 20 Strep vs. PCR	Routine diagnostic vs. PCR
Enterococcus spp.	40 (20.5)	73 (37.4)	40 (20.5)	11 (27.5)	22 (55.0)
E. avium		7			
E. faecalis		50			
E. faecium		14			
E. durans		2			

Table 2. Identification of genus Streptococcus spp. by serogrouping, API 20 Strep and PCR and the identified discrepancy (n, %).

Species	Number (%) of identified isolates				
	Routine diagnostic	API 20 Strep	PCR	Discrepancy	
				API 20 Strep vs. PCR	Routine diagnostic vs. PCR
S. agalactiae	3	7	3	0 (0.0)	0 (0.0)
S. bovis	0	5	6	4 (66.7)	6 (100.0)
S. canis	2	0	2	2 (100.0)	0 (0.0)
S. dysgalactiae	27	16	14	5 (35.7)	4 (28.6)
S. parauberis	0	0	1	1 (100.0)	1 (100.0)
S. porcinus	0	6	0	0 (0.0)	0 (0.0)
S. uberis	19	54	86	37 (43.0)	73 (84.9)
S. mutans	0	1	0	0 (0.0)	0 (0.0)
S. equinus	0	1	0	0 (0.0)	0 (0.0)
Genus *Streptococcus*	51 (26.2)	90 (46.2)	112 (57.4)	49	84

uberis, a biochemical extremely variable species. According to Lämmler (1991) and Khan *et al.* (2003) serological investigation of *S. uberis* revealed antigens of E, G, P and U. Difficulties exist also for *S. dysgalactiae*, because of its well known serological diversity (Vandamme *et al.*, 1996). This can be confirmed in our study. The percentage of *S. uberis* isolates (27.7%) detected with the API 20 STREP system is close to data published by Devriese (1999), while the frequency of *Enterococcus spp.* (37.4%) is higher in our study than reported by Gillespie *et al.* (1997). The distribution of the remaining streptococci was variable. Unfortunately, only few data from others concerning distribution of gram positive catalase negative cocci isolated from bovine mastitis milk developed with molecular based methods are available. Gillespie *et al.* (1997) found 65% *S. uberis*, 20% *S. dysgalactiae*, 6% *S. agalactiae* and only 0.6% Enterococci in 163 milk samples of dairy cows using randomly amplified polymorphic DNA (RAPD) fingerprinting method, and agreement of data with the API 20 STREP about 91%. In our study the low accordance (54.9%) between the API 20 STREP and the molecular results is confirmed by Bosshard (2004), who found 39.2% discrepancy in comparison to molecular methods. A misidentification of enterococci is reported by others (Odierno *et al.*, 2006; Fortin *et al.*, 2003; Baum *et al.*, 1998). That goes conform with our data, 24 *S. uberis* isolates were misidentified as *Enterococcus spp.* by the API 20 STREP system. *S. canis* was never detected by the API 20 STREP system, but for two times by means of PCR and serogrouping. In conclusion some reasons for misidentification in API 20 STREP system could be explained by non included species (like *S. parauberis*), biochemical variability within a species (*S. uberis*) and misinterpretation of reaction colours. A lot of molecular methods such as PCR-RFLP, DNA sequencing and other PCR based methods are able to distinguish catalase negative gram positive cocci (Zschöck *et al.*, 2005; Khan *et al.*, 2003; Gillespie *et al.*, 1997.). Compared with biochemical methods, PCR based methods are less time consuming. Some of them can give reliable results within few hours. One disadvantage is that these methods do not cover the whole range of catalase negative gram positive cocci, so they are limited by the species integrated in the kit. The most routine laboratories are not prepared for doing molecular analysis and their use is limited to reference laboratories. Additionally taxonomy of streptococcal species is still an unresolved problem (e.g. for the *S. bovis* group). Permanent changing of established species names causes disagreement between taxonomists, molecular biologists and clinical bacteriologists, and does not facilitate a reliable diagnostic (Köhler *et al.*, 2007).

It was the objective of this study to gain information about the distribution of catalase-negative mastitis pathogens in Austria, identified with molecular methods under routine conditions. At the moment no comparable data do exist. Additionally the system of serological and biochemical routine mastitis diagnostic was evaluated. This study has shown that commonly used methods to identify catalase negative and gram positive cocci from mastitis milk can result in a high number of misidentifications.

In conclusion, the correct identification of environmental mastitis pathogens like *S. uberis* and enterococci has to be developed in routine diagnostics to be able to set up control programmes for reducing the impact of these infections in the dairy herd.

Acknowledgements

The study was funded by the Federal Ministry of Health, Family and Youth (BMGF-7024/0034-IV/6/2006) and the University of Veterinary Medicine Vienna. Many thanks to the Head of the Institute of Milk Hygiene, Milk Technology and Food Science Univ. Prof. Dr. Martin Wagner and his team for the technical and scientific support.

References

Baum, H., Klemme, F.R., Geiss, H.K. and Sonntag, H.G., 1998. Comparative evaluation of a commercial system for identification of gram-positive cocci. Eur. J. Clin. Microb. Inf. Dis. 17: 849-852.

Bosshard, P.P, Abels, S., Altwegg, M., Böttger, E.C. and Zbinden, R., 2004. Comparison of conventional and molecular methods for identification of aerobic catalase-negative gram-positive cocci in the clinical laboratory. J. Clin. Microbiol. 42: 2065-2073.

Deasy, B.M., Rea, M.C., Fitzgerald, G.F., Cogan, T.M. and Beresford, T.P., 2000. A rapid PCR based method to distinguish between *Lactococcus* and *Enterococcus*. Sys. Appl. Microbiol. 23: 510-522.

Devriese, L.A., Hommez, J., Laevens, H., Pot, B., Vandamme, P. and Haesebruck, F., 1999. Identification of aesculin-hydrolyzing streptococci, lactococci, aerococci and enterococci from subclinical intramammary infections in dairy cows. Vet. Microbiol. 70: 87-94.

Facklam, R., 2002. What happened to the streptococci: Overview of taxonomic and nomenclature changes. Clin. Microbiol. Rev. 15: 613-630.

Fortin, M.S, Messier, S., Paré, J. and Higgins, R., 2003. Identification of catalase-negative, non β-haemolytic, gram-positive cocci isolated from milk samples. J. Clin. Microbiol. 41: 106-109.

Gillespie, B.E, Jayarao, B.M. and Oliver, S.P., 1997. Identification of *Streptococcus* species by randomly amplified polymorphic deoxyribonucleic acid fingerprinting. J. Dairy Sci. 80: 471-476.

Kawata, K., Anzai, T., Senna, K., Kikuchi, N., Ezawa, A. and Takahashi, T., 2004. Simple and rapid PCR method for identification of streptococcal species relevant to animal infections based on 23S rDNA sequence. FEMS Microbiol. Lett. 237: 57-64.

Khan, I.U, Hassan, A.A., Abulmawjood, A., Lämmler, C., Wolter, W. and Zschöck, M., 2003. Identification and epidemiological characterization of *Streptococcus uberis* isolated from bovine mastitis using conventional and molecular methods. J. Vet. Sci. 4: 213-223.

Köhler, W., 2006. The present state of species within the genera Streptococcus and Enterococcus. Int. J. Med. Microbiol. 297: 133-150.

Lämmler, C., 1991. Biochemical and serological properties of *Streptococcus uberis*. J. Vet. Med. B 38: 737-742.

National Mastitis Council Laboratory Handbook on Bovine Mastitis 1999, Madison WI, USA: NMC

Odierno, L., Calvinho, L., Traverssa, P., Lasagno, M., Bogni, C. and Reinoso, E, 2006. Conventional identification of *Streptococcus uberis* isolated from bovine mastitis in Argentinean dairy herds. J. Dairy Sci. 89: 3886-3890.

Tomita, T., Meehan, B., Wongkattiya, N., Malmo, J., Pullinger, G., Leigh, J. and Deighton, M., 2008. Identification of *Streptococcus uberis* multilocus sequence types highly associated with mastitis. Appl. Env. Microbiol. 74: 114-124.

Vandamme, P., Pot, B., Falsen, E., Kersters, K. and Devriese, L.A., 1996. Taxonomic studies of lancefield streptococcal groups C, G and L (*Streptococcus dysgalactiae*) and proposal of *S. dysgalactiae* subsp. *equisimilis subsp.* nov. Int. J. Syst. Bact. 46: 774-781.

Zschöck, M., Manhold-Maurer, S., Wescher, A., Merl, K., Khan, I. and Lämmler, Ch., 2005. Evaluation of tRNA intergenic spacer length polymorphism analysis as a molecular method for species identification of streptococcal isolates from bovine mastitis. J. Dairy Res. 72: 333-337.

Detection of mastitis pathogens by analysis of volatile metabolites

K.A. Hettinga[1], H.J.F. van Valenberg[1], T.J.G.M. Lam[2] and A.C.M. van Hooijdonk[1]
[1]Dairy Science and Technology group, Wageningen University and Research Centre, P.O. Box 8129, 6700 EV Wageningen, the Netherlands
[2]GD Animal Health Service Ltd, P.O. Box 9, 7420 AA Deventer, the Netherlands
Corresponding author: kasper.hettinga@wur.nl

Abstract

The possibility to detect mastitis pathogens based on their volatile metabolites was studied. The 5 most important mastitis pathogens in the Netherlands (*Staphylococcus aureus,* coagulase-negative staphylococci, *Streptococcus uberis, Streptococcus dysgalactiae,* and *Escherichia coli*) were used in this study. Using a neural network, mastitis causing pathogens were identified based on the produced pattern of volatile metabolites. The source of the metabolites is unknown; they can be formed by the pathogens, but they can also be formed by enzymes coming from e.g. the blood of the cow. By inoculating milk of healthy cows with mastitis pathogens, the formation of volatile metabolites by bacteria in milk could be separated from possible other sources of metabolite formation. In general, most metabolites were found in similar concentration in both type of samples. However, some metabolites (mainly ethyl esters of free fatty acids) were not found in inoculated samples, probably due to lack of enzyme activity related to the cows' blood. It was concluded that volatile bacterial metabolites could be used for pathogen identification, and that the metabolites were mostly formed by the pathogen and are not the result of the mastitis process in the udder.

Keywords: diagnosis, neural network, pathogens, volatile metabolites

Introduction

Determination of mastitis causing pathogens is of great interest, both for choice of treatment as well as for herd level management measures to prevent the spread of mastitis. Currently, determination of mastitis pathogens is generally done by bacteriological culturing. One of the disadvantages of this method is that it is time-consuming. Faster methods of pathogen detection are advantageous, because farmers are earlier able to choose an optimal treatment. In microbiology, screening of volatile bacterial metabolites for detection and classification purposes is frequently used (Turner and Magan, 2004). In our study, the first goal was to apply this principle to clinical mastitis samples.

The volatile metabolites detected in mastitis milk samples may be formed by the pathogen in the sample. For example, the formation of 2- and 3-methylbutanal, as well as branched free fatty acids by *Staphylococcus aureus* has been described by Ritter and Hanni (1960). In mastitis samples, other, not previously described, metabolites may also detected. Whether these components were formed by the pathogen is not known. Detected metabolites may, for example, also be formed by enzymes which travel from the blood trough the disturbed blood-milk barrier to the milk, or by enzymes associated with endothelial cells of the udder tissue. Additionally, a combination of enzymes from several sources may be involved in the formation of volatile metabolites. The second goal of this study was to determine whether the volatile metabolites originate from the pathogens, which has been studied using inoculation of pathogens in milk of healthy cows.

Materials and methods

Clinical samples

Samples from cows with clinical mastitis were selected from the bacteriological diagnostic lab of the GD Animal Health Service (GD). Samples had been screened for the presence of bacteria. If one of 5 pathogens of interest (*Staph. aureus*, coagulase-negative staphylococci (CNS), *Streptococcus uberis*, *Streptococcus dysgalactiae*, or *Escherichia coli*) was cultured, the remainder of the sample (approx. 5 ml) was frozen at -20 °C for later use. Ten samples per pathogen were collected. Also, the pathogen cultured from the clinical samples was frozen at -80 °C for inoculation.

Inoculated samples

Bacteria isolated from clinical mastitis samples were used to inoculate milk samples of healthy cows. In milk of healthy cows, somatic cell count (SCC) is low and the mammary epithelial tissue is intact. This minimises the amount of enzymes from the blood and somatic cells in the milk. By inoculating pathogens to these samples, the effect of the pathogen itself can be studied.

Fifteen milk samples of cows, without signs of clinical mastitis and with low SCC (<75,000/ml), were supplied by the 'De Ossekampen', the university farm of Wageningen University and Research Centre. Ten ml foremilk samples were taken after disinfection of the teat and forestriping, into sterile 12 ml tubes. Directly after taking these samples, they were transported to the laboratory and inoculated, in the same tube, with one of the five pathogens cultured from clinical samples (3 samples per pathogen). Inoculation was performed with broth containing 10^9 cfu/ml, diluted to a final inoculation level of 10^5 cfu/ml in the milk sample.

The inoculated samples were subsequently incubated at 37 °C for 8 hours. After incubation, the samples were cooled on ice to approximately 0 °C. Five ml of the sample was subsequently transferred to a headspace vial. The headspace vial was then frozen at -20 °C for a maximum of 1 week before analysis of volatile metabolites.

Analysis of volatile metabolites

The analysis was performed according to Hettinga *et al.* (2008) After thawing, 5 ml milk samples were preheated in 20 ml vials for 1 min at 60 °C. Volatile metabolites were extracted from the headspace for 5 min with a 75 μm PDMS-carboxen SPME fiber (Supelco, Bellefonte, PA) using the combiPAL autosampler (CTC Analytics AG, Switzerland). The volatile metabolites were thermally desorbed from the fiber. GC separation of the volatile components was performed on a Finnigan Trace GC gas chromatograph coupled to a Finnigan DSQ mass spectrometer. Volatiles were separated on an apolar BPX-5 column of 30 m length, 0.15 mm i.d., and 0.25 μm film thickness (SGE, Austin, TX). Oven temperature was held at -30 °C for 3 min, raised to 230 °C at 20°C/min, followed by 1 min holding. Helium was used as the carrier gas at a flow rate of 0.6 ml/min. The MS interface and the ion source were kept at 250 °C. Acquisition was performed in electron impact mode (70 eV) with 2 scans/s; the mass range used was m/z 33-250.

The resulting chromatograms were analysed using the AMDIS software for improved peak identification (NIST, Gaithersburg, MD). Peak integration was subsequently performed using the XCalibur software package. Finally, NeuralTools (Palisade, Ithaca, NY) was used to develop artificial neural networks (ANN). Probabilistic neural networks (PNN) were the type of ANN used for this study. Training of the neural networks was carried out using cross validation, with 70% of the samples used for training and 30% for validation.

Results and discussion

Clinical samples

The volatile metabolites which occur in clinical mastitis samples have been determined. A maximum of 19 volatile metabolites were detected. When comparing pathogens, *Staph. aureus* produced a very different pattern of volatile metabolites compared to the other samples. Samples with CNS and *E. coli* had enough dissimilarities with the other pathogens, making it possible to separate these two pathogens from each other and the other samples. The two streptococcus species did not show significant differences between each other but could be identified as a different group from the other pathogens. Due to variability between samples within a group, comparisons between pathogens were not sufficient for classification of the samples by univariate statistics. Therefore, an artificial neural network (ANN) was trained to classify the pathogen in the milk samples based on the bacterial metabolites.

The ANN was trained to identify the five pathogens. The correct classification rate in this case was 66%, with the main errors between the two *Streptococcus* species. This can be explained based on the similarity in presence of volatile metabolites. Because of this, for subsequent ANN training, the two different streptococcus species were handled as one group.

Extended biofilm susceptibility assay for *Staphylococcus aureus* bovine mastitis isolates: evidence for association between *Agr*-type and biofilm susceptibility

M.B. Melchior[1,4], M.H.J. van Osch[1], T.J.G.M. Lam[2], W. Gaastra[3] and J. Fink-Gremmels[3]
[1]Department of Veterinary Pharmacy and Toxicology, Faculty of Veterinary Medicine, University of Utrecht, P.O. Box 80152, 3508 TD Utrecht, the Netherlands
[2]Dutch Udder Health Centre (UGCN) P.O. Box 2030, 7420 AA Deventer, the Netherlands
[3]Department of Infectious Diseases and Immunology, Division of Molecular Infectiology, Faculty of Veterinary Medicine, University of Utrecht, the Netherlands
[4]current address: Central Veterinary Institute, Department of Bacteriology and TSEs, P.O. Box 65, 8200 AB Lelystad, the Netherlands
Corresponding author: marielle.melchior@wur.nl

Abstract

Staphylococcus aureus is one of the most prevalent causes of bovine mastitis. The antimicrobial treatment of this disease is currently based on antimicrobial susceptibility testing according to CLSI standards. However, various studies have shown that there is a discrepancy between the results of this standard susceptibility test and the actual cure rate of the applied antimicrobial treatment. Increasing evidence suggests that biofilm formation by *S. aureus* is associated to with this problem. Previous data obtained with a limited number of strains revealed that the extended biofilm susceptibility assay (EBS assay) allows for differentiation between strains, which cannot be derived from a standard susceptibility test or from a 24-hour biofilm susceptibility assay. Based on the results form a previous study with the same collection of strains (unpublished data, see poster presentations Mastitis control 2008) the effect of *Agr*-type and the presence of *IS257* in *Agr*-type II strains on the biofilm susceptibility was studied. The results revealed differences in biofilm susceptibility for both the *Agr*-type of the strains and for the presence of *IS257* in *Agr*-type II strains. The presence of *IS257* in *Agr*-type II strains also has a marked effect on the *in vitro* biofilm density of these strains. Furthermore, the results confirmed the decreasing antimicrobial efficacy against older biofilms, and the increased antimicrobial efficacy due to longer duration of antimicrobial challenge on biofilms was shown. The data presented here offer an explanation for the higher efficacy of early antimicrobial treatment and for treatments of longer duration in bovine mastitis *S. aureus* infections described in the literature from several epidemiological studies.

Keywords: antimicrobial susceptibility, biofilm, genotyping, *Staphylococcus aureus*, treatment

Introduction

Staphylococcus aureus is one of the major causes of subclinical, clinical, recurrent and chronic mastitis in dairy cattle. The nature of these infections in dairy cows, being often therapy-resistant, indicates that biofilm growth of *S. aureus* is related the course of these persistent infections (Melchior *et al.*, 2006a). A recent study, with a limited number of bovine mastitis *S. aureus* strains, has shown that these strains are able to form a bacterial biofilm (Melchior *et al.*, 2006b). Furthermore, comparison the of results obtained with the standard CLSI susceptibility test with those obtained in a biofilm susceptibility assay for a number of antimicrobials commonly used for mastitis therapy, it was evident that these strains were less susceptible when growing in a bacterial biofilm (Melchior *et al.*, 2006b, 2007).

In 2006 a representative collection of *S. aureus* bovine mastitis strains was gathered amongst Dutch dairy cows. Because of the low prevalence of penicillin-resistance amongst these strains, which is in concordance with the current penicillin-resistance prevalence in the Netherlands, twenty penicillin-resistant strains from the Dutch Veterinary antimicrobial resistance surveillance program were added to this collection (*MARAN*, 2003-2005).

Previous data obtained with this collection of strains, on the correlation between the biofilm forming ability and the prevalence of several genes, revealed three interesting features of these strains. First, a high correlation between the *Agr*-type of the strains and the amount of biofilm formed by the strains was found (unpublished data, see poster abstracts Mastitis control 2008). Second, a high correlation between the *Agr*-type I strains and the presence of beta-lactamase resistance genes and third a high correlation between *Agr*-type II strains and the presence of *IS257* was observed (unpublished data). The *Agr* locus of *S. aureus* which controls most of the virulence factors, encodes a two-component signaling pathway whose activating ligand is an *agr*-encoded autoinducing peptide (AIP) (Ji *et al.*, 1997; Lyon *et al.*, 2002; Kong *et al.*, 2006). A polymorphism in the amino acid sequence of the AIP and of its corresponding receptor divides *S. aureus* strains into four major groups. Within each group the strains produce a peptide that can activate the *agr* response in the other member strains, whereas the AIPs belonging to different groups are usually mutually inhibitory (Ji *et al.*, 1997; Jarraud *et al.*, 2002; Lyon *et al.*, 2002).

The role for the presence of *IS257* in *Agr*-type II strains, which is commonly associated with several resistance genes e.g. the beta-lactamase genes, was unclear, since in these strains it was typically not associated with any of the tested resistance genes (unpublished data). The aim of the present study was to investigate the relation between the extended biofilm antimicrobial susceptibility and the *Agr*-type of the strain collection, and secondly to investigate the effect of the presence of *IS257* in *Agr*-type II strains in the extended biofilm susceptibility assay.

Materials and methods

Collection of S. aureus isolates

The *S. aureus* strains tested in this study originated from two sources:

a. *Field strains.* From December 2005 until September 2006, cows from farms spread over the Netherlands were sampled. The selection of cows was based on their 4-6 week somatic cell count (SCC) patterns. Selection criterion for a *subclinical* infection was a cow SCC >120,000 cells/ml, without any other signs of infection. Milk samples were send to the GD Animal Health Service in Deventer (GD, Gezondheidsdienst voor Dieren, Deventer). During the same period, milk samples from animals with *clinical* bovine mastitis, which were send to the GD for diagnostic reasons, were randomly collected as well. All milk samples were incubated according to standard laboratory procedures of the National Mastitis Council (ISO 17025 certified laboratory) and the isolated *S. aureus* strains were stored at -70 °C. From the *S. aureus* positive samples all 58 strains from 54 farms were included in this study. Only one strain per cow was selected. These strains are designated the GD strains in this study (see Table 1).
b. *Penicillin-resistant* S. aureus *strains.* Because of the low number of penicillin-resistant strains in collection A (approx. 10%), which is in accordance with the current prevalence of penicillin-resistance in the Netherlands (*MARAN*, 2003-2005), a batch of penicillin-resistant strains was added to this collection. In total twenty penicillin-resistant *S. aureus* strains from bovine mastitis from the Dutch antimicrobial surveillance program (*MARAN*, 2003-2005) collected between 2003 and 2005 were obtained from the Central Veterinary Institute Lelystad (CVI, Lelystad). These strains are designated the Lelystad strains in this study (see Table 1).

Extended antimicrobial susceptibility assay for bacteria growing in biofilms

Measurements of the antimicrobial susceptibility of bacteria growing in biofilms were performed with the MBEC™ biofilm assay (Ceri *et al.*, 1999; Olson *et al.*, 2002; Melchior *et al.*, 2006b, 2007). In brief, biofilms are allowed to form on the surface of 96 pegs on the peg- lid in the assay. The biofilms formed on all pegs were found to be statistically equivalent (Ceri *et al.*, 1999) and

Table 1. Bacterial strains used in this study.

***Agr*-type**	**N=**	**Beta-lactamase pos (%)**	**Sample source (n)**
Agr I, III, IV	29	83	GD (9), Lelystad (20)
Agr II	26	0	GD (26)
Agr II, IS257 positive	23	0	GD (23)
Total	78		

were subsequently exposed in 96-well plates for a variable period of time to growth medium containing antimicrobials in different concentrations, to allow determination of the susceptibility of the bacteria grown in biofilm for these antimicrobial agents (Ceri *et al.*, 1999).

The assay was performed as previously described (Ceri *et al.*, 1999; Melchior *et al.*, 2006b, 2007) with some modifications. The *Agr*-type II, *IS257* positive strains (see Table 1) were also investigated with bacterial biofilms formed during 48h. Bacterial biofilms were challenged with antimicrobials during 24 h and 72 h with two-fold antimicrobial dilution plates (Sensititre plates, MSC Diagnostics BC, Swalmen, Netherlands). For the 72 h antimicrobial challenge, plates were replaced every 24 hours during three consecutive days. During this period the 96-well plates were incubated at 37 °C.

Results and discussions

To investigate if biofilm formation can explain the discrepancy between the high *in vitro* susceptibility, and the disappointing bacteriological cure after therapy in *S. aureus* bovine mastitis infections, 78 recently isolated strains were tested in an extended biofilm antimicrobial susceptibility assay. A secondary question was concerned with the genotypes of the strains associated with higher or lower biofilm susceptibility.

Previous investigations with the same strains as used in this work revealed that there is a very high association between the *Agr*-type of the *S. aureus* strains and the prevalence of beta-lactamase genes. The Accessory Gene Regulator (*Agr*-gene) is a two-component response regulator which, in coordination with other response regulators, is known to regulate the expression of multiple virulence factors during the colonisation and invasion phases of the staphylococcal infection (Bronner *et al.*, 2004; Chan *et al.*, 2004). There are indications that the genetic variability in the *agr* locus, which results in four *Agr*-types, influences the pathogenesis of several human *S. aureus* infections e.g. menstrual toxic shock syndrome (mostly *Agr*-type III) and scalded skin syndrome (mostly *Agr*-type IV) (Bronner *et al.*, 2004). However, the effect of the *Agr*-type of the strains, in relation to its effects on colonisation and invasion could not be studied in this biofilm antimicrobial susceptibility model.

When comparing the BMIC data for amoxicillin with clavulanic acid and cloxacillin between strain types, it became clear that the majority of *Agr*-type I, III and IV strains was inhibited between 1-4 μg/ml and the majority of *Agr*-type II strains between 0.25-0.5 μg/ml. If the beta-lactamase negative *Agr*I, III and IV strains would be excluded from this comparison, the differences would be even more pronounced. These data, derived with the antimicrobials most often used for *S. aureus* mastitis infections, might explain why it is more difficult to effectively cure the *Agr*-type I, III and IV beta-lactamase positive strains *in vivo*, compared to the *Agr*-type II strains, which are beta-lactamase negative.

When comparing the MBEC D1 and D3 data for all tested antimicrobials it becomes evident that often three days of antimicrobial challenge were necessary for eradication of the bacteria from the biofilm. The only exception were the *Agr*-type II, *IS257* positive strains for the 24 h biofilms, however the density of the bacteria in the biofilm in this assay (being more than one log lower compared to the other strains), makes a comparison difficult.

The extended biofilm antimicrobial susceptibility assay enables discrimination between strains which were eradicated at concentrations below CLSI breakpoints at D1, and strains which were not even eradicated at CLSI breakpoints concentrations at D3. The *in vitro* differences between these strains, might explain why some strains can only be effectively treated *in vivo* with a longer duration of therapy (Sol *et al.*, 1997; Pyorala and Pyorala, 1998; Sol *et al.*, 2000; Taponen *et al.*, 2003). The mechanisms behind these differences, whether they are caused by membrane proteins, regulatory systems or differences in metabolism, can be the subject of further study with the availability of this *in vitro* model.

The results of the 48h biofilm for the *Agr*-type II, *IS257* strains compared to the 24 h biofilm of the same strains, confirm results of previous studies from Amorena *et al* (1999) and Monzon *et al* (2001) and it is generally accepted that older biofilm are less susceptible. Our results with biofilm growing bacteria present an explanation for what is already known from epidemiological studies, namely that the duration of infection is an important parameter for prediction of the therapy outcomes. Whether *Agr*-type II, *IS257* positive strains are slower in formation of the biofilm *in vivo*, needs to be confirmed.

When comparing the efficacy for *Agr*-type II strains of the four tested antimicrobials results suggest that mastitis infections for all of these strains, with exception of one penicillin resistant strain which came out negative in the *BlaZ* genes PCR (unpublished results), should be treated with penicillin, as results give no evidence for better efficacy for the other tested antimicrobials. The very low association with penicillin resistance for these strains suggests that transformation of these strains to a penicillin resistant strain is very unlikely.

In conclusion, the extended biofilm susceptibility assay explains the findings of previous epidemiological studies in which it was concluded that duration of infection and duration of treatment are important parameters for therapy outcome. Furthermore our results support the exclusive use of the antimicrobial penicillin for penicillin susceptible *Agr*-type II strains, which is prescribed for penicillin susceptible *Staphylococcus spp.* in Scandinavian countries. However, care should be taken when *Agr*-type I, III or IV *S. aureus* are encountered, as these strains seem more susceptible for transformation into penicillin resistant strains.

Acknowledgements

This study is part of the five-year udder health program of the Dutch Udder Health Centre and was financially supported by the Dutch Dairy Board.

References

Amorena, B., Gracia, E., Monzon, M., Leiva, J., Oteiza, C., Perez, M., Alabart, J.L. and Hernandez-Yago, J., 1999. Antibiotic susceptibility assay for *Staphylococcus aureus* in biofilms developed in vitro. J. Antimicrob. Chemother. 44: 43-55.

Bronner, S., Monteil, H. and Prevost, G., 2004. Regulation of virulence determinants in *Staphylococcus aureus*: complexity and applications. FEMS Microbiol. Rev. 28: 183-200.

Ceri, H., Olson, M.E., Stremick, C., Read, R.R., Morck, D. and Buret, A., 1999. The Calgary Biofilm Device: new technology for rapid determination of antibiotic susceptibilities of bacterial biofilms. J. Clin. Microbiol. 37: 1771-1776.

Chan, W.C., Coyle, B.J. and Williams, P., 2004. Virulence regulation and quorum sensing in staphylococcal infections: competitive AgrC antagonists as quorum sensing inhibitors. J. Med. Chem. 47: 4633-4641.

Jarraud, S., Mougel, C., Thioulouse, J., Lina, G., Meugnier, H., Forey, F., Nesme, X., Etienne, J. and Vandenesch, F., 2002. Relationships between *Staphylococcus aureus* genetic background, virulence factors, *agr* groups (alleles), and human disease. Infect. Immun. 70: 631-641.

Ji, G., Beavis, R. and Novick, R.P., 1997. Bacterial interference caused by autoinducing peptide variants. Science 276: 2027-2030.

Kong, K.F., Vuong, C. and Otto, M., 2006. Staphylococcus quorum sensing in biofilm formation and infection. Int. J. Med. Microbiol. 296: 133-139.

Lyon, G.J., Wright, J.S., Muir, T.W. and Novick, R.P., 2002. Key determinants of receptor activation in the agr autoinducing peptides of Staphylococcus aureus. Biochemistry 41: 10095-10104.

MARAN, 2003-2005. Monitoring of Antimicrobial Resistance and Antibiotic usage in Animals in The Netherlands in 2003, 2004, 2005. Lelystad, CVI-Lelystad. Available at: www.cvi.wur.nl.

Melchior, M.B., Fink-Gremmels, J. and Gaastra, W., 2006b. Comparative Assessment of the Antimicrobial Susceptibility of *Staphylococcus aureus* Isolates from Bovine Mastitis in Biofilm Versus Planktonic Culture. J. Vet. Med. B Infect. Dis. Vet. Public Health 53: 326-332.

Melchior, M.B., Fink-Gremmels, J. and Gaastra, W., 2007. Extended antimicrobial susceptibility assay for *Staphylococcus aureus* isolates from bovine mastitis growing in biofilms. Vet. Microbiol. 125: 141-149.

Melchior, M.B., Vaarkamp, H. and Fink-Gremmels, J., 2006a. Biofilms: a role in recurrent mastitis infections? Vet. J. 171: 398-407.

Monzon, M., Oteiza, C., Leiva, J. and Amorena, B., 2001. Synergy of different antibiotic combinations in biofilms of *Staphylococcus epidermidis.* J. Antimicrob. Chemother. 48: 793-801.

Olson, M.E., Ceri, H., Morck, D.W., Buret, A.G. and Read, R.R., 2002. Biofilm bacteria: formation and comparative susceptibility to antibiotics. Can. J. Vet. Res. 66: 86-92.

Pyorala, S.H. and Pyorala, E.O., 1998. Efficacy of parenteral administration of three antimicrobial agents in treatment of clinical mastitis in lactating cows: 487 cases (1989-1995). J. Am. Vet. Med. Assoc. 212: 407-412.

Sol, J., Sampimon, O.C., Barkema, H.W. and Schukken, Y.H., 2000. Factors associated with cure after therapy of clinical mastitis caused by *Staphylococcus aureus.* J. Dairy. Sci. 83: 278-284.

Sol, J., Sampimon, O.C., Snoep, J.J. and Schukken, Y.H., 1997. Factors associated with bacteriological cure during lactation after therapy for subclinical mastitis caused by *Staphylococcus aureus.* J. Dairy. Sci. 80: 2803-2808.

Taponen, S., Jantunen, A., Pyorala, E. and Pyorala, S., 2003. Efficacy of targeted 5-day combined parenteral and intramammary treatment of clinical mastitis caused by penicillin-susceptible or penicillin-resistant *Staphylococcus aureus.* Acta. Vet. Scand. 44,:53-62.

Improving mastitis control programs through identification of risk factors related to the incidence of subclinical intramammary infections

S. Dufour[1,2], *I. Dohoo*[2,3], *T. Devries*[2,4] *and D. Scholl*[1,2]
[1]*Faculté de Médecine Vétérinaire,Université de Montréal, St-Hyacinthe, C.P. 5000, St-Hyacinthe, Quebec J2S 7C6, Canada*
[2]*Canadian Bovine Mastitis Research Network, C.P. 5000, St-Hyacinthe, Quebec J2S 7C6, Canada*
[3]*University of PEI, 550 University Ave, Charlottetown, PEI, C1A 4P3, Canada,*
[4]*University of Guelph, Kemptville Campus, Box 2003, 830 Prescott Street, Kemptville, Ontario K0G 1J0, Canada*
Corresponding author: simon.dufour@umontreal.ca

Abstract

The goal of this study was to determine the impact of modifiable management practices on the incidence of pathogen-specific subclinical mastitis. The relationship between bedding and feeding management and the incidence of coagulase negative *Staphylococcus* (CNS) intramammary infection (IMI) is explored in this paper. Ninety Canadian dairy herds were selected and in each herd bacteriological culture of three repeated quarter milk samples of 15 dairy cows was realised. The median herd CNS IMI incidence was 0.40 IMI/quarter-year at risk (first and third quartiles: 0.17 and 0.82). Cows that were housed on sawdust had three times less risk of acquiring a new CNS IMI. Use of straw as bedding and timing of feed delivery in relation to milking were not significant risk factors for new CNS IMI.

Keywords: CNS, bedding, control program, lying, nutrition

Introduction

Subclinical mastitis is recognised worldwide as one of the most costly health problems for the dairy industry. Numerous studies have already identified management practices and preventive measures associated with the prevalence of subclinical IMI (Barkema *et al.*, 1998; Barnouin *et al.*, 2004). However, a single measure of infection prevalence is not sufficient to distinguish the effects of risk factors on the IMI incidence rate from their effects on the duration of infection (Greenland and Rothman, 1998). To obtain a long term control, mastitis control programs should specifically target risk factors associated with IMI incidence. To ensure the success of these control programs, the field conditions that have the potential to facilitate or to limit their effectiveness should also be identified.

The primary objective of this study was to estimate the effects of modifiable management practices on the incidence of pathogen-specific lactational subclinical IMI. An important goal was to identify factors that act as confounders or effect-modifiers of known IMI prevention practices and that can therefore limit their effectiveness. Among the different management practices that have been associated with subclinical mastitis, bedding management has been frequently associated with subclinical IMI prevalence (Barnouin *et al.*, 2004, Fregonesi and Leaver, 2001). Another common practice that has been associated with a lower subclinical IMI prevalence is preventing cows from lying down after milking (Barnouin *et al.*, 2004). A very common way to keep cows standing after milking is to deliver fresh feed either shortly before or during milking to stimulate cows to feed rather than to lie down (Johansson *et al.*, 1999; Tyler *et al.*, 1997; Devries and Von Keyserlingk, 2005). In the present study, CNS was the most frequently involved pathogen. In this paper we will therefore focus on the possible association between the incidence of CNS IMI and the two previously discussed management practices.

Materials and methods

A cohort of 90 Canadian dairy farms distributed in four different regional centers was recruited for this prospective study. Herds were selected from strata of high, intermediate and low 12-months average bulk tank somatic cell count (SCC), with border of >300,000 and >150,000 cells/ml, respectively. This longitudinal study was based on four periods of repeated quarter milk sampling beginning March 2007 and ending August 2008. The results that are presented are preliminary results from the first period of intensive sampling (March-May 2007). During this time period single-quarter milk samples of five fresh and ten randomly selected lactating cows were collected in each herd once every three weeks for a total of three samplings. For each sampling the teat end was first cleaned and dried, the first streams of milk were discarded, and the teat end was scrubbed with an alcohol swab prior to milk collection. Milk samples were stored at -20 °C until processing. One one-hundredth of one ml of milk was cultured and bacterial species were identified according to National Mastitis Council (NMC) standards (Harmon *et al.*, 1990). Colony counts were recorded for each bacterial species. Samples with three or more bacterial species were considered contaminated and were not informative of CNS status. A quarter was considered to be infected if ten or more CNS colony forming units per 0.01ml of milk were found in pure culture. A new IMI was defined as a positive sample following a negative sample. Therefore, quarters had to be negative at either the first or second sampling to be considered at risk of a new IMI. Following bacteriology, bronopol was added to the milk and it was refrozen at -20 °C until SCC analysis. SCC was determined by a Fossomatic milk cell counter (Foss Electronic, Hillerod, Denmark). French and English versions of a questionnaire were developed to assess management practices implemented on farm and social characteristics of the producers. Questionnaire translation was realised using a formal process that included multiple translation-correction steps as described by Brislin (Lonner and Berry, 1986) and a pilot study was conducted. The questionnaires were then administered in person by the main author and a team of technicians. Production data were obtained from Dairy Herd Improvement programs.

Statistical analysis

A univariable analysis was first performed to detect extreme values. No observations were excluded for this reason. Occurrence or non-occurrence of a new CNS IMI was the dependant variable in all analyses. Multilevel models were fit to the data using MLwiN 2.02 (Rasbash, London, England). First order penalised quasi likelihood estimation (PQL) using a restricted generalised iterative least squares (RGILS) algorithm was used to build a three levels (quarter, cow and herd) random intercept logistic model containing a constant and center as a fixed effect. Bivariable analyses for screening of independent variables were then conducted using this model. A total of 30 variables were screened, 10 of them being related to bedding management, six to feeding management and five to milking procedures. The other variables screened were regional center, housing type, herd size, herd manager work's habits, parity, days in milk, quarter linear score, teat end callosity and roughness and concomitant *Staph. aureus* IMI. All independents variables with $P \leq 0.20$ (Wald's test) were retained for further analyses. Four management practices were then analysed in four separate models as primary independents variables:

- Model 1: Use of straw as bedding.
- Model 2: Use of sawdust as bedding.
- Model 3: Frequency at which new bedding is added (less than once a day, once a day or more than once a day).
- Model 4: Feed stimulation through delivery of fresh feed and/or concentrate and/or pushing the feed ± 45 minutes from the onset of milking (no feed stimulation, feed stimulation for one milking, feed stimulation for both milking).

Each management practice variable was first introduced in the previously described three-level logistic model. Then the previously screened independent variables were added to the model one at the time. Change in the estimate of the coefficient of the primary variable was evaluated and secondary variables causing a change of 10% or more were retained. These secondary variables were then introduced sequentially in the model to provide an adjusted estimate of the primary variable parameter. Finally, logically explainable interactions were evaluated as well as random coefficients at the different levels. The assumptions of normality and homogeneity of variance were evaluated by examining the Normal probability plots of residuals and plots of residuals vs. predicted values. Two alternative approaches were used to provide revised estimates; a first order marginal quasi likelihood estimation (MQL) using and RGILS algorithm and a Bayesian Markov chain Monte Carlo estimation (MCMC) using Metropolis-Hastings sampling with diffuse sampling, a burn-in period of 500 iterations and a run of 45,000 iterations.

Results

Two herds were not included in these analyses due to incomplete questionnaires at the time of the analysis. A total of 5,302 quarters from 1,288 cows were sampled, of these 640 were not considered at risk of a new IMI according to the previously described risk definition and were excluded. During the six week sampling period, 237 new CNS IMI were detected and the median herd incidence was 0.40 IMI/quarter-year at risk (first and third quartiles: 0.17 and 0.82). Variables retained following bivariable analysis are listed in Table 1.

Table 1. Unadjusted CNS odds-ratio (OR) estimates of fixed effects, bivariable analysis.

Factors		**OR (95% CI)**	**P**[1]
Parity: multiparous		0.73 (0.55, 0.96)	0.03
SCC linear	0	reference	<0.01
score at 1st	1	2.9 (1.9, 4.5)	
sample:	2	4.0 (2.6, 6.2)	
	≥3	5.7 (4.0, 8.1)	
Housing:	Tie-stall	reference	<0.01
	Free-stall	0.63 (0.40, 0.99)	
	Bedding pack	1.9 (0.92, 4.0)	
Herd manager works rather meticulously		0.68 (0.39, 1.2)	0.16
Feed stimulation ±45min. from milking			0.11
	No feed stimulation	reference	
	Feed stimulation for 1 milking	1.9 (1.0, 3.5)	
	Feed stimulation for 2 milkings	1.7 (0.94, 3.2)	
Concentrates fed in milking parlor		0.47 (0.17, 1.3)	0.14
Concentrates fed by self-feeder		2.5 (1.1, 5.5)	0.02
Straw as bedding		1.8 (1.1, 2.7)	<0.01
Sawdust as bedding		0.33 (0.13, 0.84)	0.02
Bedding adding frequency			<0.01
	< Once a day	reference	
	Once a day	1.9 (1.2, 3.0)	
	> Once a day	1.1 (0.72, 1.8)	
Clean:	Dirty teats only	reference	0.04
	All teats	0.25 (0.07, 0.92)	
Fore-strip all cows		0.78 (0.53, 1.1)	0.20
Post-dip		0.35 (0.08, 1.5)	0.16
Center:	Alberta	reference	0.01
	Ontario	1.4 (0.85, 2.3)	
	Quebec	0.67 (0.39, 1.1)	
	Atlantic	0.86 (0.38, 1.5)	

[1] Joint P value is given for multiple classes categorical variables.

Briefly, one quarter level variable, SCC linear score at first sampling and one cow level variable, primiparous vs. multiparous were retained. All other variables were herd level variables and were composed of one social characteristic, meticulousness of the herd manager (self-evaluation), type of housing and various management practices related to feeding, bedding and milking procedures. None of the tested interactions and random coefficients were significant.

In all models and for each level the assumption of equality of variance was reasonable. In all models, the assumption of normality was respected for the herd level but could not be assess thoroughly at the cow level due to the small number of replicates at this level. The revised MQL and MCMC estimates were in close agreement with the PQL estimates (data not shown). Penalised quasi likelihood estimates were retained since they were closer to zero and therefore more conservative. Table 2 provides estimates of the parameter for each primary variable after adjustment for confounding by covariates.

Discussion

Bedding management

It has been observed that CNS IMI prevalence can be influenced by bedding type (Ferguson *et al.*, 2007). In our study, we have found a similar association between bedding type and CNS IMI incidence. Although the use of straw bedding was not a significant risk factor for new CNS IMI, the use of sawdust bedding conversely had a strong negative association with CNS

Table 2. Adjusted CNS odds-ratio (OR) estimates of fixed effects (1st order PQL).

Primary variables	OR (95% CI)	Covariates
1. Feed stimulation ±45min. from milking	Reference	Center, housing type, sawdust bedding, bedding adding frequency, SCC linear score, concentrates fed in milking parlor
No feed stimulation	1.3 (0.71, 2.5)	
Feed stimulation for 1 milking	1.1 (0.60, 2.2)	
Feed stimulation for 2 milkings		
2. Straw as bedding	0.96 (0.52, 1.8)	Center, housing type, sawdust bedding, bedding adding frequency, SCC linear score, concentrates fed by self-feeder
3. Sawdust as bedding	0.37 (0.15, 0.93)	Center, bedding adding frequency
4. Bedding adding frequency		Center, housing type, sawdust bedding, SCC linear score, concentrates fed in milking parlor
< Once a day	Reference	
Once a day	1.2 (0.60, 2.4)	
> Once a day	0.83 (0.43, 1.6)	

IMI incidence. Cows that were housed on sawdust had three times less risk of acquiring a new CNS IMI. This effect of bedding type could be mediated through different mechanisms. First, the bedding material itself has an initial bacterial load and physical, biochemical and nutritional properties that can sustain and promote bacterial growth. Different bedding types will therefore support different types and different loads of bacteria. Bacteria types and counts found in bedding materials have a positive correlation with the bacteria types and counts present on the teat end (Zdanowicz *et al.*, 2004). It is likely that CNS species are not as well supported by sawdust bedding than by other types of bedding and this could result in lower CNS IMI incidence for cows housed on sawdust.

The observed association between sawdust bedding and CNS IMI incidence could also be mediated indirectly through improved cow cleanliness. Norring *et al.* (2008) observed that cow cleanliness is affected by bedding type even though there were no differences in stall dirtiness. Others have found that SCC is strongly associated with cow cleanliness (Renaud *et al.*, 2005). Cow cleanliness scores were not available for this first sampling period but they have been collected during the subsequent sampling periods and a more complete analysis of the interaction between bedding type, cow cleanliness and CNS infection will be done. Finally, although it seems plausible that more frequent addition of clean bedding could decrease subclinical mastitis incidence, the observed lower CNS IMI incidence ratio associated to this practice was not significant.

Delivery of fresh feed around milking time

Previous epidemiologic studies have observed an association between management practices which encourage cows to remain standing after milking and the probability of a herd having a lower herd SCC and lower clinical mastitis incidence (Barnouin *et al.*, 2004; Peeler *et al.*, 2000). Others have observed that delivery of feed around milking increase the time cows spend standing and the percentage of cows standing after milking (Johansson *et al.*, 1999; Tyler *et al.*, 1997; Devries and Von Keyserlingk, 2005). In the present study, however, there was no significant association between feed stimulation and CNS IMI incidence. It is possible that the observed lower SCC associated with this practice is not mediated through a reduction of CNS IMI incidence, but possibly by a decrease in the incidence of other species of bacteria. It has been demonstrated that CNS readily colonises the teat skin and teat canal and is commonly found in those areas (White *et al.*, 1989). Therefore it seems likely that the penetration of CNS bacteria in the teat canal would not necessarily be influenced by whether the cow is standing or lying.

Caution must be taken when making causal inference. Using a technique to keep cows standing after milking might in fact reflect overall better management practices. The lower SCC that was associated with preventing cows from lying down after milking found in other studies could in fact be the result from this superior general management. Attitudes, knowledge and motivation of the dairy producers have been shown to have a considerable impact on IMI prevalence (Jansen *et al.*, 2008) and could be an important source of heterogeneity of effect for numerous management practices on IMI incidence. A more complete evaluation of these social characteristics was not available when these analyses were realised, but these data are being collected and will be analysed.

Finally, there have been no controlled studies so far evaluating directly the association between the length of time spent standing after milking and the incidence rate of environmental IMI. Further research in this direction is needed to fully understand this association, and how delivery of fresh feed around milking time can impact this.

Conclusion

There was a preventive effect from sawdust bedding on the incidence of subclinical CNS IMI. Use of straw as bedding and frequency at which new bedding is added were not significantly associated to CNS IMI incidence. Additionally, providing fresh feed either shortly before or during milking did not influence the incidence of subclinical CNS IMI. We must stress that these preliminary analyses were realised with an incomplete set of independent variables. This could result in residual confounding bias still being present in our multivariable models.

Aknowledgements

This research was financed by NSERC, Alberta Milk, Dairy Farmers of New Brunswick, Nova Scotia, Ontario and Prince Edward Island, Novalait Inc., Dairy Farmers of Canada, Canadian Dairy Network, AAFC, PHAC, Technology PEI Inc., Université de Montréal and University of Prince Edward Island through the Canadian Bovine Mastitis Research Network.

References

Barkema, H.W., Schukken, Y.H., Lam, T.J.G.M., Beiboer, M.L., Benedictus, G. and Brand, A., 1998. Management practices associated with low, medium and high somatic cell counts in bilk milk. J. Dairy Sci. 81: 1917-1927.

Barnouin, J., Chassagne, M., Bazin, S. and Boichard, D., 2004. Management practices from questionnaire survey in herds with very low somatic cell score through a national mastitis program in France. J. Dairy Sci. 87: 3989-3999.

Devries, T.J. and Von Keyserlingk, M.A.G., 2005. Time of feed delivery affects the feeding and lying patterns of dairy cows. Journal of Dairy Science. 88:625-631.

Ferguson, J.D., Azzaro, G., Gambina, M. and Licitra, G., 2007. Prevalence of mastitis pathogens in Ragusa, Sicily from 2000 to 2006. J. Dairy Sci. 90: 5798-5813.

Fregonesi, J.A. and Leaver, J.D., 2001. Behaviour, performance and health indicators of welfare for dairy cows housed in strawyard or cubicle systems. Live. Prod. Sci. 68: 205-216.

Greenland, S. and Rothman, K.J., 1998. Modern epidemiology. Lippincott-Raven Publishers, Philadelphia, USA, 45 pp.

Harmon, R.J., Eberhart, R.J., Jasper, D.E. and Langlois, B.E., 1990. Microbiological procedures for the diagnosis of bovine udder infection. National Mastitis Council, Arlington, USA.

Jansen, J., Van den Borne, B.H.P., Renes, R.J., Van Schaik, G., Lam, T.J.G.M. and Leeuwis, C., 2008. Mastitis incidence explained by farmers' attitude and behaviour. Prev. Vet. Med. (in press).

Johansson, B., Redbo, I. and Svennersten-Sjaunja, K., 1999. Effect of feeding before, during and after milking on dairy cow behaviour and the hormone cortisol. Anim. Sci. 68: 597-604.

Lonner W.J. and Berry, J.W., 1986. Field methods in cross-cultural research. Sage, Beverly Hills, CA, USA, pp. 137-164.

Norring, M., Manninen, E., de Passillé, A.M., Rushen, J., Munksgaard, L. and Saloniemi, H., 2008. Effects of sand and straw bedding on the lying behavior, cleanliness, and hoof and hock injuries of dairy cows. J. Dairy Sci. 91: 570-576.

Peeler, E.J., Green, M.J., Fitzpatrick, J.L., Morgan, K.L., Green, L.E., 2000. Risk factors associated with clinical mastitis in low somatic cell count british dairy herds. Journal of Dairy Science. 83:2464-2472.

Renaud, J.K., Seykora, A.J., Heins, B.J., Endres, M.I., Farnsworth, R.J. and Bey, R.F., 2005. Association between hygiene scores and somatic cell scores in dairy cattle. J. Am. Vet. Med. Ass. 227: 1297-1301.

Tyler, J.W., Fox, L.K., Parish, S.M., Swain, J., Johnson, D.L., Grasseschi, H.A. and Gant, R., 1997. Effect of feed availability on post-milking standing time in dairy cows. J. Dairy Res. 64: 617-620.

White, D.G., Harmon, R.J., Matos, J.E. and Langlois, B.E., 1989. Isolation and identification of coagulase-negative *Staphylococcus* species from bovine body sites and streak canals of nulliparous heifers. J. Dairy Sci. 72: 1886-1892.

Zdanowicz, M., Shelford, J.A., Tucker, C.B. and Weary, D.M., 2004. Bacterial populations on teat ends of dairy cows housed in free stalls and bedded with either sand or sawdust. J. Dairy Sci. 87: 1694-1701.

Somatic cell count patterns in a large sample of UK dairy herds

A. Madouasse[1], J.H. Huxley[1], W.J. Browne[2], A.J. Bradley[2] and M.J. Green[1]
[1]School of Veterinary Medicine and Science, University of Nottingham, Sutton Bonington Campus, LE12 5RD Sutton Bonington, United Kingdom
[2]Bristol Veterinary School, Langford House, BS40 5DU Langford, United Kingdom
Corresponding author: Aurelien.Madouasse@nottingham.ac.uk

Abstract

Somatic cell counts (SCC) are widely used to assess mammary gland health in dairy herds and over 50% of UK dairy farms subscribe to a recording scheme. Individual cow SCC are generally used as a proxy for intramammary infection (IMI); a threshold of 200,000 cells/ml is commonly used to indicate probable IMI. The resolution of herd problems requires quantification of disease patterns for which realistic targets are necessary. The aims of this research were (1) to provide UK benchmarks of cow SCC changes for the diagnosis of herd problems and (2) to quantify the association between cow SCC changes and herd bulk milk SCC. Data consisted of 6,920,955 recordings from 1,845 herds in England and Wales carried out between January 2004 and December 2006. A threshold of 200,000 cells/ml was used to categorise cows as infected or uninfected. Based on 2 consecutive recordings, the movements between infection categories both during lactation and across the dry period were investigated. Linear mixed models were used to assess the association between herd bulk milk SCC and individual cow SCC movements. Overall 25% of recordings were above 200,000 cells/mL, and there was large variation between herds. Cures did not compensate for new infections during lactation; the prevalence rose from less than 20% in the first 30d in milk to more than 40% at the end of lactation. Mean (best 10% ile) new infections and cure rates were 12.7% (7.2%) and 32.7 % (44.1%) in lactation and 17.1% (6.3%) and 72.8% (88.9%) across the dry period respectively. Cows remaining infected between consecutive recordings during lactation had the greatest impact on herd SCC. Infection rates for the top 10% of UK herds provide useful, achievable targets for dairy herd mastitis control.

Keywords: benchmarks, milk recording, monitoring, somatic cell count

Introduction

In the UK, the largest provider of milk recording is the National Milk Records (NMR) to which over 50% of dairy herds subscribe. Individual cow SCC results are used to select cows to treat or to cull. A 200,000 cells/ml threshold is commonly applied to categorise cows as infected (Bradley and Green, 2005). However, when dealing with herd problems, there exist no recently published reference to guide UK farmers and vets in identifying individual herd strengths and weaknesses. Based on three years of NMR data, the aims of this research were to provide UK benchmarks of cow SCC changes for the diagnosis of herd problems and to quantify the association between cow SCC changes and herd bulk milk SCC.

Materials and methods

Data and data selection

The classical NMR recording scheme consists in the monthly collection of a milk sample from every lactating cow of a herd on two consecutive milkings by a trained technician. Data collected are milk quantity; somatic cell count, lactose, butterfat and protein contents. Additional cow historical data such as date of birth, date of calving and parity are collected as well. In order to reduce costs farmers have to pay, NMR has developed other recording schemes such as recordings less frequently than monthly, one milking taken into account instead of two and recordings operated by the farmer himself. Our initial dataset contained all the NMR data collected between the 1st of January 2004 and the 31st of December 2006.

The aims of the data selection process were to identify and remove recordings from the alternative recording schemes, herds which stopped or started milk recording during the study and small herds (<30 cows). This was done to ensure the homogeneity and the consistency of the data analysed. The dataset used in the analysis contained 6,950,898 recordings from 65,870 test-days in 1,845 herds.

Definition of cow infection categories

For the data analysis, cows were categorised as uninfected and infected using a fix threshold of 200,000 cells/ml. The infection prevalence was the percentage of recordings above 200,000 cells/ml. To reflect the differences in management of heifers and of dry cows, recordings were further categorised as happening after 29 days in milk (*Lactating*: L), before 30 days in milk in parity one (*Heifers Fresh*: HF) and before 30 days in milk in parity greater than one cows (*Cows Fresh*: CF). By looking at two consecutive recordings, cows could stay uninfected, stay infected (*Chronics*), becoming infected (*New infections*) or becoming uninfected (*Cures*).

Percentages of the above defined cow categories in each cow-infection category were calculated. New infections and cures rates were also calculated using a different denominator, as follows. The new infection rate was defined as the percentage of cows below the threshold going above at the following recording as a percentage of the number of cows below the threshold at the first recording considered. The cure rate was the percentage of cows above the threshold going below at the following recording as a percentage of the number of cows above the threshold at the first recording considered.

The association between the percentages of the herd moving between these categories between consecutive test-days and the estimated bulk milk somatic cell count (eBMSCC) was investigated using multilevel linear models.

Bulk milk somatic cell count estimation

BMSCC was estimated by dividing the total quantity of cells contributed by all cows (somatic cell concentration × milk yield) by the total quantity of milk.

Working with consistent estimates

As noted by (Dohoo and Morris, 1993), there is a great variability in test-to-test estimates. In order to obtain sufficient numbers of cow recordings in each SCC category that allowed robust estimates of the effect on BMSCC, we chose to work with herd-year BMSCC for these analyses rather than test day BMSCC.

Results

Our sample consisted of 6,920,955 recordings carried out in 1,845 herds from England and Wales between the 1st of January 2004 and the 31st of December 2006.

Benchmarks

The characteristics of the distributions are shown: in Table 1 for the herd-year percentages of recordings above 200,000 cells/ml, in Table 2 for the herd-year percentage of cows staying above 200,000 cells/ml between consecutive recordings, in Table 3 for the herd-year percentage of cows moving from below to above 200,000 cells/mL between consecutive recordings, in Table 4 for the herd-year percentage of cows moving from above to below 200,000 cells/ml between consecutive recordings.

Table 1. Characteristics of recordings above 200,000 cells/ml for each category of cow as a percentage of total herd recordings.

	nobs	min	max	mean	Percentiles				
					10	25	50	75	90
All	5535	2.0	78.5	25.0	14.1	18.7	24.4	30.3	36.5
Lactating	5535	2.0	79.3	25.4	14.2	18.9	24.8	30.9	37.3
Cows Fresh	5534	0.0	77.8	21.3	10.2	14.7	20.4	26.6	33.3
Heifers Fresh	5507	0.0	100.0	17.1	3.8	9.7	16.0	23.1	31.2

Table 2. Characteristics of cows staying above 200,000 cells/ml (Chronics) for the Lactating and Cows Fresh categories, as a percentage of total herd recordings.

	nobs	min	max	mean	Percentiles				
					10	25	50	75	90
% Lactating	5535	0.0	69.5	16.0	7.4	10.8	15.1	20.1	25.7
% Cows Fresh	5534	0.0	64.7	11.7	3.2	6.3	10.6	15.6	21.4

Table 3. Characteristics of the number of cows going from below to above 200,000 cells/ml (New Infections) as a percentage of the cow category (%) and as a percentage of the number of cows below 200,000 cells/ml (Rate) for the Lactating and Cows Fresh categories.

	nobs	min	max	mean	Percentiles				
					10	25	50	75	90
% Lactating	5535	1.9	22.3	9.4	6.3	7.7	9.3	10.9	12.5
Rate lactation	5535	1.9	48.6	12.7	7.2	9.4	12.2	15.1	18.7
% Cows Fresh	5534	0.0	45.5	9.6	3.3	5.9	9.1	12.7	16.7
Rate dry period	5533	0.0	85.7	17.1	6.2	10.5	15.8	22.6	29.6

Table 4. Characteristics of the number of cows going from above to below 200,000 cells/ml (Cures) as a percentage of the cow category (%) and as a percentage of the number of cows below 200,000 cells/ml (Rate) for the Lactating and Cows Fresh categories.

	nobs	min	max	mean	Percentiles				
					10	25	50	75	90
% Lactating	5535	0.4	19.1	7.0	4.6	5.6	6.9	8.1	9.5
Rate Lactating	5535	8.1	100.0	32.7	22.4	26.4	31.6	37.6	44.1
% Cows Fresh	5534	0.0	80.8	30.3	15.6	21.9	29.6	37.9	46.2
Rate dry period	5531	0.0	100.0	72.8	55.6	64.7	73.7	82.0	88.9

Models

The first model (Table 5) evaluated the impact of the percentage of the herd in each cow-infection category on the estimated ln(herd-year BMSCC). The *Lactating* represented 92% of recordings and had the highest coefficients. In this category, the *Chronics* had the biggest impact.

The second model (Table 6) assessed the impact of new infection and cure rates on the estimated ln(herd-year BMSCC). Again, the *Lactating* category had the greatest impact on BMSCC. Higher cure rates were associated with lower BMSCC.

Table 5. Results of Model 1 for the association between ln(herd-year eBMSCC) and cow SCC categories with denominators based on all cow recordings.

	β	**Std Error**	**$(e^{(intercept+\beta)} - e^{(intercept)}) \times 1,000$**		
			Estimate	**CI 2.5%**	**CI 97.5%**
Intercept	3.93683	0.02893	51,256		
Chronics L	0.05658	0.00131	2,984	2,844	3,124
Cures L	0.03728	0.00336	1,947	1,598	2,298
New Infections L	0.05032	0.00262	2,645	2,369	2,923
Chronics CF	0.00824	0.00058	424	366	483
Cures CF	0.00123	0.00042	63	20	106
New infections CF	0.00957	0.00074	493	418	568
Infected HF	0.00270	0.00032	138	106	171
Average day in milk	-0.00069	0.00010	-36	-46	-26
Milk per cow	0.00284	0.00054	146	92	200
Chronics L * New Infections L	-0.00135	0.00013	-69	-82	-56
Chronics L * Chronics CF	-0.00024	0.00002	-12	-15	-10
Chronics L * Cures CF	-0.00016	0.00002	-8	-11	-6
Chronics L * New Infections CF	-0.00027	0.00004	-14	-18	-10
Chronics L * Infected HF	-0.00008	0.00002	-4	-6	-3
Cures L * New infections L	-0.00149	0.00027	-76	-103	-49

L: Lactating, CF: Cows Fresh, HF: Heifers Fresh.

Table 6. Results of Model 2 for the association between ln(herd-year eBMSCC) and cow SCC categories with denominators based on cows eligible for each category.

	β	**Std Error**	**$(e^{(intercept+\beta)} - e^{(intercept)}) \times 1,000$**		
			Estimate	**CI 2.5%**	**CI 97.5%**
Intercept	5.63159	0.06011	279,105		
New Infection Rate L	0.03080	0.00253	8,729	7,303	10,162
Cure Rate L	-0.02528	0.00129	-6,967	-7,656	-6,277
New Infection Rate CF	0.01103	0.00051	3,095	2,811	3,380
Cure Rate CF	-0.01052	0.00068	-2,921	-3,289	-2,553
Infected HF	0.00613	0.00044	1,716	1,477	1,955
Milk per cow	0.00269	0.00062	752	413	1,091
New Infection Rate L * New Infection Rate CF	-0.00045	0.00003	-126	-143	-108
New Infection Rate L * Infected HF	-0.00028	0.00003	-79	-95	-64
New Infection Rate L * Cure Rate L	0.00032	0.00004	89	66	112
New Infection Rate L * Cure Rate CF	0.00019	0.00003	52	38	67
Cure Rate L * Cure Rate CF	0.00014	0.00001	40	32	47

L: Lactating, CF: Cows Fresh, HF: Heifers Fresh

Conclusion

If a threshold of 200,000 cells/ml is used as a proxy for intramammary infection, an average of 25% of all recordings from our sample originated from infected cows. During lactation, among the cows above the threshold, nearly two thirds were already above on the previous test-day. Each percent of increase in this *Chronics* category was associated with the highest increase in ln(BMSCC) when compared to the other categories of SCC. Interestingly, the *percentage of cures* had positive coefficients in the first model, while higher *cure rates* were associated with lower BMSCC in the second model. This means that even though they achieve lower cure rates, herds with mastitis problems still have a higher proportion of their herd cured from one month to the other because of a higher initial prevalence. This highlights the difficulty of interpreting herd test-day data. For example, let us consider two herds milking 100 cows both achieving a new infection rate of 10% and a cure rate of 30% between two consecutive test-days but with an initial infection prevalence of 10% for the first and of 30% for the second. On the second test-day, the prevalence in the first herd will be of 16%, 3 of the 10 initially infected cows having been cured and 9 of the 90 previously uninfected cows having become infected. The prevalence in the second herd will be of 28%, 3 of the 30 initially infected cows having been cured and 7 of the 70 previously uninfected cows having become infected. Hence, rates need to be considered in the light of previous situation or over sufficient periods of time.

There was a very large degree of variation in all the SCC indices in this study and this indicates that progress is needed and possible, regarding somatic cell counts in UK dairy herds. Depending on each herd situation and specific herd objectives, the performance of the best 10 or 25% percent of herds could be used as achievable target figures. Depending on herd situation and specific objectives, the top 10% or top 25% figures could be considered as appropriate achievable target figures as is presented in Table 7.

Table 7. Possible targets for herd monitoring of SCC.

	Target values	
	Top 10%	**Top 25%**
% recordings > 200,000 cells/ml	14.1	18.7
New infection rate lactation	7.2	9.4
Cure rate lactation	44.1	37.6
New infection rate dry period	6.2	10.5
Cure rate dry period	88.9	82.0
% heifers calving > 200,000 cells/ml	3.8	9.7

References

Bradley, A.J. and Green, M.J., 2005. Use and interpretation of somatic cell count data in dairy cows. In Practice 27: 310-315.

Dohoo, I.R. and Morris, R.S., 1993. Somatic cell count patterns in Prince Edward Island dairy herds. Prev. Vet. Med. 15: 53-65.

Table 3. Proportions of underlying distributions of cow-SCC in subsets of dataset A[1] and B[2], using the estimated density functions of the entire dataset B.

Subset class	Subset level	N	p_{N1} [4]	p_{N2} [4]	p_{N3} [4]	p_{N4} [4]	p_E [4]
Previous	Below[3]	488,995	0.33	0.34	0.21	0.05	0.07
record[a]	Above[3]	1,168,679	0.03	0.01	0.23	0.34	0.40
(dataset B)							
Previous 2	Below-below[3]	96,114	0.35	0.38	0.20	0.03	0.04
records[b]	Below-above[3]	79,298	0.06	0.10	0.42	0.22	0.21
(dataset B)	Above-below[3]	55,994	0.09	0.20	0.40	0.15	0.15
	Above-above[3]	85,129	0.00	0.00	0.09	0.43	0.48
Parity[c]	1	96,105	0.26	0.32	0.23	0.10	0.10
(dataset A)	2	79,282	0.22	0.26	0.26	0.13	0.14
	3	55,069	0.17	0.22	0.25	0.16	0.20
	4 or higher	85,069	0.13	0.16	0.20	0.18	0.33
Lactation	0-50 d	46,265	0.35	0.25	0.14	0.07	0.19
stage[d]	51-100 d	48,622	0.37	0.26	0.14	0.06	0.16
(dataset A)	101-150 d	46,738	0.25	0.29	0.21	0.08	0.18
	151-200 d	45,250	0.16	0.29	0.26	0.12	0.17
	201-250 d	43,235	0.11	0.26	0.29	0.17	0.18
	251-300 d	38,746	0.07	0.21	0.31	0.22	0.20
	301-350 d	23,468	0.05	0.17	0.30	0.26	0.23
	351-400 d	24,102	0.03	0.13	0.29	0.30	0.26

[1] Dataset A consists of records of 41,567 cows on 407 farms.
[2] Dataset B consists of records of 58,070 cows on 1578 farms.
[3] Previous record = SCC grouped by the previous test-day record being below or above the chosen threshold of 100,000 cells/ml. Previous 2 records = SCC grouped by the previous two test-day records being below or above the chosen threshold of 100,000 cells/ml.
[4] p_{Ni} = proportion of records in i^th^ normal distribution; p_E = proportion of records in exponential distribution.
[a b c d] Subsets with a letter in common were tested for independence and all pairs are different (*P*<0.01).

Biological interpretation

Observations in the N4 and E distribution are associated with major pathogens (Ten Napel *et al.*, 2008) and persisting infections: the proportion of these two distributions is particularly high after two previous SCC above 100,000 cells/ml (Table 3). Ten Napel *et al.* (2008) interpreted the

N1 distribution as uninfected cows, the N2 distribution as cows recovering from an infection, the N3 distribution as cows with a non-persistent infection and the N4 and E distribution as cows with persistent infections.

The parity effect on SCC is largely caused by a shift of records to the N3 and E distributions (Table 3). A possible explanation is that the number of animals infected with pathogens causing persisting infections increases with time and that these infections rarely disappear. In contrast, the effect of stage of lactation is mainly caused by a shift from the N1 and N2 to the N3 distribution and to a lesser extent to the N4 and E distribution. The effects of parity and stage of lactation on SCC do not appear to be direct effects on SCC, but indirect effects through the likelihood of an infection: uninfected animals have the same SCC distribution, regardless of their age or stage of lactation.

New traits

The estimated mixed density function of SCC can be utilised by transforming SCC observations to the probability of the observation being a response to infection and to the probability of the response being to a persistent infection. From these probabilities we defined several new SCC traits. For example, 'Mastitis suspected' is the probability that at least one SCC in a lactation originated from the N3, N4 or E distribution. These probabilities can be used in addition to, or instead of SCC as udder health indicators (De Haas *et al.*, 2008).

A novel tool for veterinary advice could be to make a yearly profile for a herd by estimating the percentage of records in each distribution for SCC collected during the preceding twelve months. Such a profile may give insight into the types of pathogens present in the herd.

Conclusions

There is more information in SCC that can be utilised for reducing clinical and subclinical mastitis than is currently utilised in animal breeding and in veterinary research and practice. SCC can be approximately described by a mixture of four normal and one exponential distributions. The N1 distribution can be interpreted as uninfected cows, the N2 distribution as cows recovering from an infection, the N3 distribution as cows with a non-persistent infection and the N4 and E distribution as cows with persistent infections. Uninfected animals have the same SCC distribution, regardless of their age or stage of lactation.

Acknowledgements

The farmers are greatly acknowledged for providing information on occurrence of cases of clinical mastitis. This study is part of the five-year udder health program of the Dutch Udder Health Center and was financially supported by the Dutch Dairy Board.

References

Agha, M. and Ibrahim, M.T., 1984. Maximum-Likelihood Estimation of Mixtures of Distributions. Appl. Stat. J. Royal Stat. Soc. C. 33:327-332.

De Haas, Y., Ouweltjes, W., Ten Napel, J., Windig, J.J. and De Jong, G., 2008. Alternative somatic cell count traits as mastitis indicators for genetic selection. J. Dairy Sci. 91: 2501-2511.

De Haas, Y., Veerkamp, R.F., Barkema, H.W., Grohn, Y.T. and Schukken, Y.H., 2004. Associations Between Pathogen-Specific Cases of Clinical Mastitis and Somatic Cell Count Patterns. J. Dairy Sci. 87: 95-105.

Detilleux, J. and Leroy, P.L., 2000. Application of a Mixed Normal Mixture Model for the Estimation of Mastitis-Related Parameters. J. Dairy Sci. 83: 2341-2349

Green, M.J., Green, L.E., Schukken, Y.H., Bradley, A.J., Peeler, E.J., Barkema, H.W., De Haas, Y., Collis, V.J. and Medley, G.F., 2004. Somatic Cell Count Distributions During Lactation Predict Clinical Mastitis. J. Dairy Sci. 87: 1256-1264.

Heringstad, B., Rekaya, R., Gianola, D., Klemetsdal, G. and Weigel, K.A., 2003. Genetic change for clinical mastitis in Norwegian cattle: a threshold model analysis. J. Dairy Sci. 86: 369-375.

Odegard, J., Jensen, J., Madsen, P., Gianola, D., Klemetsdal, G. and Heringstad, B., 2003. Detection of mastitis in dairy cattle by use of mixture models for repeated somatic cell scores: A Bayesian approach via Gibbs sampling. J. Dairy Sci. 86: 3694-3703.

Ten Napel, J., De Haas, Y., De Jong, G., Lam, T.J.G.M., Ouweltjes, W. and Windig, J.J., 2008. Characterization of distributions of somatic cell counts. J. Dairy Sci. (in Press).

Ten Napel, J., De Vries, A.G., Buiting, G.A.J., Luiting, P., Merks, J.W.M. and Brascamp, E.W., 1995. Genetics of the Interval from Weaning to Estrus in First-Litter Sows – Distribution of Data, Direct Response of Selection, Heritability. J. Anim. Sci. 73: 2193-2203.

Ten Napel, J. and Johnson, R., 1997. Genetic relationships among production traits and rebreeding performance. J. Anim. Sci. 75: 51-60.

A new method for mastitis diagnosis based on hysteresis threshold of somatic cell count

M.A. Pérez[1], R. Ortega[2], R. Muñiz[1] and M.B. Coya[1]
[1]Dpto. de Ingeniería Eléctrica. University of Oviedo, Campus de Viesques s/n 33203 Gijón, Spain
[2]Centro Técnico Veterinario La Espina S.L., La Espina, Salas, Spain
Corresponding author: maperezg@uniovi.es

Abstract

From a significant amount of data (more than 200 cases tested by the California Mastitis Test (CMT), microbiological cultures and Video microscopy-Somatic Cell Count (VMSCC)) this paper presents several matters of concern to the sector, such as the instrumental uncertainty of SCC in mastitis diagnosis, doubts about the disease threshold, a not very strong relation between pathogenic agents and counts, and the collection of samples at long intervals – every month, according to the official milk control programs – with regard to the time of the disease evolution. The threshold of 200 cells/µl – curiously, coinciding with the payment for quality in many countries – is very often considered to define whether a cow is diseased or not. This paper refers to the diagnostic capability of SCC, and shows that such a strict threshold does not have much basis. Moving this threshold up or down is not the solution because this moves the problem around. In contrast, we can use an alternative for considering disease based on a threshold with hysteresis in which the value of hysteresis is equal to the measure error. For that aim, the previous situation of the animal is taken into account: when the animal was healthy (low SCC), it would be considered to be diseased only if the SCC clearly exceeded the threshold; in the same way, when it was diseased (high SCC), it would be considered to be cured only if the count descended clearly below the threshold.

Keywords: diagnosis, economics, monitoring, somatic cell count

Introduction

Mastitis in cows is an extremely important problem for dairies and it causes very important economic losses for farmers. The total amount of economic losses can be estimated around 2 billions dollars per year in the USA (Deluyker *et al.*, 1993) and it reaches corresponding values in other countries. These losses are an important handicap in dairy and related industries. Somatic cells count (SCC) is usually an important tool for estimation of economic losses (Shoock, 1982) since total milk production loss, decrease of milk quality, induced veterinary costs and cows substitution cost are associated to high values of SCC. The relation between mastitis and high SCC is well known (Harmon, 1994). Thus, mastitis, high SCC and negative economic effects due to mastitis are related issues. Therefore, to reduce the negative economic impact of mastitis, all implied agents (farmers, veterinarians, dairy industry) try to reduce both, mastitis and SCC. Figure 1 shows the relationships between mastitis and SCC and the economic impact. However, it is interesting to separate the economic effects of mastitis from the economic effects of an increase in SCC caused by mastitis. As can be seen, in Figure 1, the first effect can be estimated at approximately 86% of the total losses for a farmer; the second one represents only a 14% of the total and, in addition, is modulated by legal restrictions and regulations. Therefore, any action to improve the economic yield should certainly take mastitis into account.

Evaluation of SCC in fresh milk has many implications for milk quality, productivity, animal health, and trade issues. The SCC value is an extremely important issue to determine the milk and cheese quality due to the fact that these cells increase levels of lipolysis and proteolysis that affect to the quality and shelf life of fluid milk (Ma *et al.*, 2000), reduce yield and quality of cheese because of the decreased curd firmness, fat and casein retention (Politis *et al.* 1988), and decrease the sensory quality. It is useful for milk industries to establish the price of milk for each farm by means of several limits, which differ per country. This is represented in Figure 2, where SCC and economic losses are a consequence of the main problem: the mastitis. In consequence, mastitis prevention and diagnosis becomes extremely important subjects in the farm monitoring; in next sections of this paper, several matters about mastitis diagnosis are discussed.

Materials and methods

Microbiological cultures of milk are a very important tool in mastitis diagnosis since they provide an identification of pathogen agent causing the problem, allowing a specific treatment. However, microbiological culture is a costly procedure and needs several days to produce results; therefore, it is not a first election for mastitis diagnosis. Only after other signs, cultures are useful to confirm and to specify the mastitis.

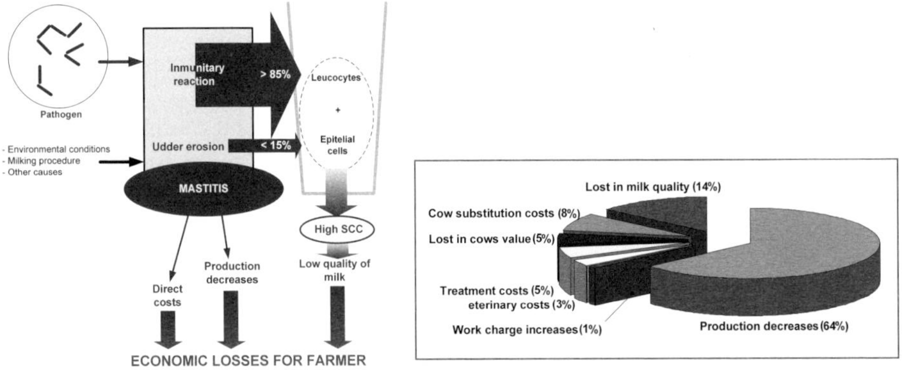

Figure 1. Economic effects of mastitis and the increase of SCC for farmer.

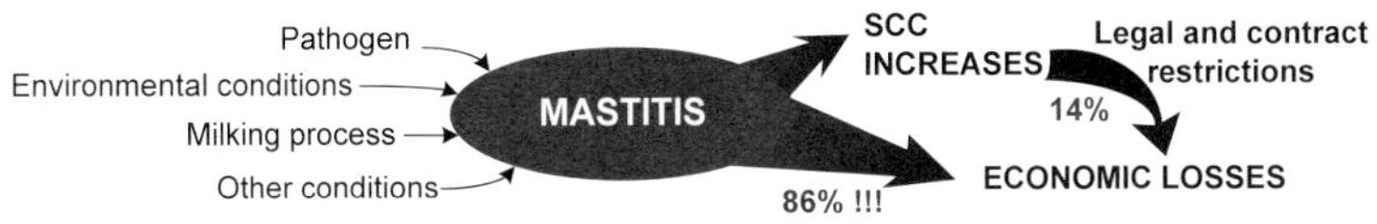

Figure 2. A new vision of mastitis economic effects where the SCC is only a consequence and it does not induced economic losses directly.

The California Mastitis Test (CMT) is a usual and universal tool for finding mastitis signs in cow milk; this test is a screening evaluation on immune system response of the animal by means of the milk viscosity after adding an agent. Although the interpretation of CMT results is subjective, depending on an operator and causing some uncertainty, trained operators can identify three or four levels without problem. Therefore, CMT is a quite simple, low-cost, mastitis diagnosis tool, but it would be interesting to know its efficiency (Pyörala, 1988; Sears *et al.*, 1990).

Somatic cells in milk represent an image of immune system situation: in normal conditions, its total number is low – it remains in physiological levels – but, under the attack of a pathogen, immune system increases the production of defensive cells, causing high values of SCC. Therefore, SCC is a robust indicator of mastitis (Harmon, 1994). Nevertheless the estimation of SCC is not a simple question, because it cannot be obtained with enough trueness on-line or in farm. Moreover, high-production laboratory methods do not provide enough trueness for diagnostic purposes (Baro *et al.*, 2005). The IDF-FIL microscopy method (IDF-FIL, 1995) could be used for a right estimation of Direct Microscopy - SCC (DMSCC) – but it has some disadvantages such as human-operator dependence, low repeatability and long analysis time since cells are manually counted; instead, a similar method with automatic image analysis will be used: VideoMicroscopy – SCC (VMSCC). Those results have full compatibility with DMSCC (Baro *et al.*, 2005; Grillo *et al.*, 2001).

Thus, relationships among the results of CMT, VMSCC and microbiological cultures were obtained from several milk samples and by following the method of Figure 3. The total study involves several samples of Holstein-Friesian cows in Asturias in Spain. The main characteristics of this study are shown in Table 1.

Looking for a threshold of SCC to mastitis diagnosis

The summarised results obtained from the study were plotted in two graphs in Figure 4, for CMT positive and for CMT negative samples. In both cases, samples positive and negative on microbiological culturing are plotted in separated bars, ordered by SCC ranges. The threshold to decide between healthy and diseased is established at 200 cells/μl. The relation CMT-SCC in mastitis diagnosis in our data revealed for CMT positive samples 37 cases of diseased cows and 59 cases of healthy cows. For CMT negative samples, SCC values defined 138 animals

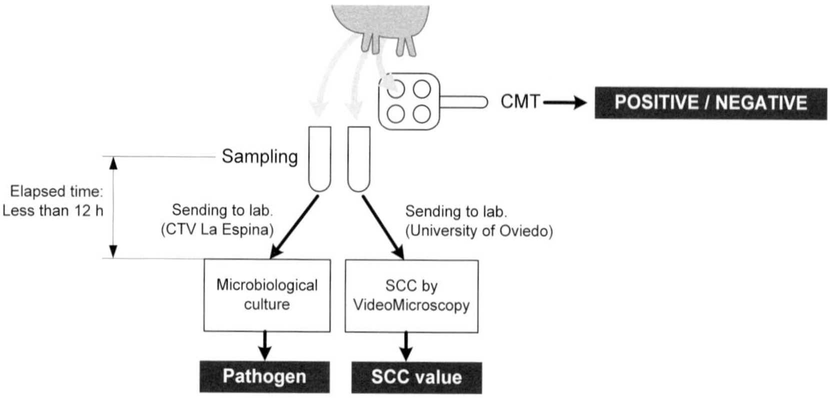

Figure 3. Methodology to compare the results from CMT, VMSCC and cultures.

Table 1. Characteristics of study.

Parameter	Value	
Area and cow type	Asturias	Holstein
Positive samples (CMT)	96	
Negative samples (CMT)	149	
Tests	VM-SCC	(University of Oviedo)
	Microbiological culture	(CTV)

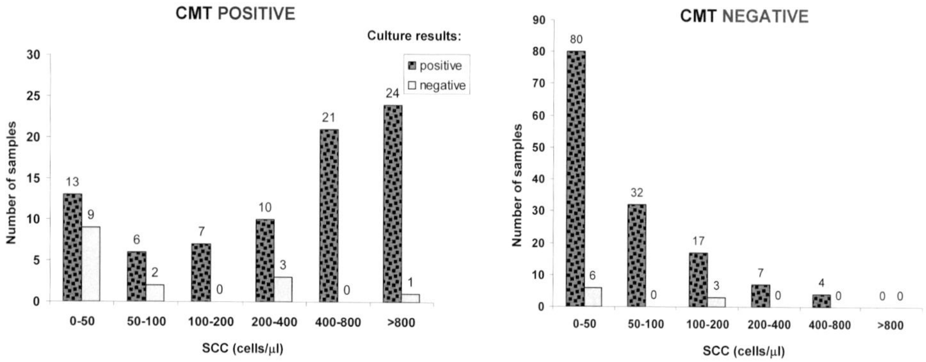

Figure 4. Results of study: left side graph represents the CMT positive cases and right side, CMT negative cases. In both graphs, positive and negative to microbiological culture are plotted for several ranges of SCC.

as healthy and 11 as diseased. This resulted in matching diagnosis around 80% of cases. Why 200 cells/µl? In several countries, this limit is used to establish the maximum count of high quality milk. Why not 400 cells/µl? This last value is used in several countries to reject milk with too high SCC. However, physiological levels of somatic cells are established below 100 cells/µl, so that a cow might be considered to be diseased when SCC reaches this threshold. Why not 100 cells/µl?

Figure 5 shows a comparison between SCC and CMT from a mastitis diagnostic point of view. As can be seen, there are no significant differences in matching diagnosis between SCC thresholds ranging from 100 cells/µl to 400 cells/µl. In all cases, concordance between SCC and CMT is higher than 75%.

Thus, CMT and SCC-threshold have similar mastitis diagnosis capability and the SCC threshold value is not critical. Nevertheless, the concordance between CMT and SCC-threshold diagnosis does not define health or disease, since both methods have uncertainty. Microbiologic cultures should constitute a better tool for mastitis diagnosis; Figure 4 includes the obtained results: for CMT positive, 81 of cultures have separated a pathogen and only 15 cases have produced negative results, matching in 84% of cases and validating the CMT positive as mastitis diagnosis. The right graph (CMT negative), however, produces surprising results, because only 9 of 149 samples were negative, causing concordance in less than 6% of cases. This result is similar in a SCC vs. culture comparison.

The culture-positive samples were classified in function of separated pathogen and the positive values were correlated to SCC values. The results for samples cultured positive to *S. aureus*,

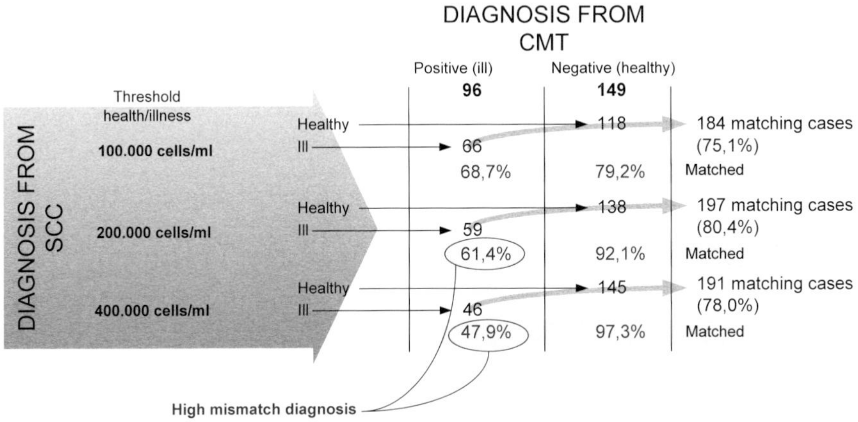

Figure 5. Mastitis diagnosis matching between SCC and CMT for 245 samples. At a glance, 200 cells/µl provides the better concordance, but 200 cells/µl produced mismatch diagnosis in 39% of CMT positives. All selected threshold produced similar results.

Corynebacterium and S. uberis are shown in Figure 6: in practice, any SCC value is feasible to be positive for *S. aureus*. The concordance of SCC diagnosis using a threshold of 200 cells/μl and microbiological cultures is approximately 50%. Similar results would be obtained if the SCC threshold ranges from 100 to 400 cells/μl. Therefore, it is unlikely that microbiological culturing is a robust tool for mastitis diagnosis.

Mastitis diagnosis by hysteresis

Results from Figures 4, 5 and 6 confirm similar behaviour of CMT and SCC as tools for mastitis diagnosis and introduce some uncertainties in microbiological cultures. However, the SCC value in those cases was a high precision measurement obtained from microscopy, an expensive and slow method not valid for high yield requirements. If a high-production somatic cell counter was used, the previous high precision would be unreachable. Is it possible to use these last SCC methods for mastitis diagnosis? With a rigid threshold, the answer will be no: Figure 7 shows a time evolution of SCC readouts for a cow, including the uncertainty of measurement and the effect over the mastitis diagnosis.

The effect over mastitis diagnosis is clear: the SCC measurement uncertainty introduces doubts if the difference between SCC and threshold is smaller than the measurement uncertainty. This consequence does not depend on method used, because any estimation of any parameter includes uncertainty. This becomes extremely important when the value of uncertainty is high. This disadvantage can be overcome by means of a comparison technique used with noisy and/or uncertainty measurement: hysteresis comparison, so that the threshold includes the value of measurement error. Thus, a healthy cow would be considered to be diseased only if the obtained SCC is higher than the SCC threshold plus the measurement uncertainty. Comparable, a diseased cow will be considered to be recovered if the obtained SCC has decreased below the SCC threshold minus the measurement uncertainty (see Figure 8).

This method may seem to have a lower precision level than the method that uses a rigid threshold, but in fact the hysteresis method provides a more secure diagnostic procedure because it takes the uncertainty of measurement into account. Therefore, precision in diagnosis

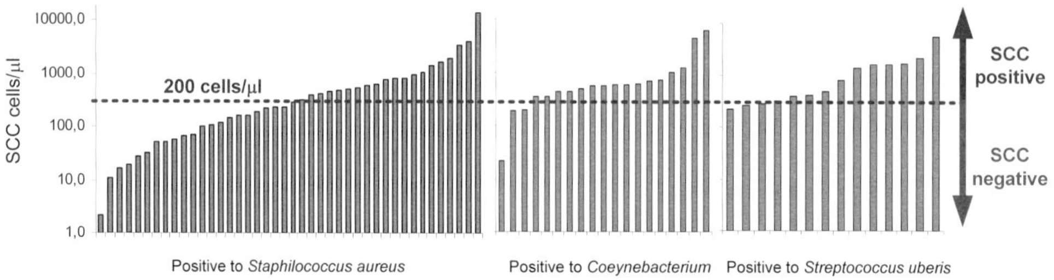

Figure 6. Mastitis diagnosis matching between SCC microbiological cultures.

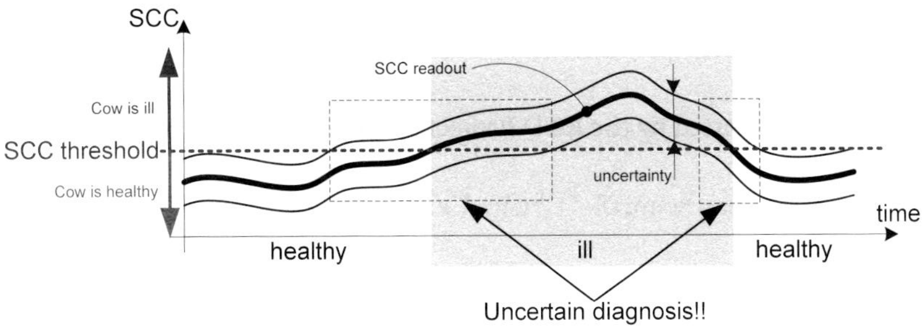

Figure 7. Effect of measurement uncertainty over the mastitis diagnosis, using a rigid threshold for SCC: there are several areas where the diagnosis is doubtful.

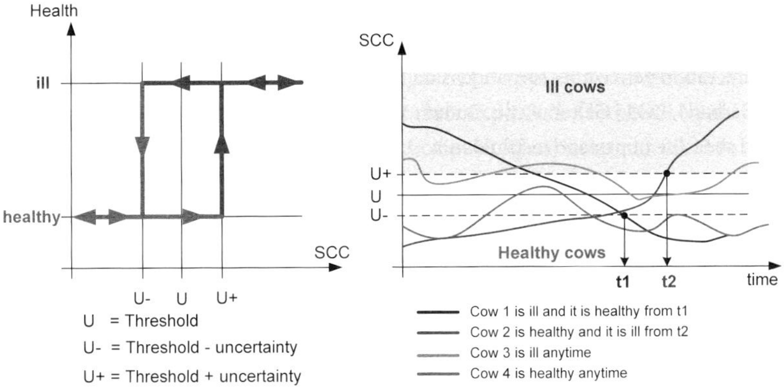

Figure 8. Hysteresis comparison of SCC to mastitis diagnosis.

depends on the measurement uncertainty. Thus, to increase diagnostic precision, it is necessary to improve the measurement trueness.

Conclusions

This paper has presented a new technique for mastitis diagnosis based upon a hysteresis threshold of SCC which includes the uncertainty in SCC estimation procedure, avoiding doubtful diagnosis (positive or negative) if SCC is close to the threshold. This new technique is the result of an extensive study of relationships between CMT, SCC and microbiological cultures that establish similar behaviour of CMT and high precision SCC (obtained by means of VM-SCC). Moreover, several uncertainties have been reported in microbiological cultures, causing important doubts about this method. Additionally, we could not find sustentation for a rigid threshold for SCC, because mastitis diagnosis results are similar for different values of that threshold.

Table 1. Diagnostic accuracy of the (non-partitioned, SCC-based) Non-P and the (partitioned-based) PART methods (example from Study I).

Study I (n=120)	**Non-P**[1]	**PART-I**[1,2]	**PART- II**[3]	**PART-III**[4]
N (%)	120 (100%)	66 (55%)	39 (32.5)	15 (12.5)
Prevalence	40.8%	36.4 %	48.7%	40.0%
Disease +	49	24	19	6
Sensitivity	63.2	95.8	91.7	100
Disease –	71	42	20	9
Specificity	84.3	88.1	100	100
Non-P dis. + (partial accuracy)	31 (49*0.632)			
Non-P dis – (partial accuracy)	60 (71*0.843)			
Non-P total accuracy	75.83% (91/120)			
PART dis + (partial accuracy)	46 (24*0.958+19*0.917+6*1.00)			
PART dis – (partial accuracy)	66 (42*0.881+20*1.00+9*1.00)			
PART total accuracy	91.7% (110/120)			

[1] Non-P: Non-partitioned testing (based on the SCC only), PART= partitioned testing (based on the indicator giving the best discrimination).

[2] Part I (groupI)= NM, EM, LM-A, LM-I.

[3] Part II (group II) =LM-I w/o I.

[4] Part III (group III).

In the tested populations, the partitioned-based method (PART, which used several indicators) revealed a greater diagnostic efficacy than the non-partitioned method (which used a single indicator, the SCC). Both in its full version (considering microbiological results and ROC analysis) and in its 'rapid' version (considering only leukocyte data for the diagnosis of disease-negative samples), the partitioned-oriented method revealed greater diagnostic ability than the Non-P. Possible explanations for the greater diagnostic ability of PART methods include: (1) a lower percentage of microbial isolations (both minor and major pathogens) in late disease stages (Figure 5), which may result in false negative results by methods that depend on only one indicator; (2) a rather lower SCC in late disease stages (Figure 4D-F), and (3) the fact that PART methods do not depend on any pre-determined indicator or indicator cut-off points but, instead, they select indicators and cut-off points after the data are collected, which are adjusted to each population. Because PART, in its 'rapid' version (not considering microbiological results but based only on leukocyte profiles), appeared to possess a greater diagnostic ability to correctly diagnose disease-negative cases than non-partitioned alternatives, and automated procedures may today rapidly assess milk leukocyte differentials, 'rapid PART' approaches could be considered to, at least, rule out which cases do not seem to be disease+ and/or do

Table 2. Assessment of disease-negative cases (example from Study II, n=500)[1].

Rapid PART (leukocyte indicators only)	Major pathogen + cultures	Minor pathogen + cultures	All pathogen+ cultures	Major/ minor pathogen ratio	Negative cultures	Diagnostic accuracy: 96.4%
NM (n=376)	9	13	22	0.69	354	
LM-T (n=28)	5	3	8	1.66	20	
LM-I (n=13)	1	3	4	0.33	9	
Non-P (SCC) (n= 500, prevalence: 15.0%)					Sp 84.7	Cut-off >446,000 cells

[1] If, in study II (without considering milk cultures and not using ROC analysis) all NM, LM-T and LM-I had been called "disease negative" ("rapid PART"), 96.4% (1-[15/417]) of the true disease-negatives (D–) would have been correctly diagnosed (considering, after such diagnosis was made, that 15 major pathogens had been diagnosed). In contrast, the non-partitioned SCC correctly identified 84.7% of the true D– samples.

not seem to require treatment (so, later, microbiologic testing could target a smaller number of samples). By partitioning the data into subsets defined by leukocyte-microbial-temporal indicators, disease stages of intra-mammary infections can be identified. When populations (e.g. herds) are tested, PART-oriented methods may offer more information to support diagnoses and diminish testing costs.

References

Hogan, J.S., Gonzales, R.N., Harmon, R.J., Nickerson, S.C., Oliver, S.P., Pankey, J.W. and Smith, K.L., 1999. Laboratory Handbook on Bovine Mastitis, 2nd edition. National Mastitis Council, Madison, WI, USA.

Chaffer, M., Rivas, A.L., Elad, D., Koren, O., Garazi, S., Chowell, G. and Schwager, S.J., 2008. Receiver operating characteristic-based accuracy assessment of a serological test used to detect Johne's disease in Israeli dairy herds. Can. J. Vet. Res. 72: 18-26.

Rivas, A.L., Quimby, F.W., Blue, J. and Coksaygan, O., 2001. Longitudinal evaluation of bovine mammary gland health status by somatic cell counts, flow cytometry and cytology. J. Vet. Diagn. Invest. 13: 399-407.

Operational use of bacteriology for mastitis control: field test of good practices

F. Sérieys[1], O. Bidaud[2] and L. Jouet-Elie[3]
[1]Filière Blanche, 12 quai Duguay Trouin, 35000 Rennes, France
[2]Intervet S.A., BP 17144, 49071 Beaucouzé, France
[3]Clinique vétérinaire, 87 rue de la Chataigneraie, 35600 Redon, France
Corresponding author: francis.serieys@wanadoo.fr

Abstract

Good practices of the veterinarian in the use of bacteriology at herd scale for mastitis prevention and treatment, were elaborated on expert sayings. In order to test them, a pilot study still in progress has been implemented in 17 farms from 9 skilled veterinary practices in France. Quarter milk samples from all the clinical cases and from the subclinical mastitis in the last lactation month and in the 1st lactation month of primipara, are aseptically taken by the farmers for bacterial identification and antibiograms. In each farm, the vet establishes 3 herd diagnosis and control plans: (1) before knowing any bacteriological result; (2) after knowing the results of a quota of analysis predetermined according to the herd situation and an acceptable cost for the farmer; (3) after knowing all the results. The aim is to precise the relevant number and kind of samples to be analysed in different epidemiological situations in order to draw reliable conclusions and recommendations. A software program was developed to help the vet to manage the herd bacteriological data. A first module allows to sort and filter the samples to be analysed and the available bacteriological results according to the kind of mastitis, the date and lactation stage of occurrence, the severity of the clinical cases. A second module provides an epidemiological and practical interpretation at herd scale by aggregation of the bacterial species according to their main reservoir (environment/udder), probable period of infection (lactation/dry period), antibiotics of choice, likelihood of cure. Results are presented in pie charts. A third module enables an interpretative reading of antibiograms and characterises each isolate towards the possible antibiotics on the market.

Keywords: control program, herd, management, prevention, veterinarian

Introduction

The evolution in the epidemiology of bovine mastitis, the new requirements of food safety and the limitations in the use of antibiotics, increase the vet practitioner needs for epidemiological diagnosis at herd scale to control the disease. However, bacteriological examination of quarter milk samples, the reference method for intramammary infections diagnosis, are not often carried out by the French practitioners, with probably no more than 5000 analysis per year performed by the official laboratories in the whole country. Most often in practice, bacteriology is considered as a strictly individual method of diagnosis helping the vet to choose a therapy for a quarter affected by clinical mastitis, particularly for recurrent case after failure of a first treatment.

This case-by-case approach without any capitalisation at the scale of the herd, only allows a poor valorisation in terms of advice given to the farmer, insufficient to justify his expense in bacteriological analysis. Moreover, if good practices for aseptic quarter milk sampling and laboratory procedures were validated a long time ago, nothing equivalent yet exists concerning the valorisation of bacteriology in terms of epidemiological diagnosis at herd scale and implementation of control measures in the farm. So, most of the vet practitioners, not precisely knowing how to cope with some scattered bacteriological results, only take into account cow milk somatic cell counts (SCC), clinical mastitis records and risk factors observed in the farm.

In this context, the objectives are the following: (1) to elaborate good practices on expert sayings about the use of bacteriology by the vet for herd-scale epidemiological diagnosis and mastitis control; (2) to test these good practices on expert sayings in the frame of a pilot-study in farms from different experienced veterinary practices; (3) to validate the positively tested good practices and integrate them in an operational tool for the vet practitioners including a software.

Good practices to be tested

Two manuals of good practices for the use of bacteriology by the vet were elaborated on expert sayings: (1) for the routine monitoring of mastitis control, apart from any particular problem; (2) for the definition of corrective control plans (prevention of new infections, treatments and culling) in farms facing a problem of clinical mastitis and/or cell counts. Only the good practices corresponding to the second purpose are presented here in their main lines. The aim was to define an operational method enabling a reliable epidemiological diagnosis by the vet at a cost acceptable by the farmer.

Bacteriology as a complement of other diagnosis methods

The use of bacteriology is not exclusive but comes as a complement of other methods bringing useful information for diagnosis, particularly somatic cell counting of cow milk at monthly intervals, systematic recording of clinical mastitis and treatments, research of mastitis risk factors in the farm (Sérieys, 1995).

Quota of bacteriological analysis and repartition of the samples to be analysed

A maximum number of bacteriological analysis is empirically fixed by the vet at the beginning of his intervention. The size of this quota has to be discussed and accepted by the farmer. It depends on the number of cows in the herd (Table 1) and may be modulated according to the economical importance of mastitis in the farm.

In the limit of the quota, the vet practitioner determines the repartition of the milk samples to be analysed according to the main patterns of the herd mastitis problem (Figure 1):
- relative importance of high somatic cell counts and clinical mastitis;
- specific problem or not of cell counts at the beginning of the first lactation;
- repartition of clinical mastitis with local or systemic signs.

If necessary, the vet can consider other criteria of repartition, for example season of occurrence of clinical mastitis.

Quarter milk sampling by the farmer

Aseptic quarter milk sampling for bacterial analysis is assumed by the farmer after demonstration and training by the vet. Samples are identified using auto-adhesive labels bearing pre-printed serial numbers in correspondence with the recorded data including at least the cow identification, quarter position, kind of mastitis (subclinical, local signs, systemic

Table 1. Indicative maximum number (quota) of bacteriological analysis according to the size of the herd for the definition of a corrective control plan.

Number of cows/herd	Quota of bacteriological analysis Number (% of number of quarters)
Up to 20	12 (>15%)
40	16 (10%)
60	20 (8,3%)
100	28 (7%)
140	36 (6,4%)

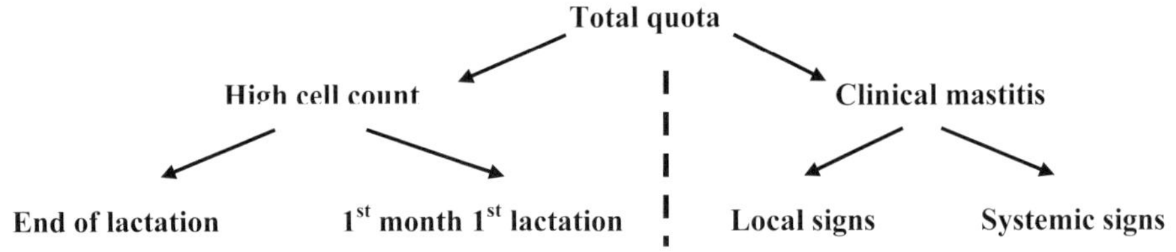

Figure 1. Repartition of the quota of bacteriological analysis according to main patterns of the herd mastitis problem.

signs) and sampling date. If milk samples are intended to be frozen, they are collected in sterile flasks containing glycerol as preservative (Cryokit®).

Incomplete identification of some pathogens

Systematic identification of the mastitis pathogens at the level of the species does not appear always justified and uselessly increases the global cost of analysis. So the pathogens are identified as follows: coagulase positive staphylococci (CPS), coagulase negative staphylococci (CNS), *Streptococcus agalactiae* (SRA), *Streptococcus dysgalactiae* (SRD), *Streptococcus uberis* (SRU), *Enterococcus* spp.(ETC), *Arcanobacterium pyogenes* (ARC), *Corynebacterium bovis* (COR), other Gram+ species (OGP), *Escherichia coli* (COL), *Pseudomonas* spp. (PSE), other Gram- species (OGN), yeasts (YEA), other micro-organisms (OTH).

Limitation in testing the sensitivity to antibiotics

Systematic testing of the sensitivity to antibiotics is limited to the CPS isolates. All are submitted to the nitrocefin test for the production of penicillinase and, if the test is positive, a complete antibiogram is carried out. For the other species, making antibiogram is only considered for severe or recurrent cases of clinical mastitis in the limit of 20% of the quota. Interpretative reading of antibiograms is carried out according to the instructions of the Comité de l'antibiogramme de la Société française de microbiologie (2007). The results, expressed as sensitive, intermediary or resistant, are given for the molecules present on the market and allowed for mastitis treatment.

Herd-scale epidemiological interpretation of bacteriology to implement the prevention plan

In complement of cow milk SCC, clinical mastitis records and identified risk factors, bacteriology results are interpreted to characterise the main epidemiological patterns of the disease in the herd by aggregation of the isolated pathogens according to their main reservoir (and the associated transfer way to the udder) and the most probable period of infection as reported by literature (Table 2).

This interpretation is made separately for subclinical and clinical mastitis isolates. COR, a contagious micro-organism transferred during lactation, but with small economic importance and CNS isolates, of various origins, are not incorporated in the aggregates. SRU isolates are taken into account only if the characteristics of the infections (subclinical, clinical, lactation stage of occurrence, SCC before clinical signs) allow the vet to hypothesise about their contagious or environmental origin. Some pathogens in high proportion may direct the vet towards more specific reservoirs or transfer ways, for example: CPS+SRD+ARC towards teat skin lesions; CPS in heifers+ARC out of lactation towards bees; PSE towards contaminated udder towels.

Table 2. Herd-scale epidemiological interpretation of bacteriology.

Epidemiological issue	Aggregation of pathogens %
Pathogen reservoir and transfer	
Udder reservoir (contagion at milking time)	CPS+SRA+SRD (+contagious SRU)[a]
Environment reservoir (few contagion)	ETC+ARC+COL+PSE+OGN (+environment SRU)[a]
Period of infection	
during lactation	CPS+SRA+SRD+PSE (+contagious SRU)[a]
during the dry period	COL+OGN

[a] Only if the distinction between contagious and environmental SRU is feasible according to the characteristics of the infections (subclinical, clinical, lactation stage of occurrence, SCC before clinical signs).

Herd scale interpretation of bacteriology for treatment plans

For the treatment in first intention of clinical mastitis, the plan distinguishes between cases without or with systemic signs (Faroult and Sérieys, 2001). For each of these mastitis forms, it considers the percentages of CPS producing penicillinase (CPS nitrocefine+), CPS not producing penicillinase (CPS nitrocefine-), SRA+SRD+SRU, ETC, COL, OGN. The first intention treatment is chosen by the vet to be active against groups of pathogens representing a great majority of the isolates, for example 75%. Antibiogram and sensitivity tests are taken into account for the choice of the antibiotic molecules, especially for contagious pathogens if they show homogeneous intra-herd profiles.

For the curative treatment of subclincal mastitis at drying off or eventually during lactation, the method is the same but only considers samples from quarters with high cell counts and the following groups of isolates: CPS nitrocefin+, CPS nitrocefin-, SRA+SRD+SRU, ETC.

Moreover, a herd prognosis of curability is established for clinical and subclinical mastitis separately, using a seven level curability scale from very low to very high with reference to the following groups of isolates: YEA+ARC+PSE; ETC+CPS nitrocefine+; CPS nitrocefine-; SRU; CNS; SRA+SRD; COL. For example, if the prognosis is bad, due for example to a high proportion of CPS nitrocefine+, culling must be rapidly considered after treatment failures of clinical mastitis and the treatment during lactation of subclinical mastitis must be inadvisable. The choice of a preventive treatment at drying off, antibiotic medicine or/and teat sealant, takes into account the bacteriological results of the samples from clinical mastitis in the first month of lactation, with particular attention to the proportion of SRU and COL.

Experimental software

A software program was developed to help the veterinarian to manage and interpret the bacteriological data at herd scale. A first module allows to sort and filter the samples to be analysed and the available bacteriological results according to the kind of mastitis, date of occurrence, lactation stage of occurrence, severity of the clinical cases. A second module provides an epidemiological and practical interpretation at herd scale by aggregation of the pathogen species according to their main reservoir, probable period of infection, treatments of choice, likelihood of cure. Results are presented in pie charts. A third module makes the interpretative reading of antibiograms and characterises each isolate towards the usable antibiotics.

Protocol of the pilot study

The aim is to assess if the epidemiological diagnosis and practical control measures drawn from the good practices in test are (1) reliable enough by comparison to a 'gold standard' consisting of the systematic bacteriological analysis of the clinical and subclinical udder infections in the herd; and (2) improve sufficiently the conclusions drawn without bacteriology to justify the extra costs for the farmer.

The pilot study has been implemented in 17 farms from 9 skilled veterinary practices in the different dairy regions of France. To be included, each farm had to call on his vet to solve a herd mastitis problem and the vet had to use the previously described good practices of bacteriology according to expert sayings in addition to the usual diagnosis means (SCC, clinical mastitis, observed risk factors). The animal phase of the study, still in progress, has been planned from October 2007 to September 2008.

The farmer aseptically collects quarter milk samples in sterile flasks with glycerol (Cryokit®): (1) from all clinical cases; (2) from all subclinical mastitis in the last month of lactation whatever the cow parity (cow milk SCC >200 000 cells/ml and CMT positive) and in the 1st month of lactation of primiparous cows (cow milk SCC >150 000 cells and CMT positive). Milk samples are frozen before posting to the Laboratoire Déparmental d'Analyses in Rennes. Boxes containing 5 frozen samples without cooling blocks are used for transportation. Pathogen identification is carried out at the level of the species except for the CNS. Antibiograms are made on all the bacterial isolates except COR and the nitrocefin test on the CPS isolates.

In each farm, the vet has to establish three successive herd diagnosis and control plans: (1) before knowing any bacteriological result; (2) after knowing, in a first time, the only bacteriological results allowed by the good practices; (3) after knowing, in a second time, all the bacteriological results constituting the 'gold standard'.

First results and discussion

The preliminary results of this study still in progress mainly concern the quality of samples and the repartition of the isolated pathogens. Among 463 milk samples collected from quarters affected by clinical (70%) or subclinical mastitis, only 23 (5%) were contaminated (Table 3). The number of contaminated samples per farm varied between 0 (7 farms) and 4 (2 farms). So, the sampling by the farmer after demonstration and short training by the vet, appears perfectly practicable as already reported (Bradley *et al.*, 2002; Houfschmitt, 2004). Basically, the default of sampling of some concerned quarters, especially from cows with high cell counts, was the main observed deficiency.

The global repartition of the isolates from clinical and subclinical mastitis (Table 4), shows that SRU is the most common pathogen (35%), followed by COL (15 %) and CPS (12%). No SRA,

Table 3. Repartition of the samples according to the number of isolates.

Nb isolates	Nb samples (%)
0 (sterile)	106 (23%)
1	315 (68%)
2	19 (4%)
>2 (contaminated)	23 (5%)
Total	463 (100%)

Table 4: Repartition of the isolates.

Pathogens isolated	Number (%)
SRU	125 (35%)
SRD	19 (5%)
CPS	44 (12%)
CNS	39 (11%)
COR	37 (10%)
ETC	7 (2%)
OGP	6 (2%)
COL	53 (15%)
OGN	16 (5%)
YEA	7 (2%)
Total	353 (100%)

PSE and ARC were found. Among CPS isolates, more than 90% were *Staphylococcus aureus* and less than 20% were positive to the nitrocefin test, a lower proportion than previously found (Sérieys and Bruneau-Gicquel, 2006). Among OGN, 50% were *Klebsiella* spp., 25% *Enterobacter* spp. and 25% other species. SRU was neatly the most frequent major pathogen in 6 herds, CPS in 1 herd, SRU + COL in 4 herds, SRU + *Klebsiella* spp. in 1 herd, SRU + CPS in 1 herd, CPS + SRD in 1 herd. In the 4 herds where CPS were relatively frequent, the isolates were entirely nitrocefin+ in 1 herd, entirely nitrocefin- in 2 herds and more than 85% of the isolates were nitrocefin- in 1 herd, confirming the high intra-herd homogeneity of this character (Sérieys and Bruneau-Gicquel, 2006).

Acknowledgements

J. Fresson (D.V.M.), J.C. Garreau (D.V.M.), L. Lafon (D.V.M.), F. Lars (D.V.M.), D. Lepoutre (D.V.M.), P. Parcollet (D.V.M.), E. Pichon (D.V.M.), O. Salat (D.V.M.), the 17 farmers of their practices and M. Bonnier of the Laboratoire Départemental d'Analyses in Rennes for their valuable contribution.

References

Bradley, A.J., Green, M.J. and Huxley, J.N., 2002. Making better use of milk samples: monitoring and investigating herd mastitis. Cattle Prac. 10: 1-8.

Comité de l'Antibiogramme de sa Société Française de Microbiologie, 2007. Recommandations 2007 du groupe de travail antibiogramme vétérinaire. Available at: http://www.sfm.asso.fr/doc/download.php?doc=DiU8C&fic=casfm_Vet-2007.pdf

Faroult, B. and Serieys, F., 2001. GTV-Partenaire: bonnes pratiques vétérinaires pour la définition d'un plan de traitement des mammites dans le troupeau. Ed. SNGTV Paris, pp. 1-27.

Houffschmitt, P., 2004. Lait de mammite: recul sur les analyses bactériologiques après congélation en élevage. Journées Nationales GTV, Tours, pp. 823-825.

Serieys, F., 1995. Les mammites des vaches laitières, 3rd edition. Ed. Institut de l'Elevage: Paris, pp. 1-64.

Serieys, F. and Gicquel-Bruneau, M., 2005. Homogénéité intra-troupeau des souches de *Staphylococcus aureus* de mammites subcliniques pour la production de β-lactamase et la résistance à la pénicilline. Rencontres Recherches Ruminants 12: 267-270.

Performance evaluation of systems for automated monitoring of udder health: would the real gold standard please stand up?

G.A. Mein[1] and M.D. Rasmussen[2]
[1]Sensortec Ltd, Hamilton, New Zealand
[2]Dept.of Agricultural Engineering, University of Aarhus, Horsens, Denmark
Corresponding author: mein@netspace.net.au

Abstract

Data from a recent field study in New Zealand and another in Denmark were analysed to illustrate some real or perceived problems with finding the 'right' reference standard to use when evaluating the performance of automated monitoring and detection systems for udder health. Our analyses imply that a robust 'gold standard' cannot be derived from observations of clots in foremilk at a single milking per month. Inclusion of cows with a few flecks in their foremilk on isolated occasions is likely to result in over-diagnosis of clinical mastitis. Addition of a criterion of raised cell count or CMT >3 in foremilk from one or more quarters of a cow reduces the likelihood of over-diagnosis of clinical mastitis or abnormal milk. However, inclusion of cell count or CMT information is not necessary if the definition of a true clinical is based on observation of clots at 2 of 3 consecutive milkings. Annex C of ISO 20966 implies that diagnosis can be based on the first squirts of foremilk. A more objective test would be to discard the first three squirts of foremilk before sampling to determine the presence of clots. Our recommended definition of a 'clinical episode' (or 'clinical case') is: 'Clots (> 2mm in average diameter) persisting beyond the first three squirts of foremilk for at least 2 of 3 consecutive milkings.' This definition would provide an effective compromise between robustness of the gold standard and the practical issues of conducting an evaluation of new sensing systems. Because the incidence of clinical cases is low and variable in most herds, a 36 h evaluation period may be too short to produce reliable data for robust statistical analyses.

Keywords: biosensors, clinical mastitis, gold standard

Introduction

The new International Standard (ISO 20966, 2007) includes an informative Annex C which attempts to deal with methods of detecting abnormal milk and interpretation of test results. A major difficulty in this field is that an independent assessment of the 'true' udder health status of a herd – even on an isolated test-day, let alone a continuous basis – is both difficult and expensive to obtain. For example, Annex C recommends that 'Sampling shall be performed in at least three herds for at least 36 h in each herd.' Another major problem is the lack of genuine agreement on the 'right' 'gold standard' against which to judge the performance of automatic monitoring and detection systems. Matters are made worse by the fact that new clinical infections are relatively infrequent events. Consequently, statistics tend to be weak. The strength of the statistics for calculation of the sensitivity depends very much on the frequency of clinical abnormalities.

Nevertheless, if automatic detection systems are to gain acceptance in the cost-conscious dairy industry, and deliver to farmers the benefits that we believe they are potentially capable of providing, these issues must be tackled. The main purpose of this paper is to invite further debate on the question: 'What is the 'right' gold standard (or standards) to use when evaluating the performance of automated monitoring and detection systems for udder health?'

Methods

Field data from New Zealand

Data obtained from a field study in New Zealand (Claycomb *et al*, personal communication, 2008) are used to illustrate some of the issues discussed in this paper. For convenience of readers, a brief description of that study is given here. In October 2006, a novel sensing system was evaluated against a quantitative 'gold standard' for clinical mastitis in a herd of 650 cows milked twice daily in a 50-stall rotary parlour. The data-set contained 26,974 cow-milking records, equivalent to an average of 642 cows milked twice daily. The 'gold standard' was based on visual observation of milk clots on a commercially-available, in-line clot filter (Mastitis detector, Ambic Equipment Ltd, UK. www.ambic.co.uk) which was installed in each milk hose of all 50 milking units. The filter consists of a stainless metal mesh with a pore size of 0.9 mm diameter. A technician was employed to check these filters for clots as soon as the cluster was removed from each cow at every milking for three weeks. The filter screen was removed and rinsed clean with running water each time that clots were found on the filter. Clots were recorded as score 1, 2 or 3 according to the sample pictures supplied with the commercial filters. Individual cow, somatic cell count (ICCC) data were obtained from the monthly herd test samples collected 1 week before the start of the 3-week experimental period and again on the final day of the field study.

Field data from Denmark

Data from a Danish study (Rasmussen and Bjerring, 2004) were re-analysed to examine relationships between the observation of clots in foremilk at successive milkings, CMT scores and the classification of quarters as true clinical or non-clinical cases. Data were reviewed for cows having at least one milking at which clots were observed in their foremilk. Cows with records from less than 3 consecutive milkings were discarded, leaving a total of 107 cows having records available for 3 to 9 consecutive milkings for the analysis.

Results

New Zealand results and implications

Clots were observed on the mastitis filter screens on 54 occasions during the New Zealand study. Of these 54 observations, 11 were scored 1, 15 were scored 2 and 28 were scored 3. For a herd of about 640 cows observed for a 3-week period, the total of 54 clot observations is equivalent to more than 11 clinical cases per 100 cows per month. By comparison, Aust-ralia's 'Countdown Downunder' warning level for a herd mastitis problem is only 2 clinical cases per 100 cows/month (Brightling *et al.*, 2000). Such a high clinical case rate could imply that the herd might be experiencing a mastitis crisis. This seemed unlikely, however, because the herd BMCC remained steady at about 150,000 cells/ml before, during and after the study.

To explore the possibility that single clot events on the filter screen might lead to over-diagnosis of clinical mastitis, one of us (GM) talked to the herd manager. His records showed that only 15 clinical cases were treated during the trial period (equivalent to a clinical treatment rate of 3.4 per 100 cows per month). The herd manager commented that he 'did not take a lot of notice of the clot results on the mastitis filter because, when he checked most of those cows, clots disappeared after a couple of squirts of their foremilk'. His comment is consistent with a practical guideline from the Australian Countdown Downunder program which helps farmers avoid over-diagnosis or over-treatment of clinical cases. According to the relevant guideline, 'a case of clinical mastitis which requires treatment occurs when there is heat, swelling and pain in the udder, or there are changes in the milk (wateriness or clots) that persist for more than three squirts of milk'. (Brightling *et al.*, 2000).

Table 1 illustrates the difficulties inherent in choosing the 'right' gold standard for monitoring clinical mastitis. Four optional benchmarks are presented in this table:

Option 1: If the presence of clots on the filter screen after milking is regarded as the 'true' gold standard for clinical mastitis, then the benchmark for comparison with results from the sensor under test would be 54 'true' clinical cows. [Note that the clot-positive filter screens could have been contaminated with clots at any stage during the milking of an individual cow].

Option 2: This 'gold standard' required the presence of clots on the filter screen after milking and ICCC > 800,000 cells/ml (equivalent to CMT score >3 as specified in Annex C of ISO 20966) at the start and/or at the end of the study. Using this option, the apparent benchmark was 34 'true' clinical cows. [Note: Because it was not possible - after the field study - to follow the precise guidelines in Annex C, this option (clots confirmed by a raised cell count) was based on ICCC data from the monthly herd test collected 1 week before, and on the final day of, the 3-wk period].

Table 1. Data derived from a 650-cow herd monitored for a 21-d period in October 2006. These data were analysed in different ways to illustrate: (a) the remarkable variation in the number of 'true clinicals' according to the gold standard used; (b) the resulting apparent variation in performance measures for the sensor that was field-tested.

Gold standard option	Number of 'true' clinical cows	Sensitivity	False Alert Rate (per 1000 cow-milkings)
1. All cows with one or more clot observations	54	37/54 (68%)	6.4
2. Discard cows with clot alerts if ICCC <800 k cells/ml	34	30/34 (88%)	6.5
3. Clot alerts at 2 consecutive milkings or 3 times in 6 milkings	21	18/21 (86%)	3.9
4. Only cows selected by herd manager for antibiotic treatment	15	12/15 (80%)	7

Note: The False Alert Rate is the number of false alert episodes per 1000 cow-milkings as defined and described in our companion paper (Sherlock *et al.*, 2008).

Option 3: This option required the presence of clots on the filter screen at 2 consecutive milkings or 3 times in 6 milkings. Cows with isolated, non-persistent observations of clots on the filter screen were ignored or discarded from the analysis. Using this gold standard, the apparent benchmark was 21 'true' clinical cows.

Option 4: If we assume that cows selected by the herd manager for treatment were the only 'true' clinical cases, then the benchmark would have been only 15 true clinicals.

In light of the difficulties of deciding which - if any - of these options was the 'true' gold standard, it is almost impossible to decide what were the 'right' performance measures for the particular sensor under test. For example, the low Sensitivity for the option with the highest number of apparently 'true' clinical cases (Option 1) might result from a fundamental problem of over-diagnosis of clinical mastitis based on a single, isolated observation of clots on the mastitis filter. At the other extreme, the 'gold' standard for Option 4, which had the lowest number of apparently 'true' clinical cases, is likely to be tarnished because the incidence of clinical mastitis often is higher than expected or found by the average herdsman.

The truth probably lies somewhere between the two extreme positions represented by Options 1 and 4. The gold standards for the two options with the highest Sensitivity (Options 2 and 3) seemed more promising and these possibilities are explored further in our next section.

Danish results and implications

Of the 107 cows having at least one milking at which clots were observed in their foremilk, 94 also had a CMT score >3 in one or more quarters. Individual cow-milkings for these two groups of 107 and 94 cows were divided into percentages of milkings at which clots were observed. In the group of 107 cows, 74% had clots in their milk at <50% of their milkings. This proportion dropped slightly, to 70% of 94 cows, when the CMT score was included as a criterion for confirming the presence of clots in milk. Thus, clots were present consistently (ie, at >50% of milkings) in only about 30% of cows with clots in their foremilk. Inclusion of a CMT criterion made no difference to the number of 'true' clinical cows if clots were present in foremilk at >50% of their milkings (60, 80 and 100% on the x-axis of Figure 1A and 1B).

The general pattern of these results is similar to those shown in Table 1 for the NZ data. The Danish group of 107 cows with clots at one or more milkings represents Option 1 in the NZ analysis. The Danish group of 94 cows (i.e. 88% of 107) with clots confirmed by CMT score >3 is similar in concept to Option 2 in which 34 clinical cases were confirmed by ICCC (i.e. 63% of 54 total clot observations in NZ). The Danish group of about 30% of cows with clots in their foremilk at >50% of their milkings is similar in concept to Option 3 (21 clinical cases, i.e. 39% of 54 clot observations in the NZ data).

Discussion

The main implication of the NZ and Danish analyses is that the classification of true clinical status needs to be confirmed either by linking a clot observation with a raised CMT score (or raised SCC) in quarter foremilk or by repeated clot observations at consecutive milkings.

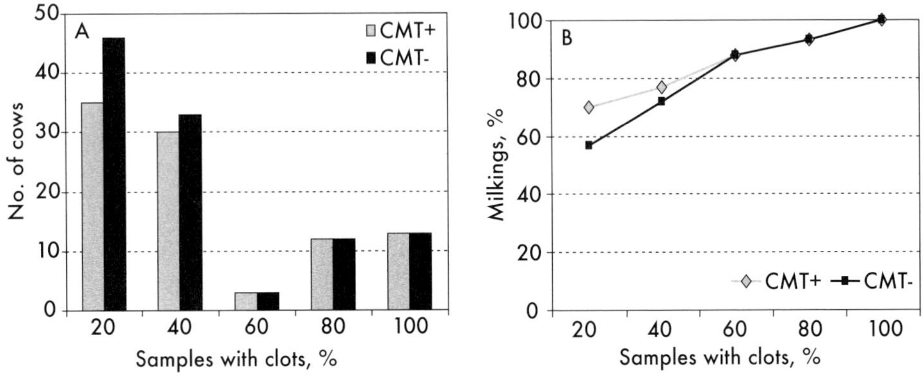

Figure 1. Frequency distribution showing the percentage of individual cow-milkings at which clots were observed in the foremilk of two groups of cows at 3 to 9 consecutive milkings for (A) number of cows (B) percent of milkings in each frequency class.

Although the CMT method is simple and convenient, CMT scoring is subjective. Some people tend to score high and others low. A further disadvantage of the CMT is that a threshold score >3 (>800,000 cells/ml) may be too low in quarter foremilk to confirm a true clinical case. According to Thurmond (1990), for example, clinical signs are not readily apparent until quarter SCC reaches 4-5 million cells/ml, although clinical symptoms have been reported for quarter milk with as few as 1-2 million cells/ml. Given the subjective nature of CMT scoring, we suggest that a more robust classification of true clinical status should be based only on observation of clots in milk on at least 2 of 3 consecutive milkings.

Annex C of ISO 20966 includes an informative note which states that 'Finding clots in the foremilk on the [specified test] filter means that the quarter and animal suffers from clinical mastitis.' In view of the previous discussion, this informative note appears likely to lead to over-diagnosis of clinical infections. This note does not include the sensible advice, given elsewhere in Annex C, to base the diagnosis on clots larger than 2 mm. Furthermore, it implies that the diagnosis can be based on the first squirts of foremilk. Because the first 10 ml of milk from each quarter is caught and discarded in most (if not all?) brands of AMS, an automatic sensor cannot monitor the first squirts of foremilk. Given that the goal of Annex C is to make objective evaluations of automatic detection systems, a more objective test would be to apply the guideline given in Australia's Countdown Downunder program for diagnosing a true clinical case, i.e. to discard the first three squirts before sampling to determine the presence of clots.

What do farmers expect from an automatic detection system?

Although we have concentrated on automated systems for detecting clinical mastitis in this paper, many farmers (and regulators) want more than this. Most farmers would like an automatic monitoring system to: detect and divert abnormal milk; to detect cows that must be treated; a system that can tell when an individual cow's milk can be included in the bulk supply following treatment; and a system that can provide a culling list. Not surprisingly, Kamphuis *et al.* (2008) found a large amount of overlap between variables selected for abnormal milk and for clinical mastitis classification. According to these authors, these two problems are unlikely to be solved with the same classification model because they 'are likely to have a different prevalence of positive cases and a different trade-off between sensitivity and specificity. For example, for abnormal milk detection, the classification model must be able to correctly discard a reasonable proportion of abnormal milk without discarding a large amount of normal milk. However, a classification model for clinical mastitis needs to identify those cows and quarters likely to have mastitis for a mastitis attention list. This list can potentially include a moderate number of cows without mastitis (false positives) but the focus must be on developing a model with a high sensitivity.'

We agree with Kamphuis *et al.* that these two problems are likely to need different classification models. In response to their proposed focus on developing a model with high sensitivity, we suggest that the target of >70% given in Annex C is a minimum requirement for a mastitis attention list. As for their key question: what is an acceptably 'moderate number' of false positives for a mastitis attention list, we suggest that the target specificity of >99% in Annex C is also a minimum requirement. This target implies that farmers must be prepared to deal with up to 10 false alerts per 1000 cow-milkings in their daily routines.

Conclusions and recommendations

Gold standard for a 'true' clinical cow

Our recommended definition of a 'clinical episode' (or 'clinical case') is: 'Clots (> 2 mm in average diameter) persisting beyond the first three squirts of foremilk for at least 2 of 3 consecutive milkings.' This definition would provide an effective compromise between robustness of the gold standard and the practical issues of conducting an evaluation of new sensing systems. A potential advantage of this definition is that its wording mirrors the classic definition of a truly infected quarter (Neave, 1975), i.e. (1) to discard the first couple of squirts before collecting a sample for culture; (2) to classify a quarter as infected if the same pathogen is isolated from that quarter at 2 consecutive or 2 of 3 consecutive culture samples.

Gold standard for a 'true' negative cow

Cows with no flakes, clots, watery, yellowish or bloody milk and with a CMT score <4 on all quarters could be used for calculation of specificity and false alert episodes per 1,000 cow-milkings. As an alternative to the subjective CMT criterion, cows could be classified as 'true negatives' if SCC is <200,000 cells/ml in composite milk of weekly samples and all foremilk samples are without any clinical signs.

Getting the numbers right

Because the incidence of clinical cases is low and variable in the majority of herds, a 36 h evaluation period is likely to be too short to produce reliable data for robust statistical analyses. As is implied in Annex C of ISO 20966, an evaluation study may require that monitoring is extended beyond 36 h until a total of at least 20 cows or quarters have been identified as true clinical cases.

References

Brightling, P., Mein, G.A., Hope, A.F., Malmo, J. and Ryan, D.P., 2000. Countdown Downunder: Technotes for Mastitis Control. Published by Dairy Research and Development Corporation, Australia.

ISO 20966, 2007. Automatic milking systems – requirements and testing. Annex C: Example of methods of evaluating detection systems for milk deemed as abnormal due to blood or to changes in homogeneity. Intl. Org. for Standardization, Geneva, Switzerland.

algorithms that generate mastitis alert lists, reporting those cows and quarters likely to have mastitis. For a CM detection model it is important to identify at least those cows with a severe udder infection. These cows need an antibiotic treatment as soon as possible that helps stop the pathogen from invading the udder. Although the sensitivity of current detection models might be improved, an additional common complaint by dairy farmers using AM considers the high number of false positive alerts on the mastitis alert lists, leading to an unwanted additional work-load (Hogeveen and Ouweltjes, 2003).

In the past, research focussed on the electrical conductivity (EC) of milk to detect CM. Variables derived from in-line EC measurements have been compared across milkings of the same quarter (Lansbergen *et al.*, 1994) or with other quarter milkings (Maatje *et al.*, 1992) to detect pattern changes possibly due to CM occurrence. Also smoothing, Kalman filters or the fuzzy logic theorem were used for CM detection (Cavero *et al.*, 2006; De Mol *et al.*, 1999; De Mol and Woldt, 2001). Most of these models used the maximum or the mean value (or a combination) measured within a cow or quarter milking. Kamphuis *et al.* (2008) suggested that not only the mean or maximum EC value showed potential for CM detection. Instead, detection performance may be improved by combining different predictive variable types, for example, combining the standard deviation of the EC measurement pattern with the slope of the measurement pattern of the colour sensor blue.

The fact that sensor data itself are noisy and often incomplete is one of the major difficulties for developing CM detection models. Furthermore, the low prevalence of CM makes modelling even more difficult. Data mining is a technique which tries to discover new knowledge in large amounts of data, and addresses the question of how to use historical data to discover general regularities to improve the process of decision making (Mitchell, 1999). Decision tree (DT) induction is a commonly used data mining technique (Quinlan, 1986) which is believed, in contrast with more traditional statistical approaches, to be capable of dealing with data that is noisy, imbalanced and/or incomplete.

The objective of this study was to explore the potential of DT induction for the automated detection of CM, using data collected in the field. The detection model should be able to deal with real on-farm data.

Materials and methods

Data collection

Data used in this study was collected from December 2006 till August 2007 at six Dutch commercial dairy herds using in total 9 AM systems (Lely Industries N.V., Maassluis, the Netherlands). The primary selection criterion for farmers to participate was a serious daily use of the mastitis alert list as criteria to check quarter visually for CM. As standard procedure, the AM system discards the first approximately 30 ml milk per quarter milking. After that, average values for each 100 ml of milk are recorded for four in-line sensors (EC, red, green and blue) for each quarter milking by the AM system. Each AM system was connected to a separate remote computer and the 100 ml measurements as well as sensor measurement values at quarter milking level were logged to this remote computer. In addition, an estimation of quarter milk yield was registered, as well as date and time registrations of when a cow entered the AM, when teat cups were attached and when milk flow started. Participating farmers were introduced to a scoring protocol (Figure 1). The protocol was set up to collect data from those cows and quarters mentioned on the mastitis alert lists and that were visually checked. In addition to the score assigned to a quarter, cow identification number, the quarter itself, and date and time of scoring were recorded. Whenever a farmer decided to start an antibiotic treatment, a milk sample (duplo) was requested for free of charge bacteriological culturing (BC) before the start of the treatment. Every four to six weeks farmers were visited to collect data from the remote computers, the scoring forms and the milk samples for BC. BC results were communicated to the farmers as soon as results were available.

Data preparation

Sensor data were collected from almost 600 cows and over 670,000 quarter milkings, and 429 quarter milkings were visually checked for CM. Sensor data and observational data were combined when the time difference between the visual check and the milking was equal to or less than 24 hours. Quarter milkings where the AM system failed to connect the teat cups were deleted from the data set together with quarter milkings where data on teat attachment and 100 ml measurements recordings were missing. A data flow diagram, described in Kamphuis *et al.* (2008), was used to define descriptive variables for sensors measurements of EC, the colours red, green and blue, milk flow (milk production in ml/second within a quarter milking), milk flow delay (time between the teat being cleaned and start of the milk flow), dead milking time (time between teat cup attachment and start of the milk flow), and milk production (total

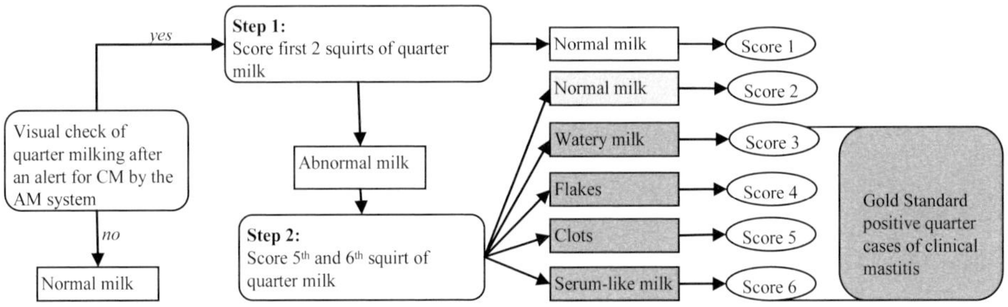

Figure 1. Scoring protocol of those quarters checked by dairy producers visually. Scoring of squirts of milk was done using a clean black CMT paddle. Scores were used to define Gold Standard positive quarter cases of clinical mastitis.

quarter milk yield divided by the time since the previous milking). A total of 1,095 independent variables were used as input for the CM detection model.

Gold standard definition of positive and negative cases of clinical mastitis

Gold standard positive (GSpos) cases were quarter milkings that received an observational score of 3 or higher (Figure 1), resulting in 100 GSpos cases. Quarter milkings that were checked and scored a 1 or 2, and quarter milkings that were not visually checked were considered as gold standard negative (GSneg) cases in first instance. However, the GSneg label was removed from all cow milkings 2 weeks prior or post a GSpos case, from quarter milkings that were separated manually or automatically, and from quarter milkings where separation details were missing. This definition resulted in 630,080 GSneg quarter milkings, from which 3,000 quarter milkings were randomly selected for further analyses.

Decision tree induction and performance analyses

A DT algorithm, using the information gain ratio to split the data set at nodes (Quinlan, 1993), was used to produce probabilities for each quarter milking to have CM. In addition to the default settings of the DT algorithm used, two important parameters were varied to study their effect on detection performance. First, a cost matrix was introduced to account for the imbalance of positive and negative cases of CM in the dataset. By introducing costs for false negative alerts, the algorithm is forced to put more emphasis on classifying quarter milking as positive for CM during training. The higher the costs the more emphasis is put on a positive classification. The confidence factor, a number that is used by the algorithm to prune developed trees to avoid over-fitting a model, was the second parameter that was varied. The lower the confidence factor, the more pruning, and the smaller the final DT is. Default values of the DT algorithm are equal costs and a confidence factor of 0.25. Ten fold cross validation (Figure 2) was used to estimate the performance of the DT classifier when applied to unseen data. To compare different DT algorithms the sensitivity (SN), the specificity (SP), the number of false positive alerts per 1,000 quarter milkings (False Alert Rate) and the positive predictive value (Success Rate) were evaluated. Receiver-operating characteristic (ROC) curves were produced to visualise the performance of several DT algorithms over the whole range of SN and SP combinations. For each of the 10 test sets of the 10fold cross validation, trade-off values ranging from 0 to 1.0 (in 40 equal steps) of the given probabilities were used to define CM. Figures for SN and SP resulting from these cut-off values were averaged to represent values of the final classifier E in Figure 2 and to create points for the final ROC-curves. Data preparation was done using SAS version 9.1 (SAS Institute Inc., Cary, NC). Development of several DTs was done in WEKA version 3.4.8 (Witten and Frank, 2005). ROC-curves were created in S-PLUS version 7.0 (Insightful Corp., Seattle, WA).

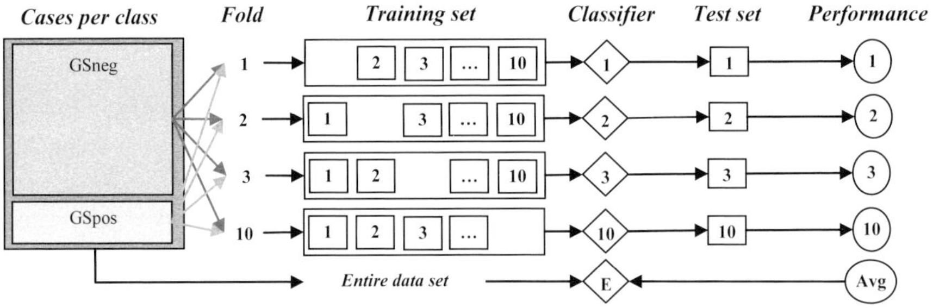

Figure 2. 10-fold cross validation to estimate expected performance of a final classifier tree E when applied to unseen data. GSNeg = gold standard negative cases of clinical mastitis. GSpos = gold standard positive cases of clinical mastitis. Avg = average detection performance of all 10 classifiers as developed on the training sets and tested on the test sets.

Results

Table 1 summarises the expected detection performance measures (SN, SP, False Alert Rate, and Success Rate) of DT algorithms with varying costs for false negative alerts and varying confidence factors and a cut-off value of 0.50 to classify CM. The default settings, marked grey, resulted in a SN of 50%, an SP of 99%, 9 False Alerts, and a Success Rate of 64%. While keeping the costs at an equal level, varying the confidence factor resulted in minor changes in SN and Success Rate. Larger effects were seen when confidence factors were fixed while costs for false negative alerts increased. For example, when the confidence factor was kept at 0.25 (default) and costs for false negative alerts increased to 100, the SN increased from 50 to 56%. At the same time, the SP decreased considerably from 99 to 95%, the False Alert Rate increased from 9 to 53, and the Success Rate decreased from 64 to 25%.

Figure 3A presents the ROC curves of a DT with default parameter settings, a DT with the highest SN (confidence factor 0.05, costs 100), and an intermediate one (confidence factor 0.05, costs 20) as presented in Table 1. Details for SP values of 90% or higher are presented in Figure 3B. The default DT has a higher SN at the same SP when compared to the other two DTs, for SP values ranging from 100 to 97%. At lower SP values, however, the figure indicates that it is possible to reach a higher SN with other DT settings.

Table 1. Sensitivity (SN), Specificity (SP), False Alert Rate and Success Rate of several decision trees at a threshold of 0.50 to classify clinical mastitis.

Costs false negative alerts	Confidence factor	SN (%)	SP (%)	False Alert Rate	Success Rate (%)
Equal costs	0.35	0.50	0.99	15	0.53
	0.25	0.50	0.99	9	0.64
	0.15	0.48	0.99	9	0.64
	0.05	0.43	0.99	7	0.68
5	0.35	0.44	0.98	22	0.39
	0.25	0.45	0.98	22	0.40
	0.15	0.45	0.98	22	0.39
	0.05	0.46	0.98	23	0.39
20	0.35	0.51	0.97	27	0.38
	0.25	0.52	0.97	27	0.39
	0.15	0.57	0.97	27	0.40
	0.05	0.58	0.97	29	0.39
100	0.35	0.55	0.95	52	0.26
	0.25	0.56	0.95	53	0.25
	0.15	0.59	0.94	58	0.25
	0.05	0.60	0.93	69	0.22

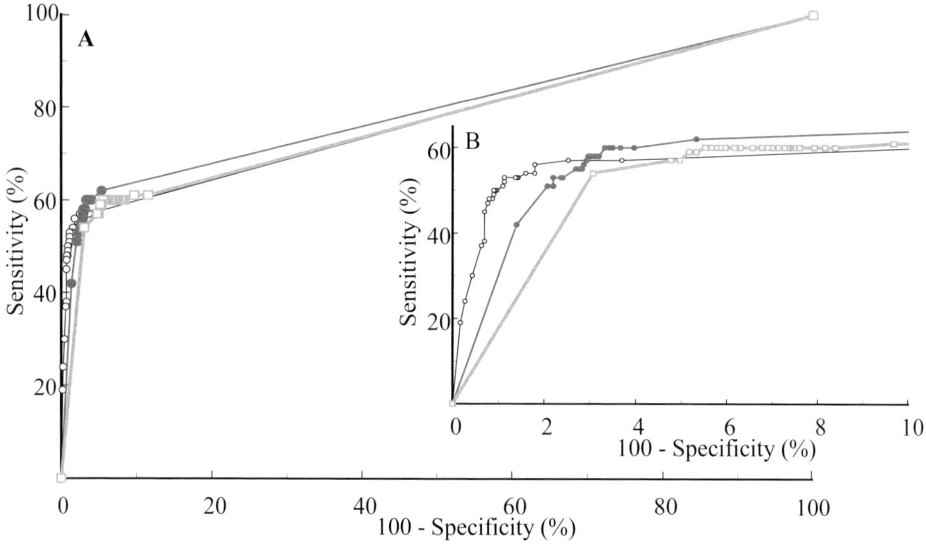

Figure 3. (A) ROC-curves of DT algorithms: default settings (○), highest sensitivity (□), and intermediate results (●); (B) Details of the curves for SP values of 90% or higher.

Discussion

The detection performances of the DT algorithms presented in the current study are comparable to the performance of the algorithm currently used by AM systems (Mollenhorst and Hogeveen, unpublished data). This may seem disappointing in first instance, but there are some points that need consideration while interpreting the results. First of all, an important issue is that rather basic DT algorithms were used here. Of course, cost matrixes and confidence factors were varied, but other more sophisticated optimising techniques like boosting or bagging are likely to improve CM detection performances. Secondly, detection performance may be improved when DTs are trained with examples where the differences in data patterns between positive and negative cases are more pronounced. For example, adding an extra restriction to the GSneg cases by including only those cows never exceeding a SCC of 200,000 cells/ml in the monthly milk production recordings may reveal data patterns that are more specific for the negative CM cases than the patterns currently present in the GSneg pool. Thirdly, the milking of interest for the DT models to alert for CM was that quarter milking to which the farmer's observation of CM was linked. This is in contrast with models described in previous studies, where different time-windows to define true positive alerts were used to detect CM. These time-windows varied from alerts 14 days preceding an actual mastitis case to be counted as a true positive alert (Maatje *et al.*, 1992) to models where a true positive alert was an alert given after the actual CM was observed (De Mol *et al.*, 1997). Wider time-windows will result in better detection performances of models, but in practice an automatic CM detection model should generate an alert within a very limited period of time before or only at the milking when CM is present. Finally, it should be remembered that data were collected at 6 commercial dairy herds such that intervention of the farmer's working routine was limited. This resulted in a large number of positive cases of CM when compared with other studies and in a data set that reflects the real on-farm situation, which includes inevitable errors and missing data. A detection algorithm should be able to deal with these types of data when implemented in practice. Therefore, results of this study gives motivation to explore DT induction for automated CM detection more extensively in the future.

The ROC-curves indicate comprehensively all possible combinations of SN and SP of a model to detect CM. Depending on what the end-user finds an acceptable level of misclassification, it would be beneficial for future models to be flexible in their threshold settings. The ROC-curve in the current study already visualised that the DT with the highest SN (60%) at a threshold of 0.50, performed worse when compared to the intermediate DT over the whole range of possible SP values. Therefore, computing the partial area under the curve would be of great interest. By doing so, worthwhile differences between models may be revealed which stay obscured when taking just one threshold value into account or when the total area under the curve is computed to compare detection models.

Conclusion

Although field data were used and the limited time-window used to define a true positive alert, results suggest that DT induction shows potential for detecting CM using AM sensor data. The default DT showed higher SN values for a SP range of 97 to 100% compared to two alternative DTs. By changing parameter settings it was possible to reach higher levels of SN for SP values lower than 97%. Main focus for future work is to optimise DT parameters, to implement boosting or bagging techniques, to study the effect of training on more strict selection of GSneg cases, and to explore the effects of different time-windows on detection performances. ROC-curves show comprehensively all possible SN and SP combinations of different DT models and computations of the partial area under the curve would make statistical comparisons between models possible. It would be beneficial for future models that they are flexible so that farmers are able to decide themselves what threshold values to use, depending on their own level of acceptance of misclassification.

References

Cavero, D., Tolle, K.H., Buxade, C. and Krieter, J., 2006. Mastitis detection in dairy cows by application of fuzzy logic. Livest. Sci. 105: 207-213.

De Mol, R.M., Keen, A., Kroeze, G.H. and Achten, J.M.F.H., 1999. Description of a detection model for oestrus and diseases in dairy cattle based on time series analysis combined with a Kalman filter. Comp. Electr. Agric. 22: 171-185.

De Mol, R.M., Kroeze, G.H., Achten, J.M.F.H., Maatje, K. and Rossing, W., 1997. Results of a multivariate approach to automated oestrus and mastitis detection. Livest. Prod. Sci. 48: 219-227.

De Mol, R.M. and Woldt, W.E., 2001. Application of fuzzy logic in automated cow status monitoring. J. Dairy Sci. 84: 400-410.

Hogeveen, H. and Ouweltjes, W., 2003. Sensors and management support in high-technology milking. J. Anim. Sci. 81 Suppl. 3: 1-10.

Kamphuis, C., Pietersma, D., Van der Tol, R., Wiedemann, M. and Hogeveen, H., 2008. Using sensor data patterns from an automatic milking system to develop predictive variables for classifying clinical mastitis and abnormal milk. Comp. Electr. Agric. 62: 169-181.

Lansbergen, L.M.T.E., Nielen, M., Lam, T.J.G.M., Pengov, A., Schukken, Y.H. and Maatje, K., 1994. Evaluation of A Prototype Online Electrical-Conductivity System for Detection of Subclinical Mastitis. J. Dairy Sci. 77: 1132-1140.

Maatje, K., Huijsmans, P.J.M., Rossing, W. and Hogewerf, P.H., 1992. The Efficacy of In-Line Measurement of Quarter Milk Electrical-Conductivity, Milk-Yield and Milk Temperature for the Detection of Clinical and Subclinical Mastitis. Livest. Prod. Sci. 30: 239-249.

Mitchell, T.M., 1999. Machine learning and data mining. Comm. ACM 42: 30-36.

Quinlan, J.R., 1986. Induction of Decision Trees. Machine Learning 1: 81-106.

Witten, I.H. and Frank, E., 2005. Data Mining; Practical Machine Learning Tools and Techniques. 2 ed. Morgan Kaufmann Publishers, San Fransisco.

Performance evaluation of systems for automated monitoring of udder health: analytical issues and guidelines

R. Sherlock[1], H. Hogeveen[2], G. Mein[3] and M. Rasmussen[4]
[1]SmartWork Systems Ltd, Christchurch, New Zealand
[2]Faculty of Veterinary Medicine, Utrecht University, Utrecht, the Netherlands
[3]Sensortec Ltd, Hamilton, New Zealand
[4]Dept. of Agricultural Engineering, University of Aarhus, Horsens, Denmark
Corresponding author: ras@smartwork.co.nz

Abstract

Previous efforts to quantify the performance of systems for automated detection of udder-health anomalies have not always been consistent. Our goal is to propose a set of definitions and procedures using time-windows to facilitate standard methods of performance measurement and comparison. In particular, we discuss or present:

- The concept of finite-duration time-windows (or *Episodes),* indicative of clinical mastitis, in both observational (gold) and automatically-generated (auto) data. These provide the basis of a matching procedure to make correct associations between occurrences identified automatically by the monitoring system (autoEpisodes) and those confirmed independently (goldEpisodes).
- Definitions of performance measures Sensitivity, Success Rate and False Alert Rate, in terms of the four outputs of a matching algorithm which identifies overlaps in sequences of autoEpisodes and goldEpisodes.

Keywords: biosensors, clinical mastitis, monitoring, time-windows

Introduction

The rapid growth in demand for automatic milking systems has generated worldwide interest in the performance of automated detection of clinical mastitis and other health conditions. To evaluate the performance of such systems, we need to decide which of the autoAlerts are valid. We also need to identify cases where an autoAlert was not issued when it should have been, and express this information in well-defined and accepted statistical measures.

The definitions and methods we propose here are applicable quite generally to the automated detection of any binary condition (e.g. clinical mastitis, oestrus). For conciseness, however, the remainder of the paper will refer only to the specific case of clinical mastitis detection.

A central difficulty is the fact that we have no continuous monitor of the mastitis infection status of a cow – just a set of observations at discrete times which are indicative of clinical mastitis (e.g. clots in foremilk, CMT, SCC, electrical conductivity measurement). Although debate persists as to which (or, more likely, what combination) of these provides a definitive 'gold-standard' for identifying the presence of a clinical infection (Mein and Rasmussen, 2008), we define goldAlerts as points in time (plus other data such as cowID, quarter, etc.) at which the chosen gold-standard test(s) indicated the presence of clinical mastitis.

Analagously, autoAlerts are generated in automatic milking systems on the basis of measurements made automatically during the milking process. Again they are, essentially, points in time at which the conditions associated with clinical mastitis are detected, along with cowID and details of those conditions. Since the times of occurrence of the (possibly multiple) autoAlerts (generated during milkings) and goldAlerts (generated by human observation) associated with the same clinical infection will not usually coincide, we associate finite-duration time-windows with the alerts and consider them to be coincident when these windows have any overlap. Although this concept has been used previously (e.g. De Mol *et al.*, 1997), the marked effect of the length of the time-window(s) on the apparent performance of the detection system has not been discussed in any detail.

This paper proposes standard nomenclature and describes a simple algorithmic procedure for generating useful statistical measures of system performance from these time-window sequences. The procedure enables meaningful comparisons to be made between different detection systems, and also facilitates comparisons of alternative potential gold-standards.

Methods

Clinical episodes

We define a clinical episode (or, where there is no ambiguity, just an episode) as a time-window of minimum width W during which the clinical mastitis status might reasonably be expected to persist. We distinguish between autoEpisodes associated with autoAlerts and having minimum widths W_a, and goldEpisodes associated with goldAlerts and having minimum width W_g. These windows (which need not be equal) give a finite range of capture for the coincidence (overlap) condition.

In the time-line diagram of Figure 1A, we illustrate this for the two extreme situations of marginal overlap when an autoEpisode precedes its associated goldEpisode and when it follows it. From the diagram it is clear that, in these simple cases of single alerts within the time window, the condition for overlap is given by:

$$t_a + W_a > t_g \text{ and } t_g + W_g > t_a \qquad (1)$$

i.e. the end-time of each window must be later than the start-time of the other.

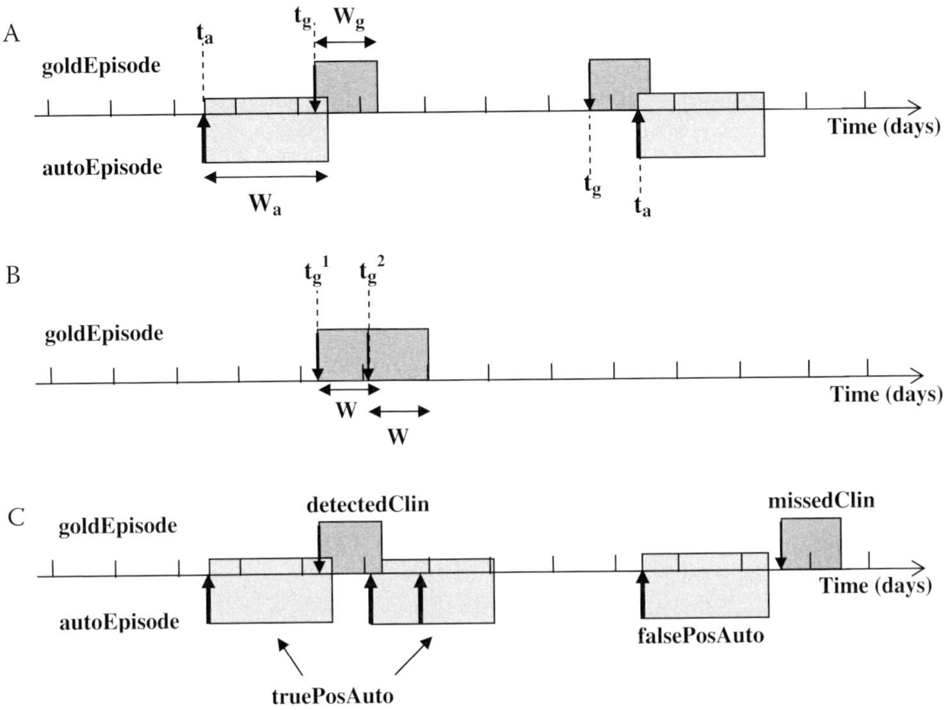

Figure 1. Illustration of definitions and relationships between the time-windows (Episodes) associated with goldAlerts (denoting observations of 'true' clinical status) and autoAlerts generated by automated clinical detection systems. (A) In the example illustrated here, the length of the goldEpisode window, W_g, is set at 24 h and that for the autoEpisode window, W_a, is set at 48 h. The alerts occur at times t_a and t_g. (B) A second alert, falling inside the initial time-window W, extends it by a further period, W. (C) The ClinEpisodes defined above can be divided into four categories based on their overlap status.

When we have a second alert of the same type (auto or gold) within the time-window of the first, that is incorporated by merging its window (W_a or W_g), as shown in Figure 1B. This procedure can be repeated as necessary for multiple alerts. The overlap condition then becomes:

$$t_a + w_a > t_g \quad \text{and} \quad t_g + w_g > t_a \tag{2}$$

where:

$$w_a = W_a + t_a^n - t_a^1,\ w_g = W_g + t_g^n - t_g^1 \tag{3}$$

and t^l and t^n denote the time of the first and the final alerts in the autoEpisode or goldEpisode. Clearly, with only a single alert $t^n = t^l$ and Equation 2 reduces to Equation 1. Thus, having lists of the times of mastitis autoAlerts from the milking system along with goldAlert observations of clinical mastitis, derived lists of autoEpisodes and goldEpisodes (defined by their start and finish times) are readily computed for any specified W_a and W_g using Equations 2 and 3. The choice of the W values is to some extent arbitrary – too small and true coincidences will be missed, too large and obviously erroneous coincidences will be formed. However, the fact that the analysis described below in Section 2.2 can be implemented in a simple algorithm means that the effects of different choices of W_a and W_g are quickly and easily explored, and in fact one finds sensible ranges (typically 1 to 4 days) over which the resulting performance measures are little changed.

As is clear from Figure 1A, the use of different values for W_a and W_g allows us to utilise any asymmetry in the 'capture range' relative to the goldAlert. This has proved useful in catering for the fact that, in a good automatic detection system, the autoAlert(s) are more likely to precede the goldAlert observation than to follow it.

Pair-match counts and performance measures

As illustrated in Figure 1C, the Episodes defined above can be divided into four categories based on their overlap status. The goldEpisodes are either detected or missed, and the autoEpisodes are either truePos or falsePos, as defined by:

- *detectedClin*: a goldEpisode which has a pair-match with one (or more) autoEpisode(s).
- *missedClin*: a goldEpisode which has no pair-match with any autoEpisode.
- *truePosAuto*: an autoEpisode which has a pair-match with one (or more) goldEpisode(s).
- *falsePosAuto*: an autoEpisode which has no pair-match with any goldEpisode.

Counts of occurrences in each of the above four categories are readily computed, and from these we can then calculate the following useful practical performance measures:

$$\textit{Sensitivity (\%)} = 100 * \textit{detectedClinCount} / (\textit{detectedClinCount} + \textit{missedClinCount}) \quad (4)$$

$$\textit{Success Rate (\%)} = 100 * \textit{truePosAutoCount} / (\textit{truePosAutoCount} + \textit{falsePosAutoCount} \quad (5)$$

$$\textit{False Alert Rate} = 1000 * \textit{falsePosAutoCount} / \textit{totalCowMilkings} \quad (6)$$

Note that we have deliberately avoided the commonly employed terms *truePos* (TP), *falsePos* (FP), *trueNeg* (TN) and *FalseNeg* (FN) because of inconsistency in their useage, e.g. consider the following three definitions of a TP as: 'a case of mastitis where one or more alerts are given' (De Mol *et al.*, 1997); 'an alert during a mastitis period' (De Mol and Woldt, 2001); and 'an alert on the day of observation' (Cavero *et al.*, 2006). Each is capable of generating a different TP list from the same basic data.

Sensitivity (Equation 4) gives a measure of the proportion of true clinical Episodes that were correctly identified as such, whereas the *Success Rate* (Equation 5) is a measure of the proportion of the autoEpisodes which were associated with a gold (true clinical) Episode. These are quite different measures.

Specificity (the converse of *Sensitivity*) is defined as the proportion of 'true nonClinical observations' correctly identified as such). In practice, however, a proper measure of this is problematic. Whereas the absence of an autoEpisode can safely be interpreted as 'non-clinEpisode' (since measurements were being made to confirm that), this is not usually the case with goldEpisodes. Apart from isolated routine herd-tests when each cow is rated as clinical or non-clinical, we cannot infer that the absence of a goldAlert implies a true non-clinical status. In Section 3 we argue that *False Alert Rate* (Equation 5) is the better measure.

To illustrate the influence of choice of window sizes on the apparent performance measures, we reproduce (with permission) in Table 1 an extract of the results of a major trial described by Kamphuis *et al.* (C. Kamphuis, personal communication, 2008). In Table 2, we compare three plausible performance scenarios from a hypothetical 1000 cow-milking trial.

Results and discussion

Effect of window sizes

In Table 1, it is evident that, with a time-window of either 24 or 48 hours, there were no goldEpisodes embracing more than a single goldAlert. This was not unexpected as the trial protocol resulted in cows being treated with antibiotics and drafted out of the milking herd immediately whenever a case clinical mastitis (i.e. a goldAlert) was confirmed. The windowing effect is seen clearly in the auto data however. With a 96 hour window the 191 autoAlerts aggregate into 50 autoEpisodes. Halving the length of the time-window (from 96 to 48 h) reduced the opportunity for aggregation of autoAlerts and thereby increased the number of autoEpisodes from 50 to 73 (~50%). This inevitably resulted in an increased *falsePosAutoCount* and the associated reduced *Success Rate* and increased *False Alert Rate.*

Comparison of performance measures

To allow comparison of the traditional *Specificity* with the measures defined in Equations 5 and 6, the scenarios represent the less-common situation where the gold status is known at every milking, and we make our episode window equal to the milking interval. Thus, at each milking we can unambiguously identify a detectedNonClin and equate a missedNonClin with a falsePosAuto so, in this special case, we can also define:

$$Specificity\ (\%) = 100 * detectedNonClinCount\ /\ (detectedNonClinCount + falsePosAutoCount)$$

Table 1. Influence of the choice of window sizes on apparent performance measures (data from C. Kamphuis, personal communication, 2008).

Wa (hour)	auto-Alerts	auto-Episodes	Wg (hour)	gold-Alerts	gold-Episodes	Sensitivity %	Success Rate %	False Alert Rate per 1000 cow-milkings
96	191	50	48	20	20	80.0	32.0	1.2
96	198	53	24	20	20	80.0	30.2	1.3
72	198	59	24	20	20	80.0	27.1	1.6
48	183	73	24	20	20	80.0	21.9	2.1

In addition to the problems of its calculation, *specificity* is a potentially confusing indicator of performance for a non-scientific audience. In scenario B of Table 2, for example, the number of false positives is half that in scenario A (which is a major improvement in performance). To a non-scientific reader, however, the improvement in specificity (from 96.9% to 98.5%) appears to be much smaller. This is a consequence of the number of clinicals being very much less than the number of non-clinicals, a situation that should always be the norm. The potential problem of 'numerical perception' of the term *specificity* is illustrated by the situation that while achieving a *sensitivity* of 90% would be considered excellent by most farmers, a *specificity* of 90% would be quite inadequate and very frustrating in most herd situations.

Table 2. Examples of performance measures evaluated for three hypothetical scenarios (A, B and C) for a 1000 cow-milking dataset with 25 goldClinicalEpisodes.

Scenario	detect-Clin-Count	false-PosAuto count	trueNeg count	Missed-Clin count	Sensitivity %	Specificity %	Success Rate %	FalseAlert Rate per 1000 c-m
A	20	30	945	5	80	96.9	40	30
B	20	15	960	5	80	98.5	57.1	15
C	20	30	940	10	66.7	96.9	40	30

Success Rate could be a more useful statistic, giving a more direct measure of the proportion of auto alerts that are likely to be correct. *Success Rate* is our alternate name for the ppv (positive predictive value). In the comparison of scenarios A & B quoted above, *Success Rate* increased from 40% to 57% while *specificity* changed only fractionally. A downside of *Success Rate* is that it is not an 'absolute' statistic. Thus, the *Success Rate* will vary with the prevalence of the condition being monitored.

This downside can be avoided by calculating the total number of false alerts over a given number of cow-milkings – eg, the total number of false alerts per 1000 cow-milkings. This expression of the '*false alert rate*' would be a simple, practical and comprehensible measure to which farmers will readily relate. In the comparison of scenarios A & B above, the *false alert rate* fell from 30 to 15 while the *specificity* change was only 1.6%. Clearly, a false alert rate of 15 per1000 c-m would provide a more realistic indication of the practical limitations of a test compared with the equivalent value for Specificity of 98.5%. The *false alert rate* is essentially 10[100% minus specificity%] per 1000 cow-milkings. This approximation should always be close enough for practical purposes since the clinical prevalence should always be very low relative to the total number of cow milkings.

Conclusions

We have presented a well-defined algorithmic scheme for calculating useful performance measures of systems implementing automated detection of clinical mastitis. 'Coincidences' of corresponding automatic alerts and gold-standard observations (both essentially points in time) are detected by allowing both to have associated time-windows. Generating counts of window overlaps and overlap failures is straightforward and system performance measures are readily expressed in terms of these counts.

Sensitivity is readily calculated and is a direct and obvious measure of the system's ability to detect clinical mastitis cases. However, *Specificity* is a potentially confusing indicator of performance for a non-scientific audience. We believe that *False Alert Rate* is a much easier term than specificity for farmers to understand when comparing promotional literature for competitive products. The *False Alert Rate* is what farmers must cope with in their day-to-day milking routines.

Although we have concentrated on automated systems for detecting clinical mastitis in this paper, the same analytical concepts, methods and expressions can be applied equally well to analyses of the performance of auto-detection systems for abnormal milk or udder infections.

References

Cavero, D., Tolle, K.-H., Buxade, C. and Krieter, J., 2006. Mastitis detection in dairy cows by application of fuzzy logic. Livest. Sci. 10: 207-213.

De Mol, R.M., Kroeze, G.H., Achten, J.M., Maatje, K. and Rossing, W., 1997. Results of a multivariate approach to automated oestrus and mastitis detection. Livest. Prod. Sci. 48: 219-227.

De Mol, R.M. and Woldt, W.E., 2001. Application of Fuzzy Logic in Automated Cow Status Monitoring. J. Dairy Sci. 84: 400-410.

Mein, G.A. and Rasmussen, M.D., 2008. Performance evaluation of systems for automated monitoring of udder health: Would the real gold standard please stand up? In: Mastitis control – From science to practice. Wageningen Academic Publishers, the Netherlands, pp. 259-266.

An investigation of factors affecting cure when treating clinical mastitis in dairy cattle with cephalosporin containing intramammary preparations

A.J. Bradley[1,2] *and M.J. Green*[3]
[1]*University of Bristol, Division of Farm Animal Science, School of Veterinary Science, Langford House, Langford, BS40 5DU Bristol, United Kingdom*
[2]*Quality Milk Management Services Ltd, Unit 1, Lodge Hill Industrial Park, Station Road, Westbury-sub-Mendip, Nr Wells, BA5 1EY Somerset, United Kingdom*
[3]*University of Nottingham, School of Veterinary Medicine and Science, Sutton Bonington Campus, Sutton Bonington, LE12 5RD Leicestershire, United Kingdom*
Corresponding author: a.j.bradley@bris.ac.uk

Abstract

Data were collated for an independent scientific analysis from a number of international, multi-centre studies that had compared the efficacy of three different, cephalosporin containing, intramammary preparations in the treatment of clinical mastitis in dairy cattle (cefalexin in combination with kanamycin (group 1); cefquinome (group 2); cefoperazone (group 3)). Quarters were assessed using standard bacteriological techniques before treatment and at 16 and 25 days post treatment. Additional data were also available on individual cows and study farms including parity, breed and cow somatic cell count histories, herd bulk milk somatic cell counts (BMSCC) and farm management regimes. Sufficient data for analysis was available from a total of 491 cases on 192 farms in 3 countries (England, France and Germany) with up to 16 cases being recruited from any one farm. Clinical cases were of diverse aetiology representing both contagious and environmental pathogens. Univariable analysis demonstrated that quarters in treatment groups 1 (88/148) and 2 (55/89) were not significantly different from each other, but were both significantly more likely to be pathogen free post treatment than quarters in group 3 (24/87), (P=0.021). Multivariable analysis using conventional random effects models indicated that country, pre-treatment rectal temperature (above normal temperature associated with increased chance of being pathogen free post treatment), individual cow somatic cell count (increased SCC associated with decreased chance of being pathogen free post treatment) and pathogen (*Staphylococcus aureus* isolation associated with decreased chance of being pathogen free post treatment) were useful predictors of pathogen free status; parity, yield, BMSCC and other farm management factors were not. The results suggest that the factors important in predicting the outcome of treatment of clinical mastitis cases may be dissimilar to those reported to affect the likelihood of cure when treating subclinical intramammary infections.

Keywords: clinical mastitis, cure, cephalosporin, treatment

Introduction

With the exception of papers reporting clinical trials, and in contrast to the treatment of subclinical mastitis, there is very little published in the peer reviewed literature about factors affecting the likely outcome of treatment of clinical mastitis cases. Whilst differences in cure rates have been demonstrated between different intramammary products (Deluyker *et al.*, 1999) the only other major factors to have been investigated and identified as being important in determining the outcome of treatment of clinical cases are the speed with which treatment is initiated and the duration of treatment, with more rapid identification and initiation of treatment (Hillerton and Semmens, 1999) and increased duration of treatment both being associated with improved cure rates (Deluyker *et al.*, 2005; Oliver *et al.*, 2004).

In contrast the factors affecting the likely outcome of treatment of sub-clinical mastitis are much better understood and have been more thoroughly investigated. It is well established that there are significant differences in cure rate associated with farm factors such as bulk milk somatic cell count (BMSCC), the pathogen involved, the duration of infection, the duration of treatment, the number of quarters affected (Deluyker *et al.*, 1999; Sol *et al.*, 1994, 1997) as well as the parity of the affected animal and the timing of treatment in the lactation cycle, with enhanced cure rates achieved in the dry period compared to lactation (Bradley *et al.*, 2003).

There are a number of ways of assessing the outcome of treatment of cases of clinical mastitis including the simple assessment of the resolution of clinical signs (treatment success as perceived by the farmer), the indirect assessment of response to treatment by measurement of post treatment somatic cell count and the 'gold standard' approach of serial bacteriological culture. Species specific cure rates based on the failure to retrieve the causal pathogen in post treatment samples are often quoted, but have the disadvantage of telling the investigator little about the overall prognostic outcome and therefore likely survival of the animal in the herd longer term. In contrast, an assessment based on the likelihood of a quarter being 'pathogen free' post treatment provides a biologically useful and robust assessment of the outcome of treatment which may better reflect the long term survival of the animal in the herd.

The primary objective of this study was to investigate factors important both in determining and predicting the outcome of treatment of clinical mastitis, in this case with intramammary products containing cephalosporins.

Materials and methods

Data were collated from two multicentre international efficacy studies which compared the use of different cephalosporin containing intramammary products in the treatment of bovine clinical mastitis occurring during lactation. Both studies followed the same protocol (with the exception of treatment regimes): Study A was conducted in the UK and France and study B in the UK and Germany. A product containing the 1st generation cephalosporin, cefalexin in combination with kanamycin (Group 1)(Ubrolexin, Boehringer Ingelheim Animal Health) was used in both studies and was compared to a 4th generation cephalosporin, cefquinome (Group 2) (Cephaguard/Cobactan, Intervet Ltd) in Study A and to a 3rd generation cephalosporin, cefoperazone (Group 3)(Pathocef, Pfizer Ltd)(Grp3) in Study B.

Cows, suffering from clinical mastitis were recruited to the studies from 192 commercial dairy farms in three countries with up to 16 cases being recruited from any one farm (Max: 16, Min: 1, Mean: 2.56, Median: 2). Herd size varied from 2 to 480 cows in milk. All animals were managed according to normal husbandry regimes for each farm and all herds followed a twice daily milking regime. The geometric mean bulk milk somatic cell count (BMSCC), in the three months prior to the study, on the farms from which cows were recruited was 211,000 cells/ml (range 48,000 and 590,000 cells/ml). There were diverse management, husbandry and milking practices across the study sites encompassing both cubicle and loose yard systems, a variety of feeding systems and significant variation in the degree of implementation of the five point plan.

Cows selected for inclusion in the study were clinically examined, by a veterinary surgeon, prior to treatment which included a detailed assessment and grading of both the affected quarter and its secretion. Cows were randomly allocated to treatment group; all treatments were applied according to the manufacturer's recommendations. Aseptic quarter milk samples were collected on days 0, 16 (±1) and 25 (±1) for bacteriological and somatic cell count analysis. Bacteriology was conducted using recognised techniques and organisms were identified and quantified using standard laboratory techniques (NMC, 1999; Quinn *et al.*, 1994).

Treatment outcomes were assessed in a number of ways. Apparent bacteriological cure of a pathogen identified on day 0 was defined as having occurred when the same pathogen was not identified in either of the post treatment samples. An outcome of 'Post Treatment No Growth' was defined for quarters which were free of any mastitis pathogen in either of the post treatment samples.

Data were collated and analysed using Microsoft access and excel (Microsoft Corp, Redmond, WA, U.S.), Minitab (Minitab Inc., State College, PA, U.S.), MLWiN (Rasbash *et al.*, 2005) and WinBUGS (Spiegelhalter *et al.*, 2004). Unvariable analysis was conducted using the chi squared test and ANOVA as appropriate. Allowances were made using a layered bonferroni correction when making multiple comparisons. Multilevel (random effects) models (Goldstein, 1995) were specified so that correlations within the data (cows within farms) were accounted for appropriately.

Results

A total of 491 cases were included in the analysis 236, 111 and 144 cases to groups 1, 3 and 2 respectively. The treated animals represented a diverse population representing 11 different dairy breeds (Holstein Friesians predominating); a wide range of parities, stages of lactation and yields. Individual cow somatic cell counts varied significantly in the month prior to treatment from $1x10^3$ to $7,679x10^3$ cells/ml. Clinical parameters at the time of presentation were also diverse.

The aetiology of the clinical mastitis cases encompassed both 'contagious' and 'environmental', gram positive and gram negative organisms. The aetiology of cases varied across the countries included in the study with contagious pathogens being most prevalent in Germany, the aetiology of cases is summarised by country of origin in Table 1. Overall, 25.4% of cases were attributed to coliform organisms, 28.3% to *S. uberis* whilst *S. aureus* was implicated in only 12.2% of cases.

Univariable analysis failed to reveal any significant differences in the apparent cure rates as summarised in Table 2. Successful treatment outcomes as measured by being 'pathogen free' post treatment are summarised in Table 3 - when comparing treatment groups using this outcome a significant difference was identified with both Groups 1 and 2 being significantly more likely to be pathogen free post treatment than the Group 3 ($P<0.05$).

Results of multivariable analysis are summarised in Table 4. Cows in the group 3 were significantly less likely to be pathogen free post treatment than quarters in treatment group 1 (OR 0.24; 95% credibility interval 0.09-0.65). Significant differences were also detected between

Table 1. Summary of aetiology of clinical cases by country.

Diagnosis	**UK**		**France**		**Germany**		**Overall**	
	n	**%**	**n**	**%**	**n**	**%**	**n**	**%**
A. pyogenes	1	0.51	0	-	3	1.95	4	0.81
Coagulase -ve *Staphylococci*	26	13.3	17	12.0	23	14.9	66	13.4
E. coli	47	24.1	31	21.8	15	9.74	93	18.9
S. uberis	71	36.4	37	26.1	31	20.1	139	28.3
S. aureus	16	8.21	13	9.15	31	20.1	60	12.2
Enterococcus spp	1	0.51	3	2.11	2	1.30	6	1.22
S. dysgalactiae	11	5.64	8	5.63	16	10.4	35	7.13
S. agalactiae	0	-	0	-	4	2.60	4	0.81
Other coliforms	8	4.10	18	12.7	6	3.90	32	6.52
Mixed aetiology	7	3.59	9	6.34	17	11.04	33	6.72
No growth	7	3.59	6	4.23	6	3.90	19	3.87
Total	195		142		154		491	

Table 2. Summary of 'apparent' cure rates by treatment group.

Diagnosis	Cefalexin and kanamycin (Group 1)			Cefquinome (Group 2)			Cefoperazone (Group 3)		
	No infected	No cured	% cured	No infected	No cured	% cured	No infected	No cured	% cured
A. pyogenes	2	2	100	1	1	100	2	2	100
Coagulase -ve *Staphs*	33	17	51.5	24	12	50.0	23	6	26.1
E. coli	45	42	93.3	38	38	100	20	16	80.0
S. uberis	70	45	64.3	54	38	70.4	36	24	66.7
S. aureus	38	14	36.8	13	2	15.4	18	6	33.3
Enterococcus spp	8	6	75.0	1	0	-	4	1	25.0
S. dysgalactiae	29	20	69.0	6	6	100	9	7	77.8
S. agalactiae	1	1	100	0	0	-	3	3	100
Other coliforms	16	10	62.5	12	11	91.7	6	5	83.3

Table 3. Summary of successful treatment outcomes as defined by 'pathogen free' status post treatment in each of the treatment groups.

	Cefalexin and kanamycin (Group 1)	Cefquinome (Group 2)	Cefoperazone (Group 3)
n	236	144	111
No. infected post treatment	148	89	87
No. pathogen free post treatment	88	55	24
% pathogen free post treatment	37.3^{a}	38.2^{a}	21.6^{b}

^{a,b} Superscripts with rows differ (P<0.05).

Table 4. Summary of the multilevel logistic regression model investigating the likelihood of being pathogen free post treatment, taking into account pre-treatment bacteriological status and post treatment somatic cell count.

Covariate	Coefficient	SE	OR	Credibility intervals	
				2.5%	97.50%
ref Treatment = 1					
2	0.390	0.428	1.48	0.63	3.48
3	-1.413	0.488	0.24	0.09	0.65
ref StudyID = B					
StudyID A	1.910	0.611	6.75	1.99	22.92
ref Country = UK					
Germany	-1.850	0.497	0.16	0.06	0.42
France	-0.402	0.440	0.67	0.28	1.61
Individual Cow SCC in the month prior to treatment					
For each unit (1.00) rise in logSCC	-0.266	0.115	0.77	0.61	0.96
ref Season = Spring					
Summer	0.471	0.571	1.60	0.51	5.02
Autumn	0.720	0.578	2.05	0.65	6.53
Winter	1.457	0.641	4.29	1.19	15.47
ref Rectal Temperature = <38.6 °C					
Rectal Temp = 38.6-39.1 °C	0.049	0.342	1.05	0.53	2.08
Rectal Temp >39.1 °C	1.150	0.525	3.16	1.11	9.03
ref Pre-treatment bacteriological status other than *Staphylococcus aureus*					
Staphylococcus aureus isolated pre-treatment	-1.199	0.566	0.30	0.10	0.94
Quarter SCC post treatment					
For each unit (1.00) rise in logQrtSCC post treatment	-0.269	0.099	0.76	0.63	0.93

countries in the odds of a quarter being pathogen free post treatment with quarters in cows in Germany being significantly less likely to experience a successful outcome compared to quarters of cows in the UK (OR 0.16; 95% credibility interval 0.06-0.42). No herd level management factors or BMSCC were found to be influential in determining the likelihood of treatment outcome. No cow level parameters were influential in the final model with the exception of individual cow SCC in the month prior to the clinical case when each unit rise in logSCC resulted in a reduced odds of being pathogen free post treatment (OR 0.77; 95% credibility interval 0.63-0.94) and elevated rectal temperature (OR 3.16; 95% credibility interval

1.11-9.03). *S. aureus* was the only pathogen, when identified in the pre-treatment sample, that had a significant impact on the outcome; *S. aureus* cases being significantly less likely to be pathogen free post treatment than other pathogens (OR 0.30; 95% credibility interval 0.10-0.94). Post treatment quarter SCC was found to be a useful indicator of a successful outcome with each unit rise in post treatment quarter logSCC resulting in a reduction in the odds of being pathogen free post treatment (OR 0.76; 95% credibility interval 0.63-0.93). In addition quarters developing a clinical case in the winter months were significantly more likely to be pathogen free than those affected in the spring (OR 4.29; 95% credibility interval 1.19-15.47).

Discussion

There was a diverse aetiology of clinical cases in the studies incorporated in this analysis, though interestingly the only pathogen to significantly affect the likelihood of a successful treatment outcome was *S. aureus*. This finding supports the findings of previous research (Barkema *et al.*, 2006), and highlights the importance of knowing the prevalence of mastitis pathogens on a unit as this will inform treatment decisions and expectations and will allow the practitioner to be more proactive in electing for more aggressive treatment regimes in an attempt to improve treatment outcomes in herd with a high prevalence of *S. aureus*.

It is interesting to speculate on the differences between the products. As one might have expected the fourth generation cephalosporin (cefquinome) performed well in the overall assessment, despite the poor cure rates against *S. aureus* reported in Table 2, highlighting the importance of multivariable analysis. Perhaps more interesting is the performance of the 1st generation cephalosporin when used in combination with the aminoglycoside kanamycin – this combination was not significantly different from cefquinome and outperformed the 3rd generation product cefoperazone. This finding demonstrates the potential usefulness of combination antibiotic therapy.

The apparent lack of similarity between our findings in this study and those of earlier researchers investigating factors impacting the likelihood of cure of sub-clinically affected quarters (Deluyker *et al.*, 2005; Milne *et al.*, 2005; Sol *et al.*, 2000, 1994, 1997) is of interest. The apparent lack of influence of parity and herd level parameters is notable, and perhaps hard to explain. Unfortunately we were unable to look at the impact of multiple infected quarters in the same cow in this study as a selection criterion was only one affected quarter per cow – it would seem likely that cows affected in multiple quarters would be less likely to cure. However, it is important to remember that clinical and sub-clinical mastitis are two very different conditions, reflected in different aetiologies and typically very different chronicity of infection by the time the disease is identified – this alone may account for the lack of similarity between the factors affecting the likely outcome of treatment.

Conclusion

The impact of treatment, cow characteristics and farm factors on the probability of a cow becoming pathogen free after antibiotic therapy for clinical mastitis was investigated. Country, season, pre-treatment rectal temperature, individual cow somatic cell count before and after treatment and mastitis pathogen were identified as useful predictors of a successful outcome but parity, milk yield, herd bulk milk cell count and other farm management factors were not.

Acknowledgements

The authors would like to acknowledge the input of the study investigators and farmers that participated in the research, but in particular the generosity of Boehringer Ingelheim Animal Health in agreeing to freely share their data to allow the analysis presented in this paper.

References

Barkema, H.W., Schukken, Y.H. and Zadoks, R.N., 2006. Invited review: The role of cow, pathogen, and treatment regimen in the therapeutic success of bovine *Staphylococcus aureus* mastitis. J. Dairy Sci. 89: 1877-1895.

Bradley, A.J., Huxley, J.N. and Green, M.J., 2003. A Rational Approach to Dry Cow Therapy II – Making Logical Treatment Decisions. In Practice 25: 12-17.

Deluyker, H.A., Chester, S.T. and Van Oye, S.N., 1999. A multilocation clinical trial in lactating dairy cows affected with clinical mastitis to compare the efficacy of treatment with intramammary infusions of a lincomycin/neomycin combination with an ampicillin/cloxacillin combination. J. Vet. Pharmacol. Ther. 22: 274-282.

Deluyker, H.A., Van Oye, S.N. and Boucher, J.F., 2005. Factors affecting cure and somatic cell count after pirlimycin treatment of subclinical mastitis in lactating cows. J. Dairy Sci. 88: 604-614.

Goldstein, H. 1995. Multilevel Statistical Models. 2nd Edition. Edward Arnold, London UK.

Hillerton, J.E. and Semmens, J.E.. 1999. Comparison of treatment of mastitis by oxytocin or antibiotics following detection according to changes in milk electrical conductivity prior to visible signs. J. Dairy Sci. 82: 93-98.

Milne, M.H., Biggs, A.M., Barrett, D.C., Young, F.J., Doherty, S., Innocent, G.T. and Fitzpatrick, J.L., 2005. Treatment of persistent intramammary infections with Streptococcus uberis in dairy cows. Vet. Rec. 157: 245-250.

NMC, 1999. Laboratory Handbook on Bovine Mastitis. National Mastitis Council Inc, Madison, WI.

Oliver, S.P., Almeida, R.A., Gillespie, B.E., Headrick, S.J., Dowlen, H.H., Johnson, D.L., Lamar, K.C., Chester, S.T. and Moseley, W.M., 2004. Extended ceftiofur therapy for treatment of experimentally-induced *Streptococcus uberis* mastitis in lactating dairy cattle. J. Dairy Sci. 87: 3322-3329.

Quinn, P.J., Carter, M.E., Markey, B. and Carter, G.R., 1994. Clinical Veterinary Microbiology. Wolfe, London.

Rasbash, J., Browne, W.J., Healy, M., Cameron, B. and Charlton, C., 2005. MLwiN Version 2.02. 2.02 ed. Mulilevel Models Project, Institute of Education, London.

Sol, J., Sampimon, O.C., Barkema, H.W. and Schukken, Y.H., 2000. Factors associated with cure after therapy of clinical mastitis caused by *Staphylococcus aureus*. J. Dairy Sci. 83: 278-284.

Sol, J., Sampimon, O.C., Snoep, J.J. and Schukken Y.H., 1994. Factors associated with bacteriological cure after dry cow treatment of subclinical staphylococcal mastitis with antibiotics. J. Dairy Sci. 77: 75-79.
Sol, J., Sampimon O.C., Snoep, J.J. and Schukken Y.H., 1997. Factors associated with bacteriological cure during lactation after therapy for subclinical mastitis caused by *Staphylococcus aureus*. J. Dairy Sci. 80: 2803-2808.
Spiegelhalter, D.J., Thomas, A. and Best, N., 2004. WinBUGS Version 1.4.1. MRC Biostatistics Unit, Cambridge UK, Cambridge.

Alternative reference method for somatic cell count based on automated video microscopy

M.A. Pérez[1], M.B. Coya[1], R. Muñiz[1], C.E. Carleos[2], J.A. Baro[3] and R. Ortega[4]
[1]Oviedo University, Ingenieria Electrica, Campus de Viesques s/n, 33203 Gijon, Spain
[2]Oviedo University, Estadística, Campus de Viesques s/n, 33203 Gijon, Spain
[3]Valladolid University, CC. Agroforestales, Campus La Yutera, Palencia, Spain
[4]CTV La Espìna, La Espina, Salas, Spain
Corresponding author: maperezg@uniovi.es

This paper presents an alternative reference method to estimate somatic cell count in cow milk. SCC is an important indicator in the detection of inflammatory reactions within the udder in cows and DM-SCC is the present IDF reference method for its evaluation, but due to its dependence on human operators, it is extremely time-consuming and subjective. In this paper, an advantageous method that involves application of a low-cost video microscopy system (VM-SCC) is analysed and discussed, including a comparison between both of them by using Bland-Altman plots, and an example of application of both methods as reference. The VM-SCC system for cow milk consists of a PC, a commercial grade photo-camera, and an optical microscope. A wide choice of commercial cameras and video processing software, allows us a flexible implementation of the method using any matching combination. The comparison between VM-SCC and DM-SCC counts has been carried out with 76 milk samples. Despite the much lower number of images analysed with VM-SCC, correlation with the reference DM-SCC method was very high, above 99.75%. The method proposed for somatic cell count in milk samples is very precise, repeatable, and does not suffer from the subjectivity of methods that rely on human operators for cell identification. Precision is maximum for the range of counts associated with sub clinical bovine mastitis. Images and the outcome of their analyses may be stored for later use. The data presented above fully support the hypothesis that VM-SCC constitutes an advantageous alternative over DM-SCC for estimation of the somatic cell count in raw milk.

Detection of clinical mastitis with help of a thermal camera

M. Hovinen[1], J. Siivonen[1,2], S. Taponen[1], L. Hänninen[1], M. Pastell[3], A.-M. Aisla[3] and S. Pyörälä[1]
[1]Department of Production Animal Medicine, P.O. Box 57, 00014 University of Helsinki, Finland
[2]MTT Agrifood Research, Vakola, 31600 Jokioinen, Finland
[3]Department of Agrotechnology, P.O. Box 28, 00014 University of Helsinki, Finland
Corresponding author: mari.hovinen@helsinki.fi

Automation of dairy farms has created a need for new health monitoring methods. In this study, thermal camera was tested for detection of clinical mastitis. Experimental mastitis was induced to six cows with 10 µg of *Escherichia coli* lipopolysaccharide (LPS). LPS was infused into the left fore quarter of each cow, and the right fore quarter served as a control quarter. Clinical examination for systemic and local signs of the cows and sampling for indicators of inflammation in milk were carried out throughout the experimental period. Thermal images of experimental and control quarters were taken at each sampling time from lateral and medial angles. First signs of clinical mastitis were seen in all cows at 2 hours post challenge, including changes in cow behaviour and local clinical signs in the affected udder quarter. Rectal temperature, milk somatic cell count and electrical conductivity increased at 4 hours post challenge. Thermal camera was successful in detecting clinical mastitis in all cows. Temperature of the udder skin of the experimental and control quarters, detected with the camera, increased parallel to the rectal temperature. However, local signs of the udder could be detected before the rise of the udder skin and body temperature. It remains to be studied how early, relative to the clinical signs of mastitis, a thermal camera would detect mastitis in field conditions. This study showed that the udder is a sensitive place for detection of any febrile disease using a non-invasive method. A thermal camera, attached to e.g. a milking or feeding parlour, could detect clinical mastitis or other febrile disease and thus enable detection of diseases in the dairy herd.

Mastitis detection: visual observation compared to inline, quarter and milking somatic cell count

H. Mollenhorst[1], P.P.J. van de Tol[2] and H. Hogeveen[1,3]
[1]Utrecht University, Dept. of Farm Animal Health, Faculty of Veterinary Medicine, Marburglaan 2, 3584 CN Utrecht, the Netherlands
[2]Lely Industries N.V., Research Dept., Software Engineering, Weverskade 110, 3147 PA Maassluis, the Netherlands
[3]Wageningen University, Business Economics, P.O. Box 8130, 6700 EW Wageningen, the Netherlands
Corresponding author: h.mollenhorst@uu.nl

Every farmer needs equipment to be able to monitor udder health. For the control of mastitis, several indicators are available. Although much research has been done on electrical conductivity, not much knowledge is available on the value of other indicators. The aim of this experiment was to explore several indicators for somatic cell count (SCC) measured during a milking that can be used best for mastitis control. Data was collected at three farms with an AMS. Four indicators were measured for each quarter; two squirts (3rd and 4th) for visual observation, inline SCC (iSCC), quarter SCC (qSCC) and one composite milking SCC (mSCC). Visual observations were categorised into normal (n=3186) and abnormal (n=22). SCC was categorised in low and high, with thresholds set at 500 kcells/ml for quarter and 200 kcells/ml for milking values. SCC data was normalised by log-transformation to calculate correlations. The correlation between iSCC and qSCC was 0.51 (n=1030) and 0.45 (n=372) for the most interesting interval (200-2000 kcells/ml). The correlation between the average qSCCs and mSCC was 0.87 and was not affected by quarter yield correction. The sensitivity/specificity of iSCC, qSCC and mSCC compared to visual observation was 55/94, 50/92 and 58/76% respectively, probably explained by the timing of observation and sample taken during the milking. The interpretation of new EU legislation states that milk with clear visual abnormalities has to be discarded. Although the correlation between iSCC and qSCC was not very high, iSCC showed the best performance compared to visual observation, especially outperforming mSCC.

Inline somatic cell counting improves clinical mastitis detection in an automatic milking system

C. Kamphuis[1], R. Sherlock[2], J. Jago[3], G. Mein[4] and H. Hogeveen[1,5]
[1]Utrecht University, Marburglaan 2, 3584 CN Utrecht, the Netherlands
[2]SmartWork Systems, P.O. Box 36515, Christchurch, New Zealand
[3]DairyNZ, Private Bag 3221, Hamilton, New Zealand
[4]Sensortec Ltd., P.O. Box 11004, Hamilton, New Zealand
[5]Wageningen University, Hollandseweg 1, 6706 KN Wageningen, the Netherlands
Corresponding author: C.Kamphuis@uu.nl

Automatic milking (AM) systems use sensor information, mainly Electrical Conductivity (EC), to generate mastitis alerts. A common complaint by farmers using AM, is the occurrence of too many false positive alerts. This study investigated the potential of a new inline SCC (ISCC) sensor for clinical mastitis (CM) detection. Data, collected at a New Zealand research farm, included EC, ISCC, laboratory testing of SCC (FSCC) and information of cows treated for CM. These treated cases were used as Gold Standard in the analyses. Three models were developed to detect these treated cases, using different time windows to define true positive, false positive and false negative alerts. Parameters of the different models were set to reach a SN of 80%. The positive predictive value (PV+) and the number of false positive attentions per 1,000 cow milkings (FP1000) were evaluated. The correlation between ISCC and FSCC for FSCC values higher than 200×10^3cells/ml was 0.82; the correlation between ISCC and EC for ISCC values higher than 200×10^3 cells/ml was 0.40. When only EC was used as detection model, PV+ was 11.9% and FP1000 was 4.6. When only ISCC was used, PV+ was 12.9% and FP1000 was 3.9. Relative performance for the third model (combining EC and ISCC data using fuzzy logic) was improved about threefold: PV+ increased to 33.3% and FP1000 decreased to 1.2. Results were consistent when different time windows were analysed. This was the first study reporting on the performance of ISCC in detecting CM. Results suggest a positive contribution in CM detection, which is promising to improve mastitis control on farms with an AM system.

A novel in-line system to manage mastitis, ketosis, reproduction and feeding in dairy herds

J.Y. Blom[1] and L.A.H. Nielsen[2]
[1]Biosens, 2 Niels Pedersens Alle, 8830 Tjele, Denmark
[2]The Danish Agricultural Advisory Center, Danish Cattle Federation, 15 Udkaersvej, 8200 Aarhus N, Denmark
Corresponding author: Biosens@agropark.dk

The Danish development company Lattec initiated the development of an automated in-line measurement system to monitor udder health, ketosis, reproduction and feeding in dairy cows. A collaborate research initiative, Biosens, was formed six years ago with the primary aim to develop models (algorithms) to process continuous in-line measurements of milk constituents in order to provide the farm manager with early warnings of disease sand conditions. Emphasis has been on delivering an early warning to the farmer, and to assess the risk of developing disease before clinical signs occur. To monitor udder health, a mastitis model was developed The model takes into consideration the in-line measurements of the intracellular enzyme Lactate Dehydrogenase (LDH), but also basic cow data, additional risk factors, and other external data. The model will become imbedded in the complete in-line solution, including software to filter and present timely and relevant information to the farmer in real-time. The system has further been supplied with a number of proposals for Standard Operations Procedures, assisting the farmer in the management of alarm cows. The mastitis model was tested on data from the Danish Cattle Research Centre. The results of the test showed a sensitivity of 82% and a specificity of 99%. The test also showed that on an average, mastitis is detected 3.5 days ahead of a clinical diagnosis. In most cases. this leaves time for considering the optimal early treatment of the cow. The system is currently being tested in a number of Danish commercial dairy farms, showing very promising results.

Acute phase proteins in milk; biomarkers for subclinical mastitis and milk quality?

M. Akerstedt[1], K. Persson Waller[2] and A. Sternesjo[1]
[1]Swedish Universtity of Agricultural Sciences, Department of Food Science, P.O. Box 7051, 750 07 Uppsala, Sweden
[2]National Veterinary Institute, Department of Pigs, Poultry and Ruminants, Department of Pigs, Poultry and Ruminants, 751 89 Uppsala, Sweden
Corresponding author: ase.sternesjo@lmv.slu.se

Mastitis is a major factor influencing milk quality due to the influx of serum components and negative effects on the synthesis of milk components. Also sub-clinical mastitis will induce unfavourable changes in the milk and it is of great importance to identify specific and sensitive biomarkers for rapid detection of affected cows. The somatic cell count (SCC) in milk is used both in mastitis diagnosis and as an indirect indicator of milk quality in bulk tank milk (BTMSCC). There is, however, no clear scientific data defining a level of BTMSCC that gives additional benefits in terms of milk quality. Since SCC is influenced by several physiological factors, much effort has been invested to find alternative biomarkers. During recent years, the potential in mastitis diagnostics of the two major bovine acute phase proteins (APP) haptoglobin (Hp) and serum amyloid A (SAA) has been studied. The overall aim of our work was to study if APP can be used as biomarkers also for raw milk quality. The occurrence of Hp and SAA in quarter, cow composite and bulk tank milk was investigated and relationships between APP and milk quality parameters such as SCC, total protein, casein, whey proteins, proteolysis, fat, and lactose were evaluated. The composition of milk samples with detectable levels of APP differed significantly from samples without detectable levels of APP, specifically in milk protein. Milk samples with detectable APP contained less of the valuable casein, more whey proteins and more protein was degraded, with economical implications for the dairy industry.

Use of DeLaval cell counter in ovine milk

C. Gonzalo and B. Linage
Facultad de Veterinaria, Universidad de León, Producción animal, Campus de Vegazana s/n, 24071-León, Spain
Corresponding author: c.gonzalo@unileon.es

This study evaluated the performance of DeLaval cell counter (DCC) when analyzing ovine milk with different soak times in diluted and undiluted milk samples in two dairy sheep breeds.A total of 101 composite ovine milk samples (50 from Assaf ewes and 51 from Churra ewes), ranging between 50×10^3 and $2,200\times10^3$ cells/ml, were divided into 10 aliquots/milk to be analysed by DCC. Four undiluted aliquots were analysed using soak times of 0, 1, 2, and 3 min, respectively; four aliquots were 1:1 diluted in PBS and analysed with the same above-mentioned soak times (0, 1, 2, and 3 min); and the other two aliquots were 1:1 diluted in propidium iodide or ethidium bromide staining solutions and analysed by DCC (0 min). The Fossomatic method was used as reference. Undiluted milk samples with soak times of 1, 2, and 3 min showed large coefficients of regression (b=0.96 to 0.98) and correlation (r>0.99) when they were compared with Fossomatic method. In these samples, DCC gave repeatability standard deviations (s_r = 35 to 51×10^3 cells/ml) lower than other DCC analytical conditions (s_r = 49 to 74×10^3 cells/ml), and their log SCC means (5.51 to 5.52) were close to the reference value (5.56). The log SCC means corresponding to samples 1:1 diluted in staining solutions (5.55) did not differ from the reference value, but these aliquots had, however, lower regression coefficients (b=0.92 to 0.93). Samples 1:1 diluted in PBS and undiluted samples with 0 min soak time showed similar or lower global accuracy than undiluted samples with soak times of 1, 2, and 3 min. Breed did not affect the results. As conclusion, results evidenced that DCC can be used in indigenous and cosmopolitan sheep breeds with different fat, protein and solid contents provided that a soak time is guaranteed before raw milk analysis for SCC.

Ability of bulk milk culture for estimating *Staphylococcus aureus* and *Streptococcus agalactiae* prevalence in dairy herds

R.G.M. Olde Riekerink[1], O.C. Sampimon[1], L.Holst Pedersen[2], J. Katholm[3] and T.J.G.M. Lam[1,4]
[1]GD Animal Health Service, Department of Ruminant Health, P.O. Box 9, 7400 AA Deventer, the Netherlands
[2]The Danish Veterinary and Food Administration, Mørkhøj Bygade 19, 2860 Søborg, Denmark
[3]Danish Dairy Board, Frederiks Allé 22, 8000 Århus, Denmark
[4]Dutch Udder Health Centre, P.O. Box 2030, 7420 AA Deventer, the Netherlands
Corresponding author: r.olderiekerink@gddeventer.com

Bulk milk culture is an easy to obtain and relatively cheap method to get an impression of the mastitis and milk quality status of a dairy herd. The objectives of this study were to estimate the ability of bulk milk culture to approximate *Staphylococcus aureus* and *Streptococcus agalactiae* prevalence in dairy herds in Danish dairy herds. In total, 50 Danish dairy herds, on which recently *Streptococcus agalactiae* was isolated from the bulk milk were selected. All quarters of all cows in lactation as well as bulk milk samples were collected. The data showed an association between isolating *Strep. agalactiae* in the tank and in quarters. Sensitivity of bulk tank culture for *Staph. aureus* was lower than for *Strep. agalactiae*. On 47 (94%) farms *Staph. aureus* was isolated from quarters, and in 29 (62%) cases *Staph. aureus* was isolated from the bulk milk. If *Staph. aureus* was isolated from the bulk milk, the natural logarithm of the colony count was correlated with the natural logarithm of quarter prevalence in a herd (correlation coefficient 0.68). Sensitivity of bulk milk culture for *Streptococcus agalactiae* is high. However, these herds were selected based on recent isolation of *Strep. agalactiae* from the bulk tank milk and might therefore have large colony counts. Colony count of *Staph. aureus* in bulk milk samples has some ability to predict the prevalence of *Staph. aureus* infected quarters in a herd. However, sensitivity of bulk milk culture is low. Sensitivity may be improved if multiple samples are taken.

Identification of mastitis-associated pseudomonads in bovine farm tank milk

J.L.W. Rademaker, Y. Xiao, J.D. Hoolwerf and M.H.J. Wells-Bennik
NIZO food research, Health & Safety, Kernhemseweg 2, 6718 ZB Ede, the Netherlands
Corresponding author: Jan.Rademaker@nizo.nl

Pseudomonas bacteria are generally not considered to be a major cause of mastitis but can create a troubling mastitis problem. Moreover, they can have a negative impact on milk quality causing flavour defects, casein breakdown and ropiness due to slime production and coagulated proteins. *Pseudomonas* species including *Pseudomonas fluorescens* can grow under refrigerated conditions (psychrotrophs) and may produce heat stable lipases and proteases. Other species such as *Pseudomonas aeruginosa* have been implicated in intramammary infection outbreaks. *P. aeruginosa* bacteria are very resistant to antibiotics. Multiple-dose bottles of antibiotics can become contaminated when the same needle is used repeatedly to draw the antibiotic from one bottle and to treat more than one animal. In a contaminated bottle *P. aeruginosa* will survive within the antibiotic for an indefinite time. In random samples from raw farm tank milk with a high somatic cell count (SCC) the dominant bacterial flora was quantified with real time PCR tests in an earlier study. Bacteria associated with mastitis such as *Staphylococcus aureus, Streptococcus uberis, Escherichia coli* and *Enterococcus* were found. Remarkably the presence of well known mastitis causing organisms was always associated with *Pseudomonas* species. To characterise the pseudomonad population in raw milk hundreds of samples with a high SCC were cultured using a *Pseudomonas* and a *P. aeruginosa* specific medium. Isolates were identified using genetic methods. The observed diversity will be discussed in relation to the possible sources of the bacteria and their ability to cause mastitis. Insight in the dominant population structure of pseudomonads from raw farm tank milk with a high SCC may enable advising farmers on hygiene measurements and specific mastitis treatments and thus aid in mastitis diagnosis and control.

Diversity of *Staphylococcus aureus* isolates from bovine milk with a high somatic cell count

J.L.W. Rademaker[1], Y. Xiao[1], J.D. Hoolwerf[1], P.H.M. Savelkoul[2] and M.H.J. Wells-Bennik[1]
[1]NIZO food research, Health & Safety, Kernhemseweg 2, 6718 ZB Ede, theNetherlands
[2]VUMC, Medical Microbiology & Infection Control, P.O. Box 7057, 1007 MB Amsterdam, the Netherlands
Corresponding author: Jan.Rademaker@nizo.nl

Staphylococcus aureus is a major pathogen causing bovine and human mastitis as well as nosocomial and community-acquired infections. Methicillin-sensitive *S. aureus* (MSSA) are widespread and methicillin-resistant variants (MRSA) emerge. MRSA became resistant to a variety of antibiotics. The human prevalence of MRSA varies from less than 1% in the Netherlands to more than 30% in other European countries. *S. aureus* is an important mastitis pathogen and causes a reduction in milk production as well as animal welfare. Moreover, MRSA is a public health risk. The presence and diversity of MRSA and MSSA was investigated in samples raw bovine tank milk. Samples were collected from Dutch dairy farms with suspected mastitis cases based on a high somatic cell count (SCC >400,000 cells/ml). Isolates from several hundreds random samples were cultured using Baird-Parker agar. The identity of the isolates was confirmed using a *S. aureus*-specific real time PCR method. All isolates were evaluated for the presence of the mecA methicillin resistance gene using two different real time PCR tests. The MRSA and MSSA isolates were characterised using spa typing, a high resolution method based on DNA sequence variations in the protein A gene. Most isolates yielded a spa PCR product. Spa typing was found a powerful tool for assessment of the diversity of *S. aureus* isolates from tank milk and may be useful for mastitis diagnosis and control including analysis of milk of individual cows. Several types were found including some novel types. Spa types of isolates under study will be discussed in comparison to those of major clonal lineages associated with human origin, antibiotic resistance profiles and animal to human transmission.

PCR-based methods for identification of *Staphylococcus* and *Streptococcus* spp. causing mastitis

K. Aulrich and K. Barth
Federal Research Institute for Rural Areas, Forestry and Fisheries, Institute of Organic Farming, Trenthorst 32, 23847 Westerau, Germany
Corresponding author: karen.aulrich@vti.bund.de

Mastitis is often caused by *Staphylococcus* (Staph.) and *Streptococcus* (Strep.) species. Especially coagulase-negative staphylococci (CNS) have become the predominant pathogens in many herds. Although CNS usually cause only subclinical or mild cases of clinical mastitis they might be important due to their ability to persist in the udder. However, CNS are often considered as one group of bacteria which arouses the same physical reactions after an infection. This approach might be lead to the contradictory results of different studies. In our opinion it is necessary to differentiate between the species of CNS and their effects on the udder. Identifying methods for all *Staph.* and also *Strep.* spp. are necessary. Currently, the species identification is mostly based on biochemical properties. However, not all CNS will be identified by these tests and misidentification may also happen. Identification methods based on molecular biology are under development. The aim of this study was to identify the most common *Staph.* and *Strep.* spp. by PCR-based methods in the institute's dairy herd. A combination of internal transcribed spacer-PCR and PCR-RFLP of 16S-23S ribosomal DNA was used for species identification. The amplicons as well as the fragments from restriction analysis were resolved in high-resolution agarose gels and visually compared with the patterns obtained for the control strains. The results of the analysed milk samples up to now showed that a combined application of both PCR methods offers the opportunity to identify *Staphylococcus* as well as *Streptococcus* spp. The identification of the following CNS: *S. epidermidis, S. xylosus, S. simulans, S. hyicus, S. chromogenes* just as *Streptococcus* spp.: *S. agalactiae, S. dysgalactiae, S. uberis and S. parauberis* just as *S. aureus* appears to be successful.

Rapid and effective method for separation for *Staphylococcus aureus* from somatic cells in mastitis milk

T. Hayashi[1,2], M. Kubota[1], K. Iwasaki[1], K. Sakaguchi[1], R. Abe[1], H. Ohtsuka[3], Y. Kiku[2], T. Ozawa[2] and H. Takahashi[2]
[1]Tokyo University of Science, Research Institute for Biological Sciences, Noda, Chiba 278-8510, Japan
[2]National Institute of Animal Health, Research Team for Production Diseases, Tsukuba, Ibaraki 305-0856, Japan
[3]Kitasato University, School of Veterinary medicine and Animal Sciences, Towada, Aomori 034-8628, Japan
Corresponding author: tomohito@rs.noda.tus.ac.jp

Early detection and treatment of *Staphylococcus aureus* (SA) mastitis is critically important for the prevention of chronic disease. Early detection of bacteria by quantitative PCR assay is one of the easiest and most sensitive methods to identify the pathogen causing mastitis. However, a major limitation of PCR-based method is the presence of inhibitors of DNA polymerase in clinical material, which can cause false-negative PCR results for the detection of target genes. To eliminate this problem, we attempted to establish methods that allow the effective separation of bacterial cells from somatic cells in mastitis milk with amino-silica. Somatic cells and SA have different sizes, surface structures, and overall electrical charges; therefore their adsorption and desorption behavior on amino-silica was also different. We found that although amino-silica could efficiently adsorb both somatic cells and SA, somatic cells were adsorbed much more strongly than bacterial cells. We identified conditions under which most of the somatic cells adsorbed and only SA desorbed from amino silica upon addition of a desorption solution. We demonstrated that this procedure effectively eliminated somatic cells in heavily contaminated milk samples, which resulted in improved clarity of the PCR band. These results indicate that the pretreatment of samples with amino silica made the PCR-based strategy for identification and quantifying disease-causing bacteria applicable for all milk samples.

DNA based bacteriological diagnosis of milk samples with no growth in conventional culturing

S. Pyörälä[1], L. Salmikivi[2], S. Taponen[1], H. Simojoki[1] and M.T. Koskinen[2]
[1]University of Helsinki, Faculty of Veterinary Medicine, Department of Production Animal Medicine, Pohjoinen pikatie 800, 04920 Saarentaus, Finland
[2]Finnzymes Oy, Keilaranta 16A, 02150 Espoo, Finland
Corresponding author: satu.pyorala@helsinki.fi

In approximately one fourth of the milk samples taken from bovine clinical mastitis, no bacterial growth can be detected in conventional culturing. Without information about the bacteriological etiology of mastitis, treatment and prevention of the disease are difficult. The aim of this study was to investigate the bacteriological etiology of these 'no growth' cases using a Real-Time PCR based commercial reagent kit (PathoProof^{TM} Mastitis PCR Assay, Finnzymes, Finland). The assay targets the DNA of 12 major mastitis species or groups and can detect and quantify viable but growth-inhibited bacteria, as well as dead bacteria. A total of 55 samples from clinical mastitis were studied. Altogether 26 out of 55 (49%) of the samples were positive for one (25 samples) or two (1 sample) of the assay's target bacteria. The positive findings included 10 *Staphylococcus* spp. (Staphylococci other than *Staph. aureus*), 8 *Streptococcus uberis*, 3 *Str. dysgalactiae*, 3 *Corynebacterium bovis*, 2 *Staph. aureus* and 1 *Escherichia coli*. By applying 'absolute quantification', based on Real-Time PCR standard curves prepared with purified DNA (dilution series of 10^6-10^2 genome copies of the target amplicons), the positive samples were calculated to contain ~10^1-10^5 bacterial copies per PCR reaction. This study demonstrates that in nearly half of the clinical mastitis cases where culture failed to detect bacteria, mastitis pathogens were still present, often in substantial quantities. We conclude that the DNA based diagnostic kit is a useful tool for bacteriological diagnosis of milk samples with no growth in conventional culturing.

Analytical specificity of the PathoProof™ mastitis PCR assay validated using culture isolates

J. Holopainen, L. Salmikivi, H. Lehmusto, S. Niskala and M.T. Koskinen
Finnzymes Oy, Diagnostics, Keilaranta 16A, 02150 Espoo, Finland
Corresponding author: mikko.koskinen@finnzymes.fi

The PathoProof Mastitis PCR Assay is a Real-Time polymerase chain reaction based reagent kit for identification of 12 mastitis causing species or groups from bovine milk. In this study, we evaluated the analytical specificity of the kit using an extensive culture collection of pathogens (including all targets of the assay) isolated from clinical mastitis cases and their phylogenetically close relatives, originating from environmental and human samples. Bacterial targets of the assay include *Staphylococcus aureus, Staph.* spp. (Staphylococci other than *Staph. aureus*), Staphylococcal penicillin resistance gene (blaZ), *Streptococcus agalactiae, Str. uberis, Str. dysgalactiae, Enterococcus faecalis, E. faecium, Corynebacterium bovis, Arcanobacterium pyogenes, Peptostreptococcus indolicus, Escherichia coli, Klebsiella pneumoniae, K. oxytoca* and *Serratia marcescens.* The assay was used for analysing a total of 630 culture isolates from ~80 species, families or groups. When considering the mastitis isolates (n=485), the specificity of the test ranged from 99.0% (*Staph.* spp.) to 100%. When including the environmental and human pathogens to the analysis (n=145), the specificity of the test ranged from 98.5% (*Staph.* spp.) to 100%. In conclusion, the PathoProof Mastitis PCR Assay had good specificity when considering pathogens isolated from bovine mastitis, as well as based on an extended sample collection including environmental and human flora. These data are highly relevant for mastitis testing laboratories now complementing or replacing bacterial culture based testing schemes with the assay.

Dairy Guard™: sensor array diagnosis of mastitis infection

R. Card[1], N. Smit[2], H. Klapproth[2] and P. Wakeley[1]
[1]Veterinary Laboratories Agency, Woodham Lane, Weybridge KT15 3NB, United Kingdom
[2]Safeguard Biosystems, 310 Front St. West Suite 305 Box 3320, Toronto, ON M5V 3B5, Canada
Corresponding author: nsmit@sgbio.com

DairyGuard™ is a diagnostic tool for the detection of bacterial causes of mastitis and is being developed by the Veterinary Laboratories Agency in collaboration with Safeguard Biosystems. It aims to provide the dairy industry with a rapid, accurate and cost-efficient procedure for the diagnosis of mastitis. Central to the DairyGuard™ platform is the use of sensor-array technology. The powerful multiplexing potential of sensor-arrays is exploited to deliver an assay that aims to complete the detection of the major causes of mastitis in one day in a single operation. The DairyGuard™ sensor-array employs a novel three dimensional gel drop technique (developed at the University of Freiburg), designed to increase its detection capability. Oligonucleotide probes that specifically target the most common causes of mastitis (including bacteria that are difficult to culture, e.g. *Mycoplasma bovis*) are present on the sensor-array. The DairyGuard™ sensor-array has already been tested for its ability to detect several of these target groups. For the species tested to date, probes have bound their target DNA specifically and with little or no cross-reaction observed. These experiments have shown that probes for the identification of several targets have been established: Eubacteria, Gram-positive bacteria, *Escherichia coli, Staphylococcus* spp., *Staphylococcus aureus, Streptococcus* spp. *Streptococcus agalactiae, Streptococcus uberis.* Future targets are *Streptococcus dysgalactiae, Corynebacteria* spp. and *Mycoplasma bovis.* When delivered to the market this will form part of the DairyGuard™ 3D SensorArray - a new system based on aseptic sampling and DNA analysis to identify the causes of mastitis.

Genotyping and biofilm formation of *Staphylococcus aureus* isolates: evidence for lack of penicillin-resistance in *Agr*-type II strains

M.B. Melchior[1], E. van Duijkeren[2], D.J. Mevius[1,2], M. Nielen[2] and J. Fink-Gremmels[2]
[1]Central Veterinary Institute, Edelhertweg 15, 8219 PH, the Netherlands
[2]Faculty of Veterinary Medicine, Yalelaan 1, 3508 TD Utrecht, the Netherlands
Corresponding author: marielle.melchior@wur.nl

The increasing evidence regarding the role of biofilm formation in bovine *Staphylococcus aureus* mastitis infections led to further investigations on biofilm formation in standard growth medium and bovine milk whey. For a collection of 99 recently isolated and historical *S. aureus* strains, the biofilm forming ability in both growth media was correlated with the presence of the ica-, bap-, and IS257 genes. These genes have previously been found to be correlated with biofilm formation in human *S. aureus* isolates. All strains were genotyped with respect to *Agr*-type and *Agr*-subtype, and the presence of the resistance genes blaZ and smr by PCR. The prevalence of *Agr*-types and investigated genes and the correlations hereof with the results of the biofilm assays were statistically evaluated. The data showed a very strong correlation between *Agr*-type I and penicillin-resistance in the bovine *S. aureus* mastitis strains. None of the *Agr*-type II strains were found to contain penicillin resistance genes. The *Agr*-type also had a significant effect on biofilm formation, however contrary to human isolates there was no significant effect for ica- and IS257 genes on biofilm formation. The bap gene was not found in any of the investigated strains. The presence of both biofilm related genes and resistance genes showed a high correlation with the *Agr*-type of the strains. These results indicate that the most prevalent *Agr*-types in *S. aureus* bovine mastitis, *Agr*-type I and II, might be regarded as different subspecies. The extremely high correlation between *Agr*-type II and penicillin susceptibility strongly suggests that these strains are not perceptive for the blaZ genes.

Molecular typing of coagulase-negative staphylococci and coliforms isolated on Flemish dairy farms

V. Piessens[1], S. de Vliegher[2], B. Verbist[1], G. Braem[3], M. Heyndrickx[1], L. Herman[1] and E. van Coillie[1]
[1]Ministry of the Flemish Community, Inst. for Agric. and Fisheries Res. Unit techn. and Food, Brusselsesteenweg 370, 9090 Melle, Belgium
[2]Ghent University, Dept. of Reprod., Obstet. and Herd Health, Fac. Vet. Med., Merelbeke, Belgium
[3]Res. Group Industr. Microbiol. and Food Biotechnol., VUB, Brussels, Belgium
Corresponding author: veerle.piessens@ilvo.vlaanderen.be

In Flanders, a shift of the distribution of mastitis pathogens towards coagulase-negative staphylococci (CNS) and coliforms has been observed and this may be the cause of the recent problems of increasing bulk milk somatic cell counts and/or decreasing milk quality. In this study the main sources of infection of CNS and the distribution of various CNS species on dairy farms are determined by molecular identification and typing techniques. CNS are isolated monthly from several farm environment samples, teat end swabs and udder quarter milk samples on six farms in total. For comparison, three farms with and three without specific coliform problems are included in the study and on each farm, ten randomly selected cows are monitored during one year. Milk samples are also analysed for coliform bacteria, in order to identify chronically infected cows shedding high levels of these pathogens in their milk and to identify the particular coliform species and strains. For rapid and reliable species identification of CNS isolates, Amplified Fragment Length Polymorphism (AFLP) is used as a molecular based identification system by including several staphylococcal type strains. For strain typing of CNS both Random Amplification of Polymorphic DNA (RAPD) and AFLP are used, for coliforms RAPD and PFGE are applied. This epidemiological study will give more insight into the infection sources of CNS and into the characteristics of CNS and coliform species causing mastitis.

Phenotypic characterisation of *Prototheca* spp. isolated from bovine mastitis

S. Marques, E. Silva, C. Kraft, J. Carvalheira, V. Huss and G. Thompson
ICBAS-UP, Rua Padre Armando Quintas, 4485-661 Vairão, Portugal
Corresponding author: saramarques@mail.icav.up.pt

Members of the genus *Prototheca* are unicellular algae related to the green algae of the genus *Chlorella*, but without chlorophyll. These pathogenic algae cause infectious diseases in humans and animals. They are very resistant, being also isolated from water treated with chloride and from pasteurised milk. The prevalent form of protothecosis in animals is bovine mastitis, which generally occurs in a chronic subclinical or a mild clinical inflammatory process of the udder affecting cows that do not respond to routine therapy, resulting on the reduction of milk production and consequently economic losses. Until recently only two species were known to be associated with disease in animals and humans, *Prototheca zopfii* and *P. wickerhamii*, respectively. A new species, *P. blaschkeae*, was described in 2006, which was isolated from a human case of onychomycosis. The objective of the present work was to phenotypically characterise *Prototheca* spp. isolated from bovine mastitis in the Northwest of Portugal. Forty seven *Prototheca* isolates obtained from mastitic milk of dairy cows belonging to 21 different farms in this region were previously identified as *P. zopfii* (43 isolates), and as *P. blaschkeae* (4 isolates). These were phenotypically characterised by morphological data analysis and biochemistry profile determination using API 20C Aux and BBL Crystal Kits systems. Our results indicated that the two *Prototheca* spp. analysed in this study, showed differences in their biochemical profiles. Nevertheless,the determination of fermentation and assimilation patterns of *P. zopfii* isolates revealed considerable differences among them, as heterogeneities for strains of this specie are well known. We conclude that despite biochemical analyses can provide useful information for the characterisation of the *Prototheca* spp., their correct identification requires genetic analyses.

Antimicrobial susceptibility of *Escherichia coli* isolated from acute bovine mastitis

L. Suojala[1], H. Simojoki[1], A.-L. Myllyniemi[2], A. Pitkälä[2] and S. Pyörälä[1]
[1]University of Helsinki, Pohjoinen pikatie 800, 04920 Saarentaus, Finland
[2]Finnish Food Safety Authority, Mustialankatu 3, 00790 Helsinki, Finland
Corresponding author: leena.suojala@fimnet.fi

The aim of this study was to determine the in vitro antimicrobial susceptibility of *Escherichia coli* isolated from acute clinical mastitis in Finland. Use of antimicrobials for food animals is generally strictly controlled in Finland. Clinical mastitis suspected to be caused by Gram-negative bacteria is often treated with broad-spectrum antimicrobials such as enrofloxacin or trimethoprim-sulfonamides. It is known that the use of antimicrobials causes selection pressure resulting in antimicrobial resistance. Minimal inhibition concentration (MIC) values of 140 *E. coli* isolates from acute bovine mastitis were determined for ampicillin, gentamicin, tetracycline, cloramphenicol, sulfametoxazol, ceftiofur, streptomycin, trimethoprim and ciprofloxacin by VetMIC™ microdilution method (SVA, Uppsala, Sweden) in Research Department of Finnish Food Safety Authority EVIRA, Helsinki, Finland. Isolates were from samples collected during years 2003-2006 from acute clinical mastitis from 64 different farms in Southern Finland. A total of 27.9% isolates showed resistance to one or more antimicrobials tested. Among them, 18.6% was resistant to ampicillin, 16.4% to streptomycin, 15.7% to tetracycline, 13.6% to sulfametoxazol and 10.7% to trimethoprim. No resistance was found for gentamicin, ceftiofur and ciprofloxacin. Antimicrobial resistance of *E. coli* isolated from mastitis in the present study is at the same level than found in the national resistance surveillance (FINRES-Vet 2005-2006) and markedly lower than reported in most other countries. In conclusion, antimicrobial resistance appears to be no problem among mastitis caused by *E. coli* in Finland. However, strict antimicrobial policy should be continued in therapy of food animals to retain this good situation.

Antimicrobial susceptibility patterns of streptococci isolated from bovine mastitis

C. Locatelli, L. Scaccabarozzi, A. Casula and P. Moroni
University of Milan, Department of Veterinary Pathology, Hygiene and Public Health, Via Celoria 10, 20133 Milan, Italy
Corresponding author: paolo.moroni@unimi.it

Mastitis is the most common disease in dairy herds and the main cause of antibiotic use. Drug therapy may exert a selective pressure towards resistant strains, so monitoring susceptibility of isolates should be of crucial importance. Epidemiology of mastitis pathogens changed in recent time shifting from contagious to environmental origin. *Streptococcus* genus represents one of the most frequently isolated. Prevalence of contagious *Str. agalactiae* diminished in favour of environmental *Str. uberis* and *Str. dysgalactiae*, responsible for large part of clinical mastitis and whose control is limited by insufficient information regarding their epidemiology. *Streptococcus canis* is infrequent but can cause subclinical mastitis with elevated somatic cell counts and reduced milk production. We determined the MICs of erythromycin, oxytetracycline, cefalonium, amoxicillin, penicillin G, cloxacillin, tilmicosin, enrofloxacin, cephapirin, and cefquinome for a total of 93 Streptococci so represented: 18 *Str. agalactia*e, 41 *Str. uberis,* 14 *Str. agalactiae,* and 20 *Str. canis.* Cefalonium, cephapirin and cefquinome revealed the most effective molecules, penicillin G and amoxicillin maintain their efficacy while erythromycin and enrofloxacin show a reduced activity. In general, *Str. agalactiae* and *Str. canis* too remain sensible to most drug, while *Str. uberis* and *Str. dysgalactiae* follow a trend of reduced susceptibility. Implications of the work for mastitis control: broth dilution is considered the method of choice for determination of susceptibility patterns of mastitis pathogens and correct therapy has to preserve antimicrobial drugs as an efficient weapon in mastitis control.

Antimicrobial susceptibility of staphylococci isolated from bovine mastitis in thirteen Estonian dairy farms 1998-1999

L. Haltia, A. Pitkälä, V. Myllys and T. Honkanen-Buzalski
Finnish Food Safety Authority Evira, Mustialankatu 3, 00790 Helsinki, Finland
Corresponding author: laura.haltia@evira.fi

Staphylococcal isolates are the most frequent finding in bovine mastitis milk samples in Estonia. We report here the antimicrobial resistance of these isolates. Antimicrobial susceptibility of 230 *Staphylococcus aureus* and 215 coagulase-negative staphylococci (CNS) was determined using agar dilution method according to NCCLS and using the breakpoints recommended by the CLSI or other investigators. Of *S. aureus* isolates, 47.4% and of CNS isolates, 34.4% were resistant to penicillin. All *S. aureus*-isolates were sensitive to oxacillin, but of CNS isolates, 39.1% were resistant to it with MIC range 0.06-2 μg/ml. Of *S. aureus* isolates, 3% were resistant to chloramphenicol, 3.5% to erythromycin, 0.9% to oxytetracycline, 1.7% to trimethoprim-sulfamethoxazole and 0.9% to lincomycin. Of CNS isolates, 6.5% were resistant to chloramphenicol, 12.5% to erythromycin, 10.2% to oxytetracycline, 23.3% to trimethoprim-sulfamethoxazole and 11.2% to lincomycin. All isolates were in vitro susceptible to cephalothin, gentamicin and neomycin. The penicillin resistance was at the same level as recorded in Finland (resp. 26.5% - 2005; 52.1% - 2004; 63.6% - 1998), and higher than recorded in Sweden (7%) or Norway (6.5%). This may reflect the different use of antimicrobials in these countries. Chloramphenicol resistance might result from its earlier use. Resistance to it is acquired and can remain for years. The use of chloramphenicol in humans might become viable if the MRSA infections increase and effect of new antimicrobials is limited. Animals can be reservoir of resistant bacteria. We suggest regular monitoring of antimicrobial resistance as a basis for appropriate medication practice.

Lincosamide resistance in Gram-positive pathogens isolated from quarters with persistent subclincal mastitis

M.D. Apparao and P.L. Ruegg
University of Wisconsin, Dept. of Dairy Science, 1675 Observatory Dr., Madison, WI 53706, USA
Corresponding author: plruegg@wisc.edu

Pirlimycin is one of the most frequently administered intramammary compounds used for treatment of mastitis. Pirlimycin is a lincosamide and resistance is often encoded by ribosomal methylase genes that also confer resistance to other antimicrobials of the macrolide-lincosamide-streptogramin group. However, the genes linA and linB encode resistance only to lincosamides. The objective of this study was to determine the prevalence of linB genes Gram positive cocci isolated from persistent cases of subclinical mastitis. CMT positive quarters (n=213) of cows allocated to a 'treatment' group received intramammary pirlimycin. No treatment was given to quarters (n=208) of cows in the control group. Aseptic milk samples were collected pretreatment and 3 weeks later. A 'persistent' infection was defined as isolation of the same bacterial species from both pretreatment and post treatment milk samples. Persistent infections (56 infections; 112 pathogens) were confirmed using a PCR based methodology. Susceptibilities of persistent pathogens were determined using broth micro-dilution. Identification of linBgenes was performed using a published PCR protocol. Statistical analysis was carried out using SAS 9.1. An association between presence of linB and genus was observed ($P<0.05$). Of persistent isolates, linB was present in 4 (3%) coagulase negative staphylococci (CNS; n=102) and 3 (33%) streptococci (n=9). The presence of linB was associated with the occurrence of phenotypic resistance ($P<0.05$). Of isolates that demonstrated phenotypic resistance to pirlimycin (n=22), 5 (22%) were positive for linB in contrast to 2 (2%) pirlimycin susceptible isolates (n=90). The presence of linB was not associated with parity, treatment or sampling period. Routine screening for linB may be a useful tool for surveillance of lincosamide resistance in bovine mastitis pathogens.

Advantage of cefalexin and kanamycin in combination to control bovine mastitis

E. Maneke[1], A. Pridmore[2] and I. Lang[1]
[1]Boehringer Ingelheim Vetmedica GmbH, Bingerstrasse, 55216 Ingelheim, Germany
[2]Don Whitley Scientific, Otley Road, BD17 7SE Shipley, United Kingdom
Corresponding author: elke.maneke@boehringer-ingelheim.com

Our objective was to investigate the in vitro efficacy of cefalexin, alone and in combination with kanamycin, against mastitis pathogens by determining fractional inhibitory concentration (FIC) and antibacterial kill kinetics (KK). Two strains per bacterial species (*Staphylococcus aureus, Escherichia coli, Streptococcus* spp.) were chosen for FIC and one strain per species for KK testing. All strains were representative of their respective species, based on MIC_{90} determinations. FIC was determined using broth microdilution technique and FIC index of the combination was calculated by adding the FICs of individual test articles obtained from equally effective concentrations of both drugs. KK data were generated for two ratios of cefalexin / kanamycin (1.25:1 and 1:2.3) and cefalexin alone, each tested at 4×MIC. Bacterial inocula were incubated for 24 h while viable counts were enumerated at hourly intervals for 12 h and finally after 24 h. CLSI guideline M26-A considers a $\geq 3\log_{10}$ reduction in bacterial counts to indicate bactericidal activity. Synergistic or additive effect (FICindex = 0.375–1.0) was observed for most of the species. KK data for both ratios of cefalexin / kanamycin demonstrated bactericidal activity against all species within <2-12 h. The reduction in viable count against *Staphylococcus aureus* and *E. coli* was very rapid (<2 h). Cefalexin alone, however, produced mainly a bacteriostatic effect except against *E. coli* and *S. agalactiae*, viable counts of which were reduced by $\geq 3\log_{10}$ after 7-9 h. In conclusion, the combination of cefalexin / kanamycin offers enhanced antibacterial activity at lower or comparable antibiotic concentrations compared with cefalexin alone. The two agents therefore exert synergistic antibacterial activity.

Field study on acute mastitis with intoxication and different treatment regimes: provisional results

L. Podstatzky[1] *and P. Winter*[2]
[1]*Agricultural research & education centre, AREC Raumberg-Gumpenstein, Austrasse 10, 4601 Wel, Austria*
[2]*Veterinary University Vienna, Clinic for ruminants, Veterinärplatz 1, 1210 Vienna, Austria*
Corresponding author: leopold.podstatzky@raumberg-gumpenstein.at

This study focuses on additional therapy with non-steroidal anti-inflammatory drugs and infusions to parenteral antibiotic treatment in coliform mastitis in the field. Until now 18 cows with typical inclusion criteria (clinical score) were involved in this study. All cows were treated with marbofloxacin (2 mg/kg once a day for three days). The cows were divided in three upper groups (no infusion, 0.9% NaCl, 7.2% NaCl) and three subgroups (without and with tolfenamin acid (2 mg/kg)). Clinical score was determined, blood and milk samples were taken at 0, 12, 24, 48, 72 hours and 3 weeks after mastitis occurrence. Blood samples were examined for acute phase proteins (serumalyoid A, haptoglobin) and milk samples were used for bacterial diagnosis. Of these 18 cows 11 were tested positive for *Escherichia coli*, 1 positive for *Klebsiella* spp., 2 negative in all milk samples and 2 positive for *Streptococcus* spp. and *Staphylococcus aureus*, respectively. Until 72 hours milk samples from cows with *S. aureus*, *Streptococcus* spp. and *Klebsiella* were positive. Number of *E. coli* positive cows reduced from 11 to 2 from hour 0 to 72. At the end of the observation period all milk samples were negative, except one sample with *Streptococcus* spp. Bacteriological cure rate was better in the group without infusion, no difference existed with or without tolfenamin acid. Clinical cure rate will be discussed. Preliminary data show that acute mastitis is mainly caused by *E. coli*, but also by other bacteria. Differences can be shown in acute phase protein due to mastitis causing bacteria.

An investigation of three approaches to dry cow therapy to prevent intramammary infection in the dry period and clinical mastitis in early lactation

A.J. Bradley[1,2], J.E. Breen[1] and M.J. Green[3]
[1]Univ of Bristol, School of Veterinary Science, BS40 5DU, United Kingdom
[2]QMMS Ltd, Somerset, BA5 1EY, United Kingdom
[3]Univ of Nottingham, School of Veterinary Science, LE12 5RD, United Kingdom
Corresponding author: a.j.bradley@bris.ac.uk

The aim of this study was to investigate 3 different dry cow therapy regimes, in low SCC herds (BMSCC <200,000 cells/ml) in SW England. 489 cows were recruited to the study and randomly allocated to receive one of three different therapies; Cephaguard Dry Cow (Cobactan DC, Intervet), Orbenin Extra Dry Cow (Pfizer Ltd) or Combination therapy comprising Orbenin Extra and the internal teat sealant Orbeseal (Pfizer Ltd). All quarters were sampled for bacteriology at drying off and again in the week immediately post calving; two quarters were also sampled two weeks before the estimated calving date to allow an interim assessment of pathogen status. Quarters were subsequently monitored for clinical mastitis for the first 100 days of lactation. Multilevel models were constructed to assess the efficacy of products in preventing intramammary infection (IMI) and survival analysis was used to examine factors that influenced the risk of clinical mastitis in the first 100 days of lactation. No significant differences were identified between the treatment groups in terms of cure of IMIs caused by the major pathogens. However, quarters in both the Combination (OR 2.01; 95% CI 1.32-3.07) and Cephaguard (OR 1.61; 95% CI 1.07-2.43) treated groups were significantly more likely to be free of a major pathogen, including *Enterobacteriacae* and *S. uberis*, post calving than quarters in the Orbenin Extra treated group. The Orbenin Extra treated group were significantly more likely to develop clinical mastitis compared to the Cephaguard treated group (HR 2.06; 95% CI 1.08-3.92), the Combination treated group were not significantly different in terms of clinical mastitis to the other treatment groups.

Effect of dry therapy using an intramammary infusion containing penethamate, penicillin, and framycetin on intramammary infections and somatic cell counts in dairy sheep

C. Gonzalo[1], B. Linage[1], M.T. Juárez[2], E. Beneitez[2], A. Martínez[2] and J.A. Asensio[2]
[1]Universidad de León, Facultad de Veterinaria, Producción Animal, Campus de Vegazana, 24071-León, Spain
[2]Consorcio de Promoción del Ovino, Camino de Canillas, 49630-Villalpando, Zamora, Spain
Corresponding author: c.gonzalo@unileon.es

The IMI dynamics during the dry period were studied in 435 half-udders of 229 Assaf ewes randomly assigned to two lots: (1) treated lot (TL) with 223 half-udders which received a complete dry therapy of an antibiotic combination containing 100 mg penethamate hydriodide, 280 mg benethamine penicillin and 100 mg framycetin sulphate (Mamyzin Secado, Boehringer Ingelheim Spain S.A.), and (2) control lot (CL) with 212 non-treated half-udders. Bacteriological samplings were carried out at drying-off and at lambing. Cure, persistent infections, reinfection, and new infection rates were 81.7%, 12.8%, 5.5%, and 7.9% respectively for TL, and 13.3%, 70.4%, 16.3% and 22.8% respectively for the CL. The prevalence of IMI decreased significantly from 48.9% at drying-off to 13.0% at lambing for the TL, but it did not vary for the CL (46.2% and 52.4%, respectively). Log SCC diminished significantly between drying-off (5.68) and lambing (5.33) in the TL, whereas log SCC did not vary in the CL (5.61 vs. 5.66). Antibiotic residues were no detected ≥54 h postpartum; and this delay may be considered as relevant to respect EU-MRL. In addition, the same antibiotic combination was used as dry therapy, in a field study, in all 10,313 dairy ewes from 25 flocks. This treatment significantly decreased bulk tank SCC in subsequent lactation. Flock, milking type, and total bacterial count were also significant factors affecting bulk tank SCC. As a conclusion, the antibiotic formulation used as dry therapy drastically diminished IMI prevalence and SCC during the dry period in dairy ewes and was also effective to reduce bulk tank milk SCC in the flocks.

Comparative synergistic activity of a cefalexin and kanamycin combination in Mueller Hinton Broth medium and in milk

J.P. Ganiere
Ecole Nationale Veterinaire de Nantes, Unité de pathologie infectieuse, Atlanpôle La Chantrerie, 44307 Nantes, France
Corresponding author: laurent.goby@boehringer-ingelheim.com

An *in vitro* investigation was performed to compare the kill kinetics of cefalexin and kanamycin alone and in fixed combination at a ratio of 1.5 to 1.0, against *Streptococcus uberis, Staphylococcus aureus* and *Escherichia coli* strains isolated from field cases of bovine mastitis. The fixed ratio of the combinations tested corresponds to the final formulation of an intramammary injector (Ubrolexin TM, Boehringer Ingelheim Animal Health) currently under development for local treatment of bovine clinical mastitis. The effect of milk as a diluent on the rate of bacterial killing was also investigated. The time-kill method of synergy testing assesses the bactericidal activity of the antibiotics being tested and offers a dynamic picture of the antimicrobial action as well as the interaction between the individual components over time. The methodology applied used the broth microdilution method following the guidelines set by the CLSI. Kill kinetics of the combination were performed comparatively in Mueller-Hinton broth (MHB) and in low-fat UHT (ultra-high temperature) milk against three isolates from each bacterial species. The kill kinetics experiment performed in MHB demonstrated that cefalexin and kanamycin combined in a fixed ratio of 1.5:1 exhibited a clear synergistic bactericidal activity against major mastitis pathogens: low kanamycin concentrations resulted in enhanced bactericidal activity of cefalexin. The combination exhibited a larger and faster rate of kill of *S. aureus, S. uberis* and *E. coli* compared to either cefalexin or kanamycin alone, while using a lower total amount of antibiotic. Although the bactericidal activity of the cefalexin and kanamycin was decreased in milk compared to that observed in MHB, the synergistic effect of the combination was maintained in this medium.

Determination of withdrawal time in milk of cows treated with dry treatament syringes

C. Acuna, M. Falletti, M. Landeira, G. Casasnovas and A. Daffner
United Milk Producers Cooperative From Route Eight, Laboratory, Ruta 41 Cuartel IV CC 164, San Antonio de Areco 2760, Argentina
Corresponding author: acunacristina@areconet.com.ar

The objective of this study was to determine the withdrawal time of milk in animals treated with intramammary syringes for dry cows (DCT) containing cloxacillin 500 mg (as benzathine salt) and ampicillin 250 mg (as trihydrate). Animals (n=24) with a dry period of 30-40 days were selected for the residues assay. Milk of each quarter was sampled at the moment of parturition and every 12 hours until 144 hours after parturition. Residues were quantificated with Agar diffusion test with *Bacillus stearotermophilus* var. *calidolactis* ATCC 10149 (DA) and Penzym S 100 (P). The latter assay is used in milking foundations in case of anticipated parturition date, so as to reduce the risk of residues. In order to validate the analytic method DA, two polinomic lineal regression models were adjusted, with the ampicillin concentration and the quadrate concentration as independent variables, and the diameter of the inhibition halo, in mm, as dependent variable. The presence of an inhibition halo of 15.5 mm indicated that the concentration of ampicillin and cloxacillin was ≤ to the MRLs; 0.004 ppm and 0.03 respectively. According to the statistical analysis for DA, 24 hours after parturition the level of residues is ≤ to MRLs ($P \leq 0.05$). With the P test, samples were negative 72 hours after parturition. Furthermore, quarters (n=4) with double syringe dry cow treatment were analysed, and the residues level were ≤ to MRLs 48 hours and 84 hours for DA and P respectively. According to the results and taking into account the normal descalostrating period of ≥ 4 days applied in the country, the is no risk of milk residues in cows with dry periods of more than 30 days.